Drug and Hormone Resistance in Neoplasia

Volume I

Basic Concepts

Editors

Nicholas Bruchovsky, M.D.
Head, Department of Cancer
Endocrinology
Cancer Control Agency of
British Columbia
Vancouver, Canada

James H. Goldie, M.D.
Head, Division of Advanced
Therapeutics
Cancer Control Agency of
British Columbia
Vancouver, Canada

CRC Press, Inc.
Boca Raton, Florida

Library of Congress Cataloging in Publication Data

Main entry under title:

Drug and hormone resistance in neoplasia.

   Bibliography.
   Includes index.
   Contents: v. 1. Basic concepts.
   1. Cancer—Chemotherapy—Complications and
sequelae. 2. Drug resistance. 3. Hormone
therapy—Complications and sequelae.
I. Bruchovsky, Nicholas. II. Goldie, James H.
[DNLM: 1. Drug resistance. 2. Hormones—
Pharmacodynamics. 3. Neoplasms—Drug therapy.
QZ 267 D793]
RC271.C5D77   1983   616.99'4061   82-4530
ISBN 0-8493-6516-3 (v. 1)   AACR2
ISBN 0-8493-6517-1 (v. 2)

Direct all inquiries to CRC Press, Inc., 2000 Corporate Blvd., N.W., Boca Raton, Florida, 33431.

© 1982 by CRC Press, Inc.

International Standard Book Number 0-8493-6516-3 (v. 1)
International Standard Book Number 0-8493-6517-1 (v. 2)

Library of Congress Card Number 82-4530
Printed in the United States

FOREWORD

I am honored to be asked to write a Foreword in this text. At this point in the development of effective means for treating disseminated cancers I can think of no area that needs careful consideration and analysis more than *Drug and Hormone Resistance in Neoplasia.*

Some years ago I wrote the following:

Cancer chemotherapy is many things. It is not just 'screening' as some seem to think, nor is it just organic chemistry, biochemistry, cell population kinetics, pharmacology, or sophisticated experimental therapeutics in model systems and in man. It is all of these things and many more, but most of all it is discovery, development, collation across disciplines, and application to man with (for good reason) a prevailing sense of urgency. We want and need and seek better guidance and are gaining it, but we cannot afford to sit and wait for the promise of tomorrow so long as stepwise progress can be made with tools at hand today.

More recently I have read that chemotherapy and adjuvant chemotherapy now cure thousands of patients bearing *certain* disseminated cancers each year. I would like to dream that improved planning with respect to selection and delivery of combinations of noncross-resistant drugs might result in significantly increased cure rates and include cancers in which only temporary responses are being achieved today. Stepwise progress is not appealing to most of us, but this is an apt description of what has happened in improving the control of about a dozen disseminated human cancers over the past two decades. If we cannot have a dramatic "breakthrough" today or tomorrow, my second choice would be continuing stepwise progress—at an accelerated pace.

New and better noncross-resistant drugs certainly are needed, but if history is repetitive new drugs also will be limited by tumor stem cells that are specifically and permanently resistant to them and often will have to be used in combination with other drugs.

The above implies my views and concerns in 1982. To me it seems clear that the inverse relationship between tumor cell burden and curability with drugs is in no small measure a reflection of the direct relationship between tumor cell burden and tumor cell heterogeneity. Large bodies of diverse experimental data support the view that the overgrowth of drug-resistant tumor stem cells during treatment is a major cause of chemotherapeutic failure. This is a stumbling block that can be attacked in a rational manner at the clinical level.

Two sentences in the Preface of this book were the first to catch my eye.

There are few phenomena in medicine more dramatic than the production of a complete or nearly complete remission of advanced malignancy. As well, there are few things more frustrating and discouraging than to observe the relentless recurrence of a malignancy that had initially responded to treatment.

These words also describe the elation and frustration experienced over the years by some experimental oncologists I know quite well. So often we have hoped that the remissions induced in cancer-bearing animals by different treatments would carry over to humans, but that the subsequent recurrences would not. All too often both did.

What are the reasons for the recurrence of neoplasms that initially respond to cytotoxic drugs? In animal cancers they often are quite simple. If treatment is stopped after remission induction, then after recurrence a second remission often can be achieved by the same doses of the same drug or drugs. When this is possible the implication is that at cessation of treatment, and at relapse, the vast preponderance of the surviving tumor cell mix still was comprised of drug-sensitive tumor cells. On the other hand, when neoplasms regress and later recur during continuing undiminished treatment, this implies that the continuing treatment had selected to the point where, say, 50% or greater of the surviving tumor cells are resistant to the doses of the drug or drugs being used. This has been a consistent observation repeatedly documented by harvesting the recurring tumor cells, passing them to other animals, and retesting their responsiveness to the same doses of the same drug or drugs. Neoplasms that regress and regrow during combination chemotherapy will show resistance to one or more of the drugs in the combination, but not necessarily to maximum tolerated doses of all of the drugs in the combination.

It seems to me, as to the authors of this book, that gaining both theoretical and pragmatic information regarding the phenomena responsible for the failure of anticancer drugs and hormone manipulation or hormone treatment is very important.

Finally, I am impressed with the organization of this book and the wealth of information presented in it. It will be of much value to many who are concerned with improving cancer treatment.

Howard E. Skipper, Ph.D.
President Emeritus
Southern Research Institute
Birmingham, Alabama

PREFACE

At the present time the most useful and effective agents for the systemic treatment of cancer are the antineoplastic drugs generally characterized as "cytotoxic" and the steroid hormones. Chemotherapeutic agents alone or in combination with hormones are capable of curing patients with a variety of disseminated malignancies. Hormones, though not curative when used by themselves, are capable of inducing significant clinical responses in those classes of tumors that are deemed hormone-dependent. Although the proportion of patients who achieve long-term remission or cure is progressively increasing, it is still apparent that the great majority of malignancies that are treated with drugs and hormones ultimately become refractory to the treatment with the resultant inevitable fatal consequences for the patient.

There are few phenomena in medicine more dramatic than the production of a complete or nearly complete remission of advanced malignancy. As well, there are few things more frustrating and discouraging than to observe the relentless recurrence of a malignancy that had initially responded to treatment. It seems self-evident that in order to improve current end results in the treatment of a great variety of neoplasms more information will be required about this process whereby tumors become resistant to the effects of systemic treatment. In these two volumes we have asked a number of investigators to review the mechanisms that are thought to underlie the development of resistance by tumors to drug and steroid hormones. From a consideration of these mechanisms we have attempted to determine to what extent current treatment protocols in a variety of malignancies are likely to be effective in overcoming resistance to treatment.

In Volume I we have reviewed the basic biological mechanisms associated with resistance in experimental systems. Similarities and differences between drug and hormone resistance are indicated. We have chosen to put some emphasis on spontaneous mutations to drug resistance as an important mechanism, as we feel that this is a process that has received insufficient attention in the past. In Volume II the clinical aspects of drug and hormone resistance are discussed. We have concentrated on malignancies of the breast, endometrium, and prostate as relevant clinical examples because these common solid tumors of adults illustrate both drug sensitivity and resistance as well as hormone dependency and hormone resistance.

In the final two chapters we have attempted to bring together a set of unifying concepts as to how resistance and treatment failure arises and from these derive inferences as to how future therapy might be more effectively directed.

The editors would like to express their thanks to the following investigators who through discussions and correspondence have provided us with many ideas and insights, and as well have permitted us to see data from studies in prepublication form: Dr. Howard E. Skipper, Southern Research Institute, Dr. Frank M. Schabel Jr., Southern Research Institute, Dr. R. W. Brockman, Southern Research Institute, Dr. J. W. Meakin, Ontario Cancer Treatment and Research Foundation, Dr. Douglass C. Tormey, Wisconsin Clinical Cancer Center.

We would as well like to thank Barbara Williams, Cynthia Wells, and Linda Wood for secretarial assistance in the preparation of these two volumes.

The editors also wish to gratefully acknowledge the support of the Cancer Control Agency of British Columbia.

N. Bruchovsky
and
J. H. Goldie

THE EDITORS

Nicholas Bruchovsky, M.D., is Head of the Department of Cancer Endocrinology at the Cancer Control Agency of British Columbia.

Dr. Bruchovsky received his M.D. from the University of Toronto in 1961 and his Ph.D. in Medical Biophysics in 1966. He served as an intern at the Toronto General Hospital from 1961 to 1962 and as a resident at Parkland Memorial Hospital, Southwestern Medical School from 1966 to 1968. During this time his work with Dr. J. D. Wilson led to the proposal that dihydrotestosterone is the action form of testosterone.

Dr. Bruchovsky subsequently joined the Department of Medicine at the University of Alberta where he was promoted to the rank of Professor in 1976. In 1979 he moved to Vancouver to assume his present position with the Cancer Control Agency of British Columbia, and also as Professor of Medicine at the University of British Columbia.

Dr. Bruchovsky is a Fellow of the Royal College of Physicians and Surgeons of Canada, and a member of the Canadian Society for Clinical Investigation, the Canadian Society of Endocrinology and Metabolism, the Canadian Oncology Society, the Endocrine Society and the International Study Group for Steroid Hormones.

His present research concerns the mechanism of action of testosterone, and the control of neoplastic growth by androgens and other hormones. He has published over 50 articles on these and related topics.

James H. Goldie, M.D., F.R.C.P.(C) is Head of the Division of Advanced Therapeutics, Cancer Control Agency of British Columbia, Vancouver, B.C. and is Clinical Associate Professor of Medicine, University of British Columbia.

Dr. Goldie received his M.D. from the University of Toronto in 1961, and was made a Fellow of the Royal College of Physicians of Canada in 1966. His postgraduate studies in the cancer field were done at the Ontario Cancer Institute, Toronto and the Chester Beatty Institute, London, England.

Dr. Goldie has served as a member of a number of national and international committees of organizations in the cancer field. He was chairman of the investigational drug subcommittee of the National Cancer Institute of Canada and a member of the scientific grants panel of the N.C.I.C. He is also a consultant to the Division of Cancer Treatment, U.S. National Cancer Institute.

Dr. Goldie's main areas of interest include clinical practice as a medical oncologist at the Cancer Control Agency of British Columbia, and has a major research interest in anticancer drug resistance with especial emphasis on antifolate drugs and is the author of more than 60 papers and abstracts in this field.

CONTRIBUTORS

Pierre R. Band, M.D.
Professor of Medicine
Universite de Montreal
Director of Clinical Research
Institut du Cancer de Montreal
Centre Hospitalier Notre-Dame
Montreal, Canada

Pierre-Paul Baskevitch, Ph.D.
Attache de Recherches Agrege
Centre National de la Recherche
  Scientifique
Montpellier, France

Suzanne Bourgeois, Ph.D.
Director of Regulatory Biology
  Laboratory
The Salk Institute
Adjunct Professor
Biology Department
University of California
San Diego, California

Nicholas Bruchovsky, M.D.
Head, Department of Cancer
  Endocrinology
Cancer Control Agency of British
  Columbia
Professor of Medicine
University of British Columbia
Vancouver, Canada

Andrew J. Coldman, M.A.
Senior-Statistician
Division of Epidemiology
Cancer Control Agency of British
  Columbia
Vancouver, Canada

C. M. L. Coppin, D. Phil.
Division of Medical Oncology
Cancer Control Agency of British
  Columbia
Vancouver, Canada

Michele Deschamps, R.N., M.Sc.
Institut du Cancer de Montreal
Centre Hospitalier Notre-Dame
Montreal, Canada

J. M. Elwood, M.D.
Professor and Chairman
Department of
  Community Health
University of Nottingham
Nottingham, England

Judith C. Gasson, Ph.D.
Research Associate
The Salk Institute
San Diego, California

James H. Goldie, M.D.
Head, Division of Advanced
  Therapeutics
Cancer Control Agency of British
  Columbia

Bridget T. Hill, Ph.D.
Head, Laboratory of Cellular
  Chemotherapy
Imperial Cancer Research Fund
  Laboratories
Honorary Senior Lecturer
Institute of Urology
London, England

Marianne Huet-Minkowski, Ph.D.
Chargee de Recherches
Centre National de La Recherche
  Scientifique
Paris, France

John Tod Isaacs, Ph.D.
Assistant Professor of Oncology
Assistant Professor of Urology
Johns Hopkins Hospital
Baltimore, Maryland

Victor Ling, Ph.D.
Associate Professor
Department of Medical Biophysics
University of Toronto
Staff Scientist
The Ontario Cancer Institute
The Princess Margaret Hospital
Toronto, Canada

Robert L. Noble, M.D.
Senior Research Scientist
Department of Cancer Endocrinology
Cancer Control Agency of British
  Columbia
Vancouver, Canada

Paul S. Rennie, Ph.D.
Research Scientist
Department of Cancer Endocrinology
Cancer Control Agency of British
  Columbia
Associate Professor of Surgery
University of British Columbia
Vancouver, Canada

Henri Rochefort, M.D.
Professor of Biochemistry
University of Montpellier
Montpellier, France

K. D. Swenerton, M.D.
Clinical Assistant Professor
Faculty of Medicine
University of British Columbia
Medical Oncologist
Division of Medical and Gynecologic
  Oncology
Cancer Control Agency of British
  Columbia

DRUG AND HORMONE RESISTANCE IN NEOPLASIA

Volume I
Basic Concepts

Genetic Basis of Drug Resistance in Mammalian Cells
Victor Ling

Biochemical and Cell Kinetic Aspects of Drug Resistance
Bridget T. Hill

A Mathematical Model of Drug Resistance in Neoplasms
Andrew J. Coldman and James H. Goldie

Glucocorticoid Resistance in Lymphoid Cell Lines
Marianne Huet-Minkowski, Judith C. Gasson, and Suzanne Bourgeois

Biochemical Aspects of Androgen Resistance
Paul S. Rennie

Biochemical Aspects of Estrogen Resistance in Mammary Tumors
Pierre-Paul Baskevitch and Henri Rochefort

Cellular Factors in the Development of Resistance to Hormonal Therapy
John T. Isaacs

Tumor Progression Endocrine Regulation andControl
Robert L. Noble

Volume II
Clinical Concepts

Drug and Hormone Resistance in the Management of Breast Cancer
Pierre R. Band and Michele Deschamps

The Importance of Early Diagnosis and Prompt Institution
of Treatment in Reducing Mortality from Breast Cancer
J. M. Elwood

The Treatment of Advanced Prostatic Cancer with Drugs and Hormones
C. M. L. Coppin

The Treatment of Early and Advanced Endometrial Carcinoma
with Drugs and Hormones
K. D. Swenerton

Clinical Implications of the Phenomenon of Drug Resistance
James H. Goldie and Andrew J. Coldman

Basis for the Use of Drug and Hormone Combinations in
the Treatment of Endocrine Related Cancer
Nicholas Bruchovsky and James H. Goldie

TABLE OF CONTENTS

Volume I

Chapter 1

GENETIC BASIS OF DRUG RESISTANCE IN MAMMALIAN CELLS

Victor Ling

TABLE OF CONTENTS

I. INTRODUCTION

It is now recognized that drug-resistant neoplastic cells do arise during the course of the disease, and they present a major obstacle in the management of cancer. What is the origin of these cells? How rapidly do they arise? By what mechanisms do they mediate resistance? The answers to these questions will undoubtedly be required for us to be ultimately successful in chemotherapeutic treatment of cancer.

Consideration of these questions forms the theme of this chapter. The viewpoint taken is that drug-resistant neoplastic stem cells often do arise from *mutations*. Implicit in this view is that the drug-resistant phenotype is inherited and propagated; thus the well-established notion that the survival of a single drug-resistant cancer cell in vivo could prove fatal[1] is based on such a premise. This view does not exclude the importance of nongenetic events but rather it emphasizes the aspect of *hereditability* associated with genetic changes which is of overriding importance in the present context.

An attempt will be made in this chapter to present evidence that drug-resistant mammalian cells do arise from mutations and have a genetic basis. Selected examples will be taken from studies with cells in culture since they are the best characterized from this perspective. Tissue culture systems offer a number of advantages for genetic analysis which have been exploited in recent years.[2,3] For example, clonal populations can be established, rare variants can be selected, cells can be maintained under defined growth conditions, and a number of genetic manipulations can be more easily conducted. Representative mutants with different mechanisms of drug resistance will be described along with approaches for the characterization of the resistant phenotype. Three major mechanisms have been delineated and characterized: overproduction of the drug target (e.g., gene amplification), reduced drug permeability, and altered interacion of the drug with its target.

Of course, not all drug-resistant phenotypes characterized in culture systems will necessarily be represented in neoplastic cells in human; nevertheless, one can anticipate that the fundamental processes operative in generating drug-resistant mutants in culture will be universal, and that their investigation will provide tools and concepts to facilitate understanding of the in vivo situation.

II. CRITERIA ASSOCIATED WITH A GENETIC ORIGIN

Evidence in support of a genetic origin for a drug-resistant phenotype include: the phenotype is stably inherited in the absence of selection; it is spontaneously generated with a rate consistent with mutation rates in natural populations; the frequency of appearance is induced with known mutagens; an altered gene product can be demonstrated; chromosomal localization of the determinant is associated with the drug-resistance trait; and an altered gene can be demonstrated at the DNA level. Such criteria have been used in the past for differentiating between genetic changes and epigenetic modulations in bacterial systems. In mammalian cells, similar considerations applied to a number of well-characterized systems have resulted in the conclusion that most stable drug-resistant phenotypes generally do have a genetic basis.[2-6]

This conclusion is supported by data presented in Table 1. The examples presented in this table have been limited to drug-resistant mutants isolated from cultured hamster cells. The intention here is to illustrate the large repertoire of resistant phenotypes involving a wide variety of cell targets that can be obtained within a single species. Equivalent results have been obtained in other systems. This table is by no means exhaustive but some of the better characterized drug-resistant mutants are represented.

A. Frequency of Drug-Resistant Cells and Response to Mutagens

The proportion of resistant cells in a tumor or cell culture at any given moment denotes the *frequency* of the variant phenotype in question. Measurements of this sort are easily accomplished in systems where clonogenic assays have been established and a comparison of the number of surviving colonies in the presence and absence of an appropriate concentration of drug can be made. As can be seen in Table 1, in established cell cultures, typical spontaneous frequencies of mutations for a variety of stably drug-resistant phenotypes occur at 10^{-5} to 10^{-7}. These frequencies can be influenced by a number of factors such as the selective conditions used for detection (i.e., concentration of drug), age of the culture, growth conditions, and exposure to mutagens. Nevertheless, this type of data confirms that the frequency of heritable drug-resistant phenotypes is usually low. Classical epigenetic modulations are thought generally to affect a greater proportion of a population, say 10% or more. It should be emphasized however that the frequency of a particular phenotype does not implicate any particular mechanism by which the phenotype is generated. The consideration so far simply indicates that in general, genetically based mechanisms are associated with relatively low frequencies of drug resistance in a nonselective environment.

If the frequency of a drug-resistant phenotype in a cell population is significantly increased (10 to 100-fold) after exposure to known mutagens, then this behavior is consistent with a genetic origin for the phenotype (Table 1). Nonresponse to a mutagen however is usually not definitive as not all mutagens are effective for inducing a particular phenotype. That mutagens could appreciably increase the frequency of drug-resistant mutants merits consideration from a clinical viewpoint, at least at the theoretical level, since some therapeutic agents (for example radiation and alkylating drugs) have mutagenic capability.

B. Luria-Delbrück Fluctuation Analysis of Mutation Rate

As noted above, the tacit assumption of a genetic origin for a drug-resistant phenotype is that resistant variants arise *spontaneously* at a defined *rate* in the absence of selecting agent. The Luria-Delbrück fluctuation analysis provides a means of testing the stochastic nature of generation of the phenotype.[37] This is illustrated in Figure 1 where subclonal cultures of a cell population are allowed to replicate for an appropriate defined number of generations and then each subclone is analyzed for the frequency of drug-resistant colonies. As illustrated, in situations where the resistant cells are spontaneously generated, different subclonal cultures will contain very different numbers of resistant colonies since this number will be dependent on when during the growth of the subclone to a defined size the resistant variant first appeared. Because of the spontaneous nature of generation of mutants, the fluctuation among subclonal populations will be large; thus the ratio of variance compared with the mean number of resistant colonies will be large. A rate for the generation of drug-resistant mutants can be calculated from such data.[37,38]

It is useful to keep in mind that the proportion or frequency of mutants in each subclonal population will increase as the population continues to grow until some equilibrium level is established. This is so since once a mutant is generated in a population it will also grow and divide; at the same time, new mutants are generated at a defined rate, the equilibrium level will be dependent on among other things, the mutation rate, relative growth rate of the mutants compared with the rest of the population, and reversion rate. Thus as noted above, while a frequency measurement of resistant cells in a population is not indicative of genetic origin, a rate measurement along with indications of spontaneous generation as provided by a Luria-Delbrück fluctuation test is.

Table 1
DRUG-RESISTANT HAMSTER CELL MUTANTS

Resistance to selecting drug[a]	Approximate spontaneous frequency (response to mutagens)	Luria-Delbrück analysis: mutation per cell per generation	Hybrid phenotype[b]	Altered gene product identified	DNA-Mediated transfer of resistance	Ref.
*Asparaginase	1×10^{-5} (positive)	$\sim 10^{-6}$	Dominant	Asparagine synthetase	yes	7
*β-Aspartylhydroxamate	1×10^{-7} after mutagen treatment	NR	Dominant	Asparagine synthetase	yes	8,9
*Ara A (3 classes)	4×10^{-5} (positive)	1×10^{-7}	NR	Ribonucleotide reductase (for one class)	NR	10
*Hydroxyurea (2 classes)	$\sim 10^{-5}$ (positive)	5×10^{-6}	Dominant	Ribonucleotide reductase	NR	11—13
*Ara C (2 classes)	1×10^{-6} after mutagen treatment	NR	Dominant (1 class) Recessive (1 class)	dC kinase CTP synthetase?	NR	14—16
*Melphalan	1×10^{-7} (NR)	NR	NR	Localized in the nuclear fraction	NR	17
*Methotrexate (3 classes)	3×10^{-7} (positive)	2×10^{-9} (for 1 class)	Dominant (2 classes) Recessive (1 class)	Dihydrofolate reductase drug transport	yes	18—20
*Colchicine (resistant to: adriamycin, daunomycin, vinblastine, melphalan)	5×10^{-6} (positive)	NR	Dominant	Membrane P-glycoprotein	yes	21—25
Colcemid	1×10^{-7} (positive)	NR	Dominant	Tubulin	NR	26—28
Podophyllotoxin	3×10^{-7} (positive)	4×10^{-7}	Dominant	Tubulin (probably)	NR	29
α Amanitin	$\sim 10^{-7}$ (positive)	NR	Dominant	RNA polymerase II	yes	30—32
Emetine	2×10^{-7} (positive)	5×10^{-8}	Recessive	40S Ribosomal subunit	NR	33, 34
Ouabain	1×10^{-5} (positive)	5×10^{-8}	Dominant	Membrane Na$^+$/K$^+$ AT-Pase	yes	3, 25, 35
Phytohemagglutinin	5×10^{-5} (positive)	1.5×10^{-6}	Recessive	Glycosyl transferase	NR	36

a Mutants resistant to cancer chemotherapeutic drugs are marked by an asterisk. NR = not reported.
b Classification of a dominant phenotype includes incomplete dominant and co-dominant phenotypes.

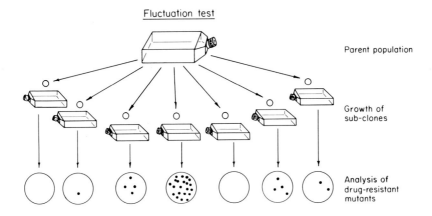

FIGURE 1. A fluctuation test to demonstrate the spontaneous generation of drug-resistant mutants.

The spontaneous mutation rate for a drug-resistant phenotype can be relatively constant for different cell lines, for example resistance to ouabain has been determined at approximately 5×10^{-8} mutations per cell per generation for mouse L-cells, hamster CHO cells, and human diploid fibroblasts[3] (see Table 1). This rate however can be significantly increased under certain circumstances such as in mutant lines where "mutator genes" have been generated,[39-41] in some virally transformed lines[42] and in certain metastatic tumor cells.[43] It is perhaps significant that the mutation rates to drug-resistance in Bloom syndrome fibroblasts are also elevated compared with fibroblasts from normal individuals.[44,45] Thus it is possible that in genetically altered neoplastic cells in vivo that the mutation rate to drug-resistance may be different from those presently observed in cultured cells.

C. Hybrid Phenotype

The technique of cell:cell hybrid formation[2,3,46] and subsequent analysis of hybrid clones offers an important genetic tool for studying the expression of a drug-resistant phenotype in a cell containing other genomes specifying different traits. A dominant or recessive nature of the resistant phenotype can be determined and this can be useful for identifying different mechanisms of resistance (c.f., Table 1, and discussion of mutants resistant to methotrexate IIIB). In the case of recessive markers, hybrids can be used to delineate complementation groups revealing different alterations giving rise to a similar phenotype. With dominant markers, hybrids can be used to study the effects of gene dosage or different genomic combinations on the expression of a resistant phenotype. Chromosome loss occurs in hybrid cells especially with crosses between cells of different species.[46,47] Such reduced hybrids have been used to map the determinants of drug-resistant phenotypes on specific chromosomes. Thus analysis of a variety of hybrid cells has provided strong evidence for a chromosomal origin and a genetic basis for many drug-resistant phenotypes.

It is pertinent to ask whether a particular drug-resistant phenotype is dominant or recessive since in principle, recessive mutations would not be expressed at frequencies readily observable in fully diploid cells where two or more mutations at the same locus would be required before the phenotype could be expressed. In this context it is significant that highly malignant tumors are often aneuploid with a tendency to maintain a hyperdiploid state.[48] However, from Table 1, it is seen that many phenotypes resistant to chemotherapeutic drugs identified in culture cells are dominant, and in theory at least, they can be expressed in polyploid cells as a result of only a single mutation. It has been postulated that some pseudodiploid cells in culture are functionally hemizygous and hence recessive mutations are readily detected.[5,49] Whether or not such a functionally hemizygous state exists in aneuploid tumor cells in vivo is not known at present, but it obviously has important implications with respect to the variety and types of drug-resistant mechanisms that could occur in patients.

D. Chromosome and DNA Transfer

Development of gene transfer systems in bacteria provided a major tool for elucidating in detail the genetics of a wide variety of phenotypes including drug-resistant markers. Recent advances in mammalian cell genetics involving chromosome- and DNA-mediated gene transfer[50-53] should also facilitate investigations of higher organisms along the same lines. This approach applied to drug-resistant phenotypes in mammalian cells provides unequivocal evidence of a genetic basis for these phenotypes. As can be seen in Table 1, such evidence have been obtained in a number of well-characterized systems. In practice dominant resistant phenotypes are easier to work with since recipient cells expressing the appropriate marker can be selected directly. Also, it has been observed that unlinked markers in the genome are generally not cotransferred, thus coexpression of different phenotypes in a transformant is likely due to the pleiotropic nature of the mutant gene (for example, multiple resistance to different drugs expressed in colchicine-resistant mutants IIIC).

The ability to transfer a drug-resistant phenotype via DNA also provides an approach for isolating the gene(s) in question by molecular cloning.[53,54] The potential of using purified genes for investigating drug resistance in mammalian cells has not yet been fully exploited.

E. Summary

It is quite clear from the data presented in Table 1 that a very wide variety of stable drug-resistant phenotypes with properties completely consistent with a genetic origin can be isolated from mammalian cells. Although consideration of drug-resistant lines has been limited here only to well-characterized cells in culture, it would be surprising if the basic mechanisms generating such mutants were not also operative in cells in vivo. Of course the type and variety of mutants represented could be different, but the process of generating variants from mutations and enrichment of subpopulations by selection would be universal.

III. PROPERTIES OF DRUG-RESISTANT MUTANTS

A. General Considerations

In this section, properties of mutants resistant to some anticancer drugs are considered along with approaches used to delineate their mechanisms of resistance. With respect to the drug-resistant phenotype itself, three aspects deserve further discussion.

1. Stability

The mutants listed in Table 1 all display stable drug-resistant phenotypes, maintaining their resistance in the absence of selecting agents for one month or longer in culture. This aspect is consistent with the heritability of genetic mutations. Unstable resistant phenotypes are sometimes observed and investigation of the origin and mechanism of such phenotypes is more difficult. Instability could of course implicate an epigenetic mechanism; however, in our experience it is not uncommon to observe that in the absence of drug, drug-resistant mutants have appreciably slower growth rates. Thus if the "fitness" of drug-sensitive revertant cells for growth is better than the mutant cells, then they could quickly take over the culture with the end result of the resistant phenotype appearing unstable. It should also be appreciated that certain genetic events could occur at high rates such as that associated with chromosome segregation in hybrids, and loss of acentric chromosomal fragments (double minutes, discussed in IIIB) resulting in phenotypic instability.

2. Degree of Resistance

In some mechanisms, resistance to a cytotoxic drug is essentially complete as a result of a single alteration. A particularly good example of this is resistance to phytohemagglutinin (Table 1) where mutants isolated in a single step are resistant to concentrations of drug more than two hundred fold higher than the selecting dose.[36] In contrast, high resistance to some drugs requires multiple changes since a series of selection steps is required usually with each step yielding resistant variants with a frequency characteristic of mutation frequencies, in the 10^{-4} to 10^{-7} range. Colchicine resistance is an example of this class (see IIIC). This mechanism of generating highly resistant phenotypes likely involves multiple genes or alleles. Mutants with this mechanism of resistance are very unlikely to be selected in a single-step using a *high* concentration of drug since simultaneous multiple alterations would be required for such a mutant to survive the selection. This has obvious implications in chemotherapeutic strategies.

3. Cross-Resistance

Determination of resistance to other drugs expressed by a mutant could provide useful information concerning the nature of the resistant phenotype. Cross-resistance to compounds related to the selecting drug is usually expected and this can be used in some cases to differentiate between different classes of mutant. In some cases, such as in the colchicine-resistant mutants described below, a very wide-ranging cross-resistance to unrelated drugs is observed. This pleiotropic phenotype readily distinguishes membrane-altered mutants from the tubulin-altered ones which are resistant only to tubulin-binding compounds.[26] Wide-ranging cross-resistant phenotypes can present special problems in chemotherapeutic treatments since neoplastic cells acquiring such a mutation could be particularly refractile even to a combination of drugs.

B. Methotrexate-Resistance (Mtx^R)

Methotrexate is one of the most useful antineoplastic agents presently available and its mechanism of action has been well-studied.[55] Resistance to this compound has been observed in a number of systems including animal tumor cells and human cell lines (see References 55-58, 60). One of the systems characterized genetically is that of Flintoff and co-workers[18,19] using Chinese hamster ovary cells in culture. By using clonal selections in single-step drug treatments, they have been able to isolate stable mutants possessing different mechanisms of resistance and three mechanisms have been clearly delineated by biochemical, genetic, and physiological analyses. The three mechanisms of resistance currently recognized are increased level of drug target enzyme dihydrofolate reductase (DHFR); decreased affinity of DHFR for Mtx; and decreased uptake of Mtx by resistant cells. Properties of these three classes of mutants are charted in Table 2 where it can be seen that members of the different classes can be distinguished in a number of ways. First, Class II is recessive whereas Classes I and III are dominant in cell:cell hybrids. Second, Class II is more resistant to aminopterin than methotrexate, while the other two classes express a level of resistance to aminopterin similar to their response to methotrexate. Third, the responses of the three classes to diaminopyrimidines, low molecular weight lypophilic inhibitors of dihydrofolate reductase, are particularly revealing. The Class I mutants do not cross-react to these compounds

Table 2
CHO CELL MUTANTS RESISTANT TO METHOTREXATE

Mutant class	Defect	Hybrid phenotype	Relative resistance to:		
			Methotrexate	Aminopterin	Diaminopyrimidines
I	Reduced Mtx binding to DHFR	Dominant	16—19	8—12	~ 1.0
II	Reduced Mtx uptake by whole cells	Recessive	38—58	205—290	0.08—0.24
III (selected in a second step from Class I)	Increased DHFR activity or level	Dominant	375—540	350	10—33

Note: Data for this table compiled from studies of Flintoff and co-workers.[18,19,59] The diaminopyrimidines tested were pyrimethamine, metoprine, and trimethoprin. Relative resistance is expressed as the ratio of the D_{10} value (drug concentration required to reduce the colony-forming ability to 10% of control without drug) for the Mtx^R lines to the D_{10} value for drug-sensitive wild-type line. A ratio greater than 1.0 indicates cross-resistance while one less than 1.0 denotes collateral sensitivity.

while Class II mutants display a 4 to 10-fold increased sensitivity and Class II mutants a 10 to 30-fold increased resistance.

The collateral sensitivity of Class II mutants to diaminopyrimidine has been further exploited for selection of revertants which display wild-type response to these compounds.[59] Such revertants were obtained with a frequency of 10^{-4} to 10^{-5}, and this frequency can be increased by prior treatment of the cells with mutagen. Analysis of these revertants indicates that their resistance to methotrexate and aminopterin has also reverted towards wild-type response. Taken together, this study clearly shows the genetic basis of resistance to methotrexate displayed by the Class II mutants. Moreover, the pleiotropic phenotype of cross-resistance to aminopterin and collateral sensitivity to disminopyrimidine is clearly the result of the same mutation. Understanding of the basis of this collateral sensitivity could have important clinical applications.

This study of methotrexate resistant mutants in CHO cells is significant in that it demonstrates that different mechanisms of resistance could be operative either independently or in combination in a single cell line giving rise to the resistant phenotype. Resistant clones from Classes I and II occur at approximately equal frequencies in *mutagenized* cultures[18,19] but in untreated cultures, only Class I mutants were observed from greater than 3×10^7 cells tested, suggesting that the spontaneous occurrence of Class II mutants is relatively rare compared with Class I mutants. Class III mutants were observed in second-step selections for increased resistance. This work illustrates the importance of single-step selections and clonal isolation of mutant populations since without such an approach some mechanisms of resistance could easily be masked. This is true for example in cases where continuous selection is applied to allow outgrowth of a resistant population and the resulting resistant phenotype could develop from a combination of mechanisms.[2,3]

The class of Mtx^R mutant possessing increased levels of DHFR is perhaps the most intensively investigated (for review see Schimke et al.[60]). The molecular mechanism responsible for this increased level of DHFR enzyme has been studied in some detail in a number of systems. The increased enzyme level seems to result from an amplification in copy number of the gene resulting in a concordant increase in messenger RNA production and enzyme synthesis. Cells with highly amplified genes (e.g., 200 copies) can be selected by subjecting the culture to increasing concentrations of methotrexate. Two classes of resistant cells have been obtained under these conditions. One is a relatively stable class in which the amplified DHFR genes appear to reside in homogeneously staining regions (HSRs) detected in metaphase chromosomes. The localization of these genes has been verified by *in situ* hybridization of metaphase cells with radioactive DNA complementary to DHFR messenger RNA.[61] The second class is relatively unstable and loses its resistant phenotype when cultured under nonselective conditions. In this case the amplified DHFR genes appear to be associated with the presence of acentric chromosomal fragments called double minute (dmin) chromosomes.[62] The dmin chromosomes apparently have a high probability of being eliminated from the cells under nonselective conditions. The relationship between dmin and HSR is not yet clear but it is possible that HSRs are generated from dmins.

The genomic organization of both the wild-type DHFR gene and the amplified genes in resistant mutants has been investigated at the molecular level by restriction enzyme mapping in different mouse cell lines.[63] It appears that the wild-type gene is localized within a region of DNA which spans 42,000 base pairs or larger and that the gene itself is discontinuous with several large intervening sequences. This is a remarkable observation since DHFR is a small protein coded for by only several hundred nucleotides of its messenger RNA. The amplified genes appear to be organized structurally in an identical manner as the wild-type gene in that the restriction enzyme mapping patterns of the amplified DNA is similar. This suggests that the resistant phenotype results from merely increasing the level of the normal gene and enzyme. The mechanism by which this amplification of the DHFR gene is mediated continues to be an area of intensive study.

The Class I mutation where the binding affinity of DHFR enzyme for methotrexate is significantly reduced has been characterized in both hamster and mouse cell lines.[64-66] It is perhaps significant that this altered enzyme is also observed to be overproduced when Class I mutants are subjected to further selection with increasing drug concentration.[66]

DNA-mediated transfer has been employed to unequivocally demonstrate the involvement of the DHFR gene in the methotrexate resistant phenotype.[52,67] This approach has been further extended to using cloned DHFR genes from prokaryotes inserted in an appropriate vector.[68] Thus in this respect, the genetic basis of methotrexate resistance is well understood.

C. Colchicine Resistance

Mutants resistant to the antimitotic compound colchicine and its analogues have been isolated in CHO cells in our laboratory. Two classes of mutants have been identified: one is a membrane-altered class with reduced drug permeability characterized by a pleiotropic phenotype of extensive cross-resistance to unrelated drugs; the other is microtubule-altered with reduced drug-binding affinity and displays only limited cross-resistance to related antimitotic compounds (Table 3). The membrane-altered (CH^R) class occurs at a frequency appreciably higher than the microtubule (CM^R) class and the CH^R class were the only mutants obtained in our selections with colchicine.[21,26] The microtubule-altered class was obtained when colcemid, an analogue of colchicine, was used as selective agent in the presence of nonionic detergent Tween® 80 to make the cells more permeable.[26]

In each case increased resistance can be obtained by further selective steps with increased drug concentrations; however, the degree of resistance after three selection steps is quite different, the CH^R class being more than 10 fold more resistant than the CM^R class. This stepwise increase in resistance in the CH^R class has been shown to correlate with decreased drug permeability[21,69] and an increased expression of a surface glycoprotein of 170,000 daltons, called the P-glycoprotein.[23,24] This is illustrated in Figure 2 where an antibody specific for the P-glycoprotein used to label membrane

Table 3
CHO CELL MUTANTS RESISTANT TO ANTI-MITOTIC COMPOUNDS

	Mutants selected for resistance to:	
	Colchicine	Colcemid
Spontaneous frequency	$\sim 5 \times 10^{-6}$	1×10^{-7}
Resistance to selecting drug after three steps	100—200 fold	6—10 fold
Hybrid phenotype	Dominant	Dominant
Cross-resistance	Wide-ranging to unrelated compounds	Limited to antitubulin compounds
Mechanism of resistance	Reduced drug uptake	Reduced drug binding
Altered gene product	Cell surface P-glycoprotein	Tubulin subunit protein

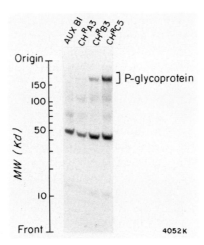

FIGURE 2. Plasma membrane components stained by a radiolabelled antiserum. Membrane vesicles were prepared from various CHO cell lines, fractionated by SDS gel electrophoresis, and subsequently transferred to nitrocellulose paper for staining by antiserum and radiolabeled protein A.[24,70] The antiserum was obtained from a rabbit immunized with membranes from highly colchicine-resistant cells. AuxB1 is the parental drug-sensitive line. CH^{R}A3, CH^{R}B3 and CH^{R}C5 is a series of related clones selected for increased resistance to colchicine.[21] The increased staining of P-glycoprotein (approximate molecular weight of 170,000) in this series of mutants is indicated. P-glycoprotein is not observed in the parental line. Other stained bands are membrane components common to all the cell lines.

components from parental cells, and mutants isolated in first, second, and third steps shows a progressive increase in that surface components. Moreover, the association of the P-glycoprotein expression with the resistant phenotype is further confirmed in analyses of cell:cell hybrids[22] and drug-sensitive revertants.[3,24] The stepwise increase in resistance in the CM^R class is associated with reduced drug-binding affinity of purified tubulin protein.[26,28] The level of tubulin in mutant cells appears not to be significantly altered. However, a variant α-tubulin subunit has been identified by two-dimensional gel electrophoresis.[28] In a similar system, Gottesman and co-workers[27] have identified altered β-tubulin subunits.

The fact that increased resistance can be obtained by multiple selection steps implicates the involvement of multiple genes or alleles in the resistant phenotype. In the case of the microtubule-altered mutants this hypothesis is completely consistent with our current understanding at the molecular level of the number and organization of tubulin genes. There is now good evidence from a number of systems including CHO cells (Elliott, Sarangi, and Ling, unpublished) that the α and β tubulin subunit proteins of microtubules are coded for by multigene families.[71,72] Thus it seems possible that progressive resistance in the CM[R] mutants is associated with alterations in different functional tubulin genes.[26,28] The CH[R] resistance associated with increased levels of P-glycoprotein expression however is more consistent with a gene amplification mechanism similar to DHFR enzyme overproduction in methotrexate resistance described above. Definitive evidence to support or eliminate this hypothesis has not yet been obtained although double minute chromosomes have recently been observed in unstable uptake mutants displaying a pleiotropic phenotype of resistance to multiple drugs.[73]

The pleiotropic phenotype displayed by the CH[R] membrane-altered mutants has important clinical implications since it is obvious that neoplastic cells possessing such an alteration could prove refractory even to treatment with combination chemotherapy. In this context it is significant that the cross-resistance of the CH[R] mutants include anticancer drugs of different classes as seen in Table 4. Collateral sensitivity however is also observed; and this may prove exploitable.[74,75] The notion that such a wide ranging pleiotropic phenotype can arise from a single mutation is supported by various lines of evidence: (1) independent clones selected for colchicine resistance in a single step all display this pleiotropy, (2) the frequency of appearance of such clones is similar to other drug-resistant phenotypes (Table 1), (3) revertant cells isolated in a single step without prior treatment with mutagens express a concomitant reversion of the pleiotropic phenotype,[3] (4) hybrid cells displaying dominance for colchicine resistance are also dominant for the pleiotropic phenotype,[22] (5) DNA-mediated transfer of colchicine resistance also results in the pleiotropic phenotype.[25] This latter result is significant since unlinked genes are not normally co-transferred in such experiments. In each of these cases (1-5), the level of cell surface P-glycoprotein expressed was concordant with the degree of resistance. Taken together, these observations provide compelling evidence that the CH[R] pleiotropic phenotype involves the expression of P-glycoprotein. By what molecular mechanism is the reduced drug permeability mediated is a question of interest and is currently being investigated.

It seems clear that the mechanism of resistance resulting in the CH[R] phenotype affects a wide variety of drugs. It is relevant to ask whether or not cells selected directly for resistance to any one of the compounds affected by the CH[R] mutation (Table 4) also yielded mutants possessing the same mechanism of resistance, i.e., reduced drug permeability, as the CH[R] mutants. In general this has proven to be the case. Mutants selected in vitro for resistance to daunomycin, adriamycin, vinblastine, actinomycin D, puromycin, etc. in a variety of animal and human cell lines all appear to possess a membrane-altered phenotype.[3,76-78] In many cases reduced drug permeability, cross-resistance to unrelated drugs, and expression of membrane-altered components have all been demonstrated. The pattern of resistance however to different drugs may differ depending on the cell type and selecting drug used. In light of these results our current bias is to assume that the mechanism of resistance associated with a multidrug resistant phenotype resides at the membrane level. In this context, it is noteworthy that resistances to unrelated drugs have been reported for a number of transplantable animal tumors.[79] Moreover, this phenotype has been observed in biopsy effusion samples from patients with breast or ovarian cancer.[80] Thus it would appear that the general class of mutations typified by the CH[R] mutation resulting in multidrug resistance is relatively common.

Table 4[a]
MULTIDRUG RESISTANCE OF A COLCHICINE-RESISTANT MUTANT CH^{R}C5

Drug	Relative resistance[b]
Colchicine	180
Puromycin	$\sim$ 100
Daunorubicin	76
Vinblastine	30
Emetine	29
Adriamycin	25
Melphalan	4—15
Chlorambucil	2
Nitrogen mustard	3
Bleomycin	$\sim$ 1
Cytarabine	$\sim$ 1
5-Fluorouracil	$\sim$ 1
Cyclophosphamide	0.3
Deoxycorticosterone	0.1
1-Dehydrotestosterone	0.1
Acronycine	< 0.06

[a]   Data compiled from work published previously.[17,74,75]
[b]   Relative resistance was determined by the concentration of drug required to inhibit growth or colony formation in the mutant line compared to the drug-sensitive parental line. A value greater than 1.0 indicates cross-resistance while one less than 1.0 denotes collateral sensitivity.

Exceptions to this general rule have been observed indicating that the membrane-altered mutation is not always the most frequent for the drugs listed in Table 4. For example in selecting for melphalan-resistant CHO cell mutants we found that the two stable clones characterized displayed only limited cross-resistance to nitrogen mustards and that the site of resistance was at the level of the cell nucleus.[17] Unstable clones were also observed but the nature of their resistance was not characterized.

Recently we have raised an antiserum against the cell surface P-glycoprotein expressed in the membrane-altered CH^R mutants (Riordan, Kartner, and Ling, unpublished results) and used this antiserum to probe for the expression of this surface antigen (c.f., Figure 2) in a variety of cell lines expressing multidrug resistance.[70] In each case, we were able to demonstrate the presence of high molecular weight (approximately 170,000 dalton) membrane components in resistant mutants from hamster, mouse, and human cells which cross-reacted with this antiserum. Such components were not observed in drug-sensitive lines. Such a finding suggests the intriguing idea that the P-glycoprotein, first identified in the CH^R mutants, is in fact a highly conserved protein which could be a functionally important constituent of the normal mammalian cell surface. Its predominance in the drug-resistant cell may be due to some mechanism resulting in the overproduction of this gene product. Moreover the expression of P-glycoprotein may be universally associated with a multidrug resistant phenotype. Whether or not such an antigen is expressed in neoplasms resistant to combination chemotherapy is a question of intense interest.

D. L-Asparaginase Resistance

The basis for the therapeutic effectiveness of the enzyme L-asparaginase for certain malignancies has received considerable attention.[81,82] It apparently stems from the nutritional requirement of the neoplastic cells for L-asparagine thus the enzymatic depletion of this amino acid in the environment results in killing of sensitive auxotrophic cells. Other mechanisms have also been proposed.[83,84] Resistant tumors are frequently observed and analysis of these cells generally indicated that an increased level of asparagine synthetase activity accompanied the onset of resistance.[81,82] In order to understand in greater detail the origin and mechanism of resistance to this novel therapeutic agent, a genetic approach involving isolation of relevant mutants in CHO cells and characterization of their sensitivity to asparaginase has been carried out.[7,8,85]

The approach taken by Waye and Stanners[7] was to isolate asparaginase-sensitive mutants from wild-type cells which were normally resistant. They observed that the primary defect was a reduced level of asparagine synthetase activity. Revertants could be isolated from these mutants which expressed a coordinate increase in the asparagine synthetase activity. A different approach taken by Arfin and co-workers[8] was to isolate mutants resistant to the compound β-aspartylhydroxamate in which the mechanism of resistance stemmed from an increased production of the asparagine synthetase enzyme. These mutants were more resistant to L-asparaginase than the wild-type cells.[85] Resistance to β-aspartylhydroxamate could be conferred on drug-sensitive recipients using DNA-mediated transfer and at the same time, an increased level of asparagine synthetase activity was observed in these transformants.[9] Waye and Stanners[86] have recently been able to transfer a cloned prokaryotic asparagine synthetase gene into rat Jensen sarcoma cells which are asparagine auxotrophs. Transformants are resistant to asparaginase and can be adapted to grow in more stringent selective medium with a resultant increase in the number of copies of the asparagine synthetase gene. Taken together, these experiments clearly implicate the involvement of asparagine synthetase in the L-asparaginase-resistant phenotype and demonstrate that the level of asparagine synthetase activity in a cell plays an important role in determining the level of the sensitivity of the cell to L-asparaginase.

A similar approach was taken to evaluate the role that asparagyl-tRNA synthetase plays in determining a sensitivity of the cell to L-asparaginase. Waye and Stanners[85] concluded from studies with mutants temperature sensitive for this enzyme that a defect in this enzyme could result in a cell being highly sensitive to low levels of asparagine in the medium. Thus it appears that two enzymes have been identified which could determine a response of the cell to L-asparaginase.

E. Summary

There is every indication from the mutants surveyed in this section that mechanisms of resistance to antineoplastic drugs can be elucidated in some detail. Therefore it seems evident that studies of well-defined drug-resistant lines isolated in vitro deserve continued innovation and emphasis in order to generate an arsenal of tools to better investigate the problem of drug resistance in patients. Future prospects for this approach appear promising in light of the modern biological techniques such as gene cloning and transfer which are currently available for application.

IV. CONCLUSIONS AND FUTURE PROSPECTS

From the studies described in this chapter, it is apparent that a very wide variety of drug-resistant phenotypes can be obtained from mutants isolated in culture. Properties associated with many of these resistant phenotypes such as dominance of expression, rate of formation, frequency of occurrence, and stability of propagation indicate that such mutations could be expressed in naturally occurring tumors. Thus it is reasonable to assume that a similarly wide variety of drug-resistant malignant cells will be found in patients.

Drug-resistant tumors have been identified in vivo although in general, they have not been characterized genetically. With our present understanding, a sound working hypothesis would be to assume that stable resistant phenotypes arise from *bona fide* mutations. Based on the premise that the presence of drug-resistant mutants could be a major obstacle limiting successful chemotherapy of neoplastic diseases, Goldie and Coldman[87] have proposed a model outlining therapeutic strategies to avoid failure due to spontaneous occurrence of such mutations. It is likely that refinement and evaluation of this model will require measurement, at the in vivo level, of the rates of mutation leading to drug resistance in various neoplasms. Most tumors would have grown to at least 10^8 cells by the time they are detected clinically, and the likelihood that some drug-resistant mutants would have already been generated is high, if one assumes mutation rates of the order observed for cells in culture (Table 1). As noted earlier, mutation rates to drug resistance can be affected under a variety of conditions (IIB). In the context of our current understanding that genetic instability and karyotypic diversity are intimately associated with malignant transformation and tumor progression,[88-90] it seems entirely possible that mutations to drug resistance could arise in spontaneous tumors at a rate much higher than previously anticipated.

The task of identifying and isolating drug-resistant mutants for investigation from spontaneous human tumors is admittedly a difficult one. Experimental tools generated from in vitro studies may be useful in this regard. For example, in a number of instances, the gene products associated with particular drug-resistant mechanisms have been identified unequivocally, and in principle, antibodies raised against such gene products could be used to detect and classify resistant tumor subpopulations. In this manner, the observation that antiserum raised against drug-resistant hamster cell surface P-glycoprotein also cross-reacts with the presumptive human P-glycoprotein[70] could be exploited. Moreover, the prospect of using specific (e.g., monoclonal) antibodies to precisely direct cytotoxic agents against drug-resistant cells is an exciting one.[91,92]

The fact that resistance to multiple drugs can result from a single mutation (see IIIC) and that the phenotype generated from such mutations is rather complex emphasizes the importance of understanding the basis of this mode of resistance. As can be appreciated, a cell acquiring a multidrug resistant mutation could be relatively refractory even to combination chemotherapy. Studies of this important drug-resistant phenotype require efforts in at least two areas. First, it would be important to delineate in more detail the role of P-glycoprotein in mediating the aspect of multidrug resistance. Isolation of the P-glycoprotein gene (currently underway) and DNA-mediated transfer of the gene to test for function[25] should provide a powerful approach towards this objective. Second, from a therapeutic viewpoint, the question of whether such mutations are found in neoplasms in man must be tackled directly. The use of anti-P-glycoprotein antibody as outlined above could provide one approach to this question. Isolation and growth of drug-resistant cells from patient biopsy samples will also be required, particularly with respect to determining the cross-resistance patterns from such putative mutants. Special emphasis should be made to screen for compounds to which mutants of this class are collaterally sensitive (Table 4). Information from this area of investigation may provide a better basis to formulate drug combinations for therapy.

A recurrent theme among the mutants reviewed in this chapter is that resistance to a number of drugs result from increased production of particular enzymes or gene products. This was demonstrated for methotrexate resistance (IIIB), asparaginase resistance (IIID), hydroxyurea resistance (Table 1), and for the multidrug resistance phenotype associated with increased P-glycoprotein expression (IIIC). The molecular mechanisms associated with increased expression of these drug-resistant associated gene products are not understood in all cases; however, increased copy number of the relevant DHFR gene has been observed in methotrexate resistant cells. This gene amplification is accompanied by the appearance of double minute chromosomes or homogeneously staining regions in metaphase chromosomes. How such chromosomal aberrations are generated is currently not understood, but they have been observed in certain forms of malignancies.[93,94] although not proven, it is assumed that some gene products are overproduced in those cells. Moreover, the concept that increased production of certain genes could lead to malignancy has gained wide support as a general mechanism for carcinogenesis.[95-97] It seems possible therefore that in some instances, modifications in the cellular genome leading to malignant transformation could also lead to the increased production of particular proteins resulting in drug-resistance and that studies of drug-resistant mutants in cancer cell populations may in fact provide insights into the process of malignant development and progression. We should be prepared for surprises.

ACKNOWLEDGMENTS

I thank Norbert Kartner, Mary Waye, and Ann Chambers for helpful discussions during the preparation of this chapter. This work is supported by the Medical Research Council of Canada, the National Cancer Institute of Canada, and the Ontario Cancer Treatment and Research Foundation.

REFERENCES

1. Brockman, R. W., *Pharmacological Basis of Cancer Chemotherapy*, Williams & Wilkins, Baltimore, 1975, 691.
2. Thompson, L. H. and Baker, R. M., Isolation of mutants of cultured mammalian cell, in *Methods in Cell Biology*, Vol. 6, Prescott, D. M., Ed., Academic Press, New York, 1973, 209.
3. Baker, R. M. and Ling, V., Membrane mutants of mammalian cells in culture, in *Methods in Membrane Biology*, Vol. 9, Korn, E. D., Ed., Plenum Press, New York, 1978, 337.
4. Demars, R., Resistance of cultured fibroblasts and other cells to purine and pyrimidine analogues in relation to mutagenesis detection, *Mutation Res.*, 24, 335, 1974.
5. Siminovitch, L., On the nature of hereditable variation in cultured somatic cells, *Cell*, 7, 1, 1976.
6. Clement, G. B., Selection of biochemically variant, in some cases mutant, mammalian cells in culture, *Adv. Cancer Res.*, 21, 273, 1975.
7. Waye, M. M. Y. and Stanners, C. P., Isolation and characterization of CHO cell mutants with altered asparagine synthetase, *Somatic Cell Genet.*, 5, 625, 1979.
8. Gantt, J. S., Chiang, C.-S., Hatfield, G. W., and Arfin, S. M., Chinese hamster ovary cells resistant to β-aspartylhydroxamate contain increased levels of asparagine synthetase, *J. Biol. Chem.*, 255, 4808, 1980.
9. Andrulis, I. L. and Siminovitch, L., DNA-mediated gene transfer of β-aspartylhydroxamate resistance into Chinese hamster ovary cells, *Proc. Natl. Acad. Sci. USA*, 78, 5724, 1981.
10. Chan, V. L. and Juranka, P., Isolation and characterization of 9-β-D-arabinofuranosyladenine-resistant mutants of baby hamster cells, *Somatic Cell Genet.*, 7, 147, 1981.
11. Lewis, W. H. and Wright, J. W., Genetic characterization of hydroxyurea-resistance in Chinese hamster ovary cells, *J. Cell. Physiol.*, 97, 73, 1978.

12. Lewis, W. H. and Wright, J. A., Ribonucleotide reductase from wild type and hydroxyurea-resistant Chinese hamster ovary cells, *J. Cell. Physiol.*, 97, 87, 1978.
13. Lewis, W. H. and Wright, J. A., Isolation of hydroxyurea-resistant CHO cells with altered levels of ribonucleotide reductase, *Somatic Cell Genet.*, 5, 83, 1979.
14. Dechamps, M., Robert de Saint-Vincent, B., Evrard, C., Sassi, M., and Buttin, G., Studies on 1-β-D-arabinofuranosylcytosine (Ara C) resistant mutants of Chinese hamster fibroblasts. II. High resistance to Ara C as a genetic marker for cellular hybridization, *Exptl. Cell Res.*, 86, 269, 1974.
15. Robert de Saint Vincent, B. and Buttin, G., Studies on 1-β-D-arabinofuranosyl-cytosine-resistant mutants of Chinese hamster fibroblasts. III. Joint resistance to arabinofuranosylcytosine and to excess thymidine - a semi-dominant manifestation of deoxycytidine triphosphate pool expansion, *Somatic Cell Genet.*, 5, 67, 1979.
16. Robert de Saint Vincent, B. and Buttin, G., Studies on 1-β-D-arabinofuranosylcytosine-resistant mutants of Chinese hamster fibroblasts. IV. Altered regulation of CTP synthetase generates arabinosylcytosine and thymidine resistance, *Biochim. Biophys. Acta*, 610, 352, 1980.
17. Elliott, E. M. and Ling, V., Selection and characterization of Chinese hamster ovary cell mutants resistant to melphalan (L-phenylalanine mustard), *Cancer Res.*, 41, 393, 1981.
18. Flintoff, W. F., Davidson, S. V., and Siminovitch, L., Isolation and partial characterization of three methotrexate-resistant phenotypes from Chinese hamster ovary cells, *Somatic Cell Genet.*, 2, 245, 1976.
19. Flintoff, W. F., Spindler, S. M., and Siminovitch, L., Genetic characterization of methotrexate-resistant Chinese hamster ovary cells, *In Vitro*, 12, 749, 1976.
20. Flintoff, W. F., personal communication, 1981.
21. Ling, V. and Thompson, L. H., Reduced permeability in CHO cells as a mechanism of resistance to colchicine, *J. Cell. Physiol.*, 83, 103, 1974.
22. Ling, V. and Baker, R. M., Dominance of colchicine resistance in hybrid CHO cells, *Somatic Cell Genet.*, 4, 193, 1978.
23. Juliano, R. L. and Ling, V., A surface glycoprotein modulating drug permeability in Chinese hamster ovary cell mutant, *Biochem. Biophys. Acta*, 455, 152, 1976.
24. Riordan, J. R. and Ling, V., Purification of P-glycoprotein from plasma membrane vesicles of Chinese hamster ovary cell mutants with reduced colchicine permeability, *J. Biol. Chem.*, 254, 12701, 1979.
25. Debenham, P. G., Kartner, N., Siminovitch, L., Riordan, J. R., and Ling, V., DNA-mediated transfer of multiple drug resistance and plasma membrane glycoprotein expression, *Molec. Cell. Biol.*, in press, 1982.
26. Ling, V., Aubin, J. E., Chase, A., and Sarangi, F., Mutants of Chinese hamster ovary (CHO) cells with altered colcemid-binding affinity, *Cell*, 18, 423, 1979.
27. Cabral, F., Sobel, M. E., and Gottesman, M. M., CHO mutants resistant to colchicine, colcemid, or griseofulvin have an altered β-tubulin, *Cell*, 20, 29, 1980.
28. Keates, R. A. B., Sarangi, F., and Ling, V., Structural and functional alterations in microtubule protein from Chinese hamster ovary cell mutants, *Proc. Natl. Acad. Sci. USA*, 78, 5638, 1981.
29. Gupta, R. S., Resistance to the microtubule inhibitor podophyllotoxin: selection and partial characterization of mutants in CHO cells, *Somatic Cell Genet.*, 7, 59, 1981.
30. Chan, V. L., Whitmore, G. F., and Siminovitch, L., Mammalian cells with altered forms of RNA polymerase II, *Proc. Natl. Acad. Sci. USA*, 69, 3119, 1972.
31. Ingles, C. J., Guialis, A., Lam, J., and Siminovitch, L., α-amanitin resistance of RNA polymerase II in mutant Chinese hamster ovary cell lines, *J. Biol. Chem.*, 251, 2729, 1976.
32. Ingles, C. J., and Shales, M., DNA-mediated transfer of an RNA polymerase II gene: reversion of the temperature-sensitive hamster cell cycle mutant TsAF8 by mammalian DNA, *Molec. Cell. Biol.*, in press, 1982.
33. Gupta, R. S. and Siminovitch, L., The isolation and preliminary characterization of somatic cell mutants resistant to the protein synthesis inhibitor - emetine, *Cell*, 9, 213, 1976.
34. Gupta, R. S. and Siminovitch, L., The molecular basis of emetine resistance in Chinese hamster ovary cells: alteration in the 40S ribosomal subunit, *Cell*, 10, 61, 1977.
35. Baker, R. M., Brunette, D. M., Mankovitz, R., Thompson, L. H., Whitmore, G. F., Siminovitch, L., and Till, J. E., Ouabain-resistant mutants of mouse and hamster cells in culture, *Cell*, 1, 9, 1974.
36. Stanley, P. and Siminovitch, L., Selection and characterization of Chinese hamster ovary cells resistant to the cytotoxicity of lectins, *In Vitro*, 12, 208, 1976.
37. Luria, S. E. and Delbrück, M., Mutations of bacteria from virus sensitivity to virus resistance, *Genetics*, 28, 491, 1943.
38. Lea, D. E. and Coulson, C. A., The distribution of the numbers of mutants in bacterial populations, *J. Genet.*, 49, 264.

39. Meuth, M., L'Heureux-Huard, N., and Trudel, M., Characterization of a mutator gene in Chinese hamster ovary cells, *Proc. Natl. Acad. Sci. USA*, 76, 6505, 1979.

40. Weinberg, G., Ullman, B., and Martin, D. W., Jr., Mutator phenotypes in mammalian cell mutants with distinct biochemical defects and abnormal deoxyribonucleoside triphosphate pools, *Proc. Natl. Acad. Sci. USA*, 78, 2447, 1981.

41. Chan, V. L., Guttman, S., and Juranka, P., Mutator genes of baby hamster kidney cells, *Mol. Cell Biol.*, 1, 568, 1981.

42. Goldberg, S. and Defendi, V., Increased mutation rates in doubly viral transformed Chinese hamster cells, *Somatic Cell Genet.*, 5, 887, 1979.

43. Cifone, M. A. and Fidler, J. I., Increasing metastatic potential is associated with increasing genetic instability of clones isolated from murine neoplasms, *Proc. Natl. Acad. Sci. USA*, 78, 6949, 1981.

44. Gupta, R. S. and Goldstein, S., Diphtheria toxin resistance in human fibroblast cell strains from normal and cancer-prone individuals, *Mutation Res.*, 73, 331, 1980.

45. Warren, S. T., Schultz, R. A., Chang, C.-C., Wade, M. H., and Trosko, J. E., Elevated spontaneous mutation rate in Bloom syndrome fibroblasts, *Proc. Natl. Acad. Sci. USA*, 78, 3133, 1981.

46. Giles, R. E. and Ruddle, F. H., Production and characterization of proliferating somatic cell hybrids, in *Tissue Culture - Methods and Application,* Kruse, P. F., Jr. and Patterson, M. K., Jr., Eds., Academic Press, New York, 1973, 475.

47. Ruddle, F. H., Linkage analysis using somatic cell hybrids, *Adv. Hum. Genet.*, 3, 172, 1972.

48. Sandberg, A. A., *The Chromosomes in Human Cancer and Leukemia,* Elsevier, New York, 1980.

49. Campbell, C. E. and Worton, R. G., Evidence obtained by induced mutation frequency analysis for functional hemizyosity at the *emt* locus in CHO cells, *Somatic Cell Genet.*, 5, 51, 1979.

50. McBride, O. W. and Peterson, J. L., Chromosome-mediated gene transfer in mammalian cells, *Annu. Rev. Genet.*, 14, 321, 1980.

51. Klobutcher, L. A. and Ruddle, F. H., Chromosome mediated gene transfer, *Annu. Rev. Biochem.*, 50, 533, 1981.

52. Lewis, W. J., Srinivasan, P. R., Stokoe, N., and Siminovitch, L., Parameters governing the transfer of the genes for thymidine kinase and dihydrofolate reductase in mouse cell using metaphase chromosomes or DNA, *Somatic Cell Genet.*, 3, 333, 1980.

53. Wigler, M., Sweet, R., Sim, G.-K., Wold, B., Pellicer, A., Lacy, E., Maniatis, T., Silverstein, S., and Axel, R., Transformation of mammalian cells with genes from procaryotes and eukaryotes, *Cell,* 16, 777, 1979.

54. Pellicer, A., Robins, D., Wold, B., Sweet, R., Jackson, J., Lowy, I., Roberts, J. M., Sim, G. K., Silverstein, S., and Axel, R., Altering genotype and phenotype by DNA-mediated gene transfer, *Science,* 209, 1414, 1980.

55. Bertino, J. R., Ed., Folate antagonists as chemotherapeutic agents, *Annals of the New York Academy Science,* Vol. 186, New York Academy Science, New York, 1971.

56. Harrap, K. R. and Jackson, R. C., Biochemical mechanisms of resistance to antimetabolites, *Antibiot. Chemother.*, 23, 228, 1978.

57. Morandi, C. and Attardi, G., Isolation and characterization of dihydrofolic acid reductase from methotrexate-sensitive and -resistant human cell lines, *J. Biol. Chem.*, 256, 10169, 1981.

58. Bertino, J. R., Dolnick, B. J., Berenson, R. J., Scheer, D. I., and Kamen, B. A., Cellular mechanisms of resistance to methotrexate, in *Molecular Actions and Targets for Cancer Chemotherapeutic Agents,* Sartorelli, A. C., Lazo, J. S., Bertino, J. R., Eds., Academic Press, New York, 1981, 385.

59. Flintoff, W. and Saya, L. The selection of wild-type revertants from methotrexate permeability mutants, *Somatic Cell Genet.*, 4, 143, 1978.

60. Schimke, R. T., Kaufman, R. J., Alt, F. W., and Kellems, R. F., Gene amplification and drug resistance in cultured murine cells, *Science,* 202, 1051, 1978.

61. Nunberg, J. H., Kaufman, R. J., Schimke, R. T., Urlaub, G., and Chasin, L. A., Amplified dihydrofolate reductase genes and localized to a homogeneously staining region of a single chromosome in a methotrexate-resistant Chinese hamster ovary cell line, *Proc. Natl. Acad. Sci. USA*, 75, 5553, 1978.

62. Kaufman, R. J., Brown, P. C., and Schimke, R. T., Amplified dihydrofolate reductase genes in unstably methotrexate resistant cells are associated with double minute chromosomes, *Proc. Natl. Acad. Sci. USA*, 76, 5669, 1979.

63. Nunberg, J. H., Kaukman, R. J., Chang, A. C. Y., Cohen, S. N., and Schimke, R. T., Structure and genomic organization of the mouse dihydrofolate reductase gene, *Cell,* 19, 355, 1980.

64. Flintoff, W. F. and Essani, K., Methotrexate-resistant Chinese hamster ovary cells contain a dihydrofolate reductase with an altered affinity for methotrexate, *Biochemistry,* 19, 4321, 1980.

65. Goldie, J. H., Krystal, G., Hartley, D., Gudauskas, G., and Dedhar, S., A methotrexate insensitive variant of folate reductase present in two lines of methotrexate-resistant L5178Y cells, *Eur. J. Cancer,* 16, 1539, 1980.

66. Haber, D. A., Beverley, S. M., Kiely, M. L., and Schimke, R. T., Properties of an altered dihydro-folate reductase encoded by amplified genes in cultured mouse fibroblasts, *J. Biol. Chem.*, 256, 9501, 1981.

67. Wigler, M., Perucho, M., Kurtz, D., Dana, S., Pellicer, A., Axel, R., and Silverstein, S., Transformation of mammalian cells with an amplifiable dominant-acting gene, *Proc. Natl. Acad. Sci. USA*, 77, 3567, 1980.

68. O'Hare, K., Benoist, C., and Breathnack, R., Transformation of mouse fibroblasts to methotrexate resistance by a recombinant plasmid expressing a prokaryotic dihydrofolate reductase, *Proc. Natl. Acad. Sci. USA*, 78, 1527, 1981.

69. See, Y. P., Carlsen, S. A., Till, J. E., and Ling, V., Increased drug permeability in Chinese hamster ovary cells in the presence of cyanide, *Biochim. Biophys. Acta*, 373, 242, 1974.

70. Kartner, N., Riordan, J. R., and Ling, V., Cell surface P-glycoprotein is associated with multi-drug resistance in mammalian cells, submitted for publication.

71. Cleveland, D. W., Lopata, M. A., MacDonald, R. J., Cowan, N. J., Rutter, W. J., and Kirschner, M. W., Number and evolutionary conservation of α- and β-tubulin and cytoplasmic β- and γ-actin genes using specific cloned cDNA probes, *Cell*, 20, 95, 1980.

72. Firtel, R. A., Multigene families encoding actin and tubulin, *Cell*, 24, 6, 1981.

73. Baskin, F., Rosenbeg, R. N., and Dev, V., Correlation of double-minute chromosomes with unstable multidrug cross-resistance in uptake mutants of neuroblastoma cells, *Proc. Natl. Acad. Sci. USA*, 78, 3654, 1981.

74. Bech-Hansen, N. T., Till, J. E., and Ling, V., Pleiotropic phenotype of colchicine-resistant CHO cells: cross-resistance and collateral sensitivity, *J. Cell. Physiol.*, 88, 23, 1976.

75. Ling, V., Genetic aspects of drug resistance in somatic cells, *Antibiot. Chemother.*, 23, 191, 1978.

76. Ling, V., Drug resistance and membrane alteration in mutants of mammalian cells, *Can. J. Genet. Cytology*, 17, 503, 1975.

77. Biedler, J. L. and Peterson, R. H. F., Altered plasma membrane glycoconjugates of Chinese hamster cells with acquired resistance to actinomycin D, daunorubicin, and vincristine, in *Molecular Actions and Targets for Cancer Chemotherapeutic Agents*, Sartovelli, A. C., Lazo, J. S., Bertino, J. R., Eds., Academic Press, New York, 1981, 453.

78. Beck, W. T., Mueller, T. J., and Tarzer, L. R., Altered surface membrane glycoproteins in vinca alkaloid-resistant human leukemic lymphoblasts, *Cancer Res.*, 39, 2070, 1979.

79. Skipper, H. E., Hutchinson, D. J., Shabel, F. M., Schmidt, L. H., Goldin, A., Brockman, R. W., Venditti, J. M., and Wodinsky, I., A quick reference chart on cross resistance between anti cancer agents, *Cancer Chemo. Rep.*, part 1, 56, 493, 1972.

80. Bech-Hansen, N. T., Sarangi, F., Sutherland, D. J. A., and Ling, V., Rapid assays for evaluating the drug sensitivity of tumor cells, *J. Natl. Cancer Inst.*, 59, 21, 1977.

81. Wriston, J. C. and Yellin, T. O., L-asparaginase: a review, *Adv. Enzymol.*, 39, 185, 1973.

82. Cooney, D. A., King, V. D., Cable, R. G., Taylor, B., and Wodinsky, I., L-asparaginase synthetase in serum as a marker for neoplasia, *Cancer Res.*, 36, 3238, 1976.

83. Dods, R. F., Essner, E., and Barclay, M., Isolation and characterization of plasma membranes from L-asparaginase-sensitive strain of leukemia cells, *Biochem. Biophys. Res. Commun.*, 46, 1074, 1972.

84. Lavietes, B. B., Regan, D. H., and Demopoulos, H. B., Glutamate oxidation in 6C3HED lymphoma: effects of L-asparaginase on sensitive and resistant lines, *Proc. Natl. Acad. Sci. USA*, 71, 3993, 1974.

85. Waye, M. M. Y. and Stanners, C. P., The role of asparagine synthetase and asparagyl-tRNA synthetase in the cell killing activity of L-asparaginase in Chinese hamster ovary cell mutants, *Cancer Res.*, 41, 3104, 1981.

86. Waye, M. and Stanners, C. P., personal communication, 1981.

87. Goldie, J. H. and Coldman, A. J., A mathematic model for relating the drug sensitivity of tumors to their spontaneous mutation rate, *Cancer Treat. Rep.*, 63, 1727, 1979.

88. Nowell, P. C., The clonal evaluation of tumor cell populations, *Science*, 194, 23, 1976.

89. Straus, D. S., Somatic mutation, cellular differentiation, and cancer causation, *J. Natl. Cancer Inst.*, 67, 233, 1981.

90. Cairns, J., The origin of human cancer, *Nature (London)*, 289, 353, 1981.

91. Krolick, K. A., Isakson, P. C., Uhr, J. W., and Vitetta, E. S., Selective killing of normal or neoplastic B cells by antibodies coupled to the A chain of ricin, *Proc. Natl. Acad. Sci. USA*, 77, 5419, 1980.

92. Gilliland, D. G., Steplewski, Z., Collier, R. J., Mitchell, K. R., Chang, T. H., and Kaprowski, H., Antibody-directed cytotoxic agents: use of monoclonal antibody to direct the action of toxin A chains to colorectal carcinoma cells, *Proc. Natl. Acad. Sci. USA*, 77, 4539, 1980.

93. Mark, J., Double minutes — a chromosomal aberration in Rous carcinomas in mice, *Hereditas*, 57, 1, 1967.

94. Biedler, J. L., Chromosome abnormalities in human tumor cells in culture, in *Human Tumor Cells in Vitro*, Fogh, J., Ed., Plenum Press, New York, 1975, 359.

95. **Pall, M. L.**, Gene-amplification model of carcinogenesis, *Proc. Natl. Acad. Sci. USA*, 78, 2465, 1981.

96. **Varshavsky, A.**, On the possibility of metabolic control of replicon "misfiring": relation to emergence of malignant phenotypes in mammalian cell lineages, *Proc. Natl. Acad. Sci. USA*, 78, 3673, 1981.

97. **Erikson, R. L., Purchio, A. F., Erikson, E., Collett, M. S., and Brugge, J. S.**, Molecular events in cells transformed by Rous sarcoma virus, *J. Cell Biol.*, 87, 319, 1980.

Chapter 2

BIOCHEMICAL AND CELL KINETIC ASPECTS OF DRUG RESISTANCE

Bridget T. Hill

TABLE OF CONTENTS

I. INTRODUCTION

Successful chemotherapy requires the development of effective antitumor drugs which, when administered according to an optimal schedule result in tumor eradication with minimal host toxicity. Although this objective is rarely achieved cures are now possible in a few human malignancies, notably the childhood tumors and testicular teratomas[1,2] and encouraging results are available from the treatment of ovarian carcinomas[3] and small cell lung cancer.[4] This provides further impetus to try and improve therapy and the prognosis for other common "solid" tumors such as those of breast, bladder, prostate, stomach, and head and neck. The development or expression of drug resistance is considered a major reason for many treatment failures, although a lack of response may also ensue from suboptimal use of chemotherapy. This chapter reviews some cell kinetic and biochemical factors associated with drug resistance and discusses ways in which it may be minimized or circumvented, emphasizing studies of potential clinical relevance.

II. CELL KINETIC FACTORS CONTRIBUTING TO THE FAILURES OF CHEMOTHERAPY

Many authors dismiss the subject of cell cycle kinetics when considering either valuable past contributions to effective therapies or potential new approaches.[5-8] The fact that this attitude currently prevails may be attributed, at least in part, to an inability to distinguish between measurements of traditional cell kinetic parameters on heterogenous cell populations and concepts of "stem cell" kinetics as originally described by the Toronto School.[9,10] While the, as yet fruitless, search for major biochemical differences between "tumor" and "normal" cells continues, the kinetic difference between normal and malignant stem cell populations first demonstrated in tumor-bearing animals over 25 years ago remains to be exploited fully. The application of *certain* specific aspects of cell cycle kinetics has been shown clinically markedly to increase the safety and selectivity of cancer chemotherapy (discussed in Section IV), although the value of this approach is often misinterpreted.[5,7,8,11]

Our knowledge of the growth characteristics of human tumors and of normal proliferating tissues at risk of damage from cytotoxic agents remains incomplete. However, certain factors are known to influence not only response to chemotherapy but also the timing and scheduling of treatment. Therefore by suitable application of our present knowledge in conjunction with information from other fields such as biochemistry, pharmacology, and toxicology, improvements in the treatment of human malignancies can *now* be achieved. This section concentrates on those specific cell kinetic factors which need to be considered when designing more effective treatment strategies. The irrelevance of some of the more traditional cell cycle kinetic parameters will be mentioned, although these have been discussed in detail in a recent review.[12]

A. Tumor Size and Growth Rate

Studies with tumor-bearing animals have provided evidence that (1) chemotherapy is most effective against small rather than large or advanced tumours,[13,14] and (2) rapidly proliferating cell populations are most sensitive to the cytotoxic effects of drugs.[9,15] While extrapolation of experimental data to the clinic is often highly speculative and can be disappointing or even misleading, this is not invariably so, as discussed below.

Current methods of investigation fail clinically to detect most tumors until they are at least two thirds of the way through their life span as illustrated in Figure 1. This shows the relationship between the number of population doublings, the increase in

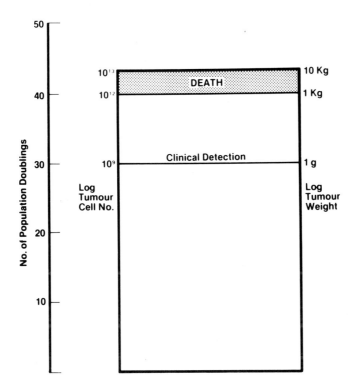

FIGURE 1. The relationship between the number of population doublings and the increase in cell number and weight during a tumor's development, clinical detection of the tumor and the death of the patient. Current methods of investigation allow detection of the tumor only when about 1 g of tumor is present and the tumor is already at least two-thirds of the way through its lifespan (reproduced from Hill,[12] with the permission of the editor of *Cell Biology International Reports*).

cell number and weight during tumor development, the level of clinical detection, and the death of the patient. Biologically most human tumors are late or advanced at the time of presentation. Failure to "cure" patients with chemotherapy alone should therefore not be unexpected. This same point applies to detection of secondary deposits, i.e., it is possible for a patient with an apparently "local" tumor to have many undetectable distant micrometastases. Fortunately this fact is now accepted by many clinicians and taken into account in treatment planning. Chemotherapy provides the systemic component in combination with optimal local therapy for adjuvant trials now being used for several human "solid" tumors notably those of the breast, lung, and ovary.[3,4,16-18]

Clinical assessment of response to therapy is based mainly on gross measurements of tumor size. The inherent inaccuracy of defining a complete remission as the absence of clinically detectable disease is apparent from Figure 1. The accepted definition of a partial response also fails to take into account the lack of uniformity of tumor growth rates, so that a 50% reduction in tumor volume may or may not be meaningful. A characteristic feature of the growth of a tumor is a progressive increase in cell number. In simple model systems such as suspension cultures of tumor cells or even experimental animal ascitic tumors, a constant relationship between cell division and time is observed and these cells are considered to grow exponentially. In many solid tumors in animals the logarithm of tumor volume increases linearly with time especially during the early period of a tumor's development. However, as the tumor mass increases, its inner and outer portions become subject to different physiological conditions which affect its growth pattern; there is a tendency for the growth rate to slow and then the growth curve can be described by a Gompertzian function.[19] For most human "solid" tumors, where estimations of tumor growth are of necessity restricted to a short period near the end of their life span, any attempt to use these measurements as a basis for future treatment planning must be approached cautiously. For example, extrapolation may be attempted to determine when the risks of local recurrence are likely to be minimal or when total tumor eradication is likely, so that chemotherapy may be stopped. When such extrapolation is made over a long time interval the chance of error increases, since the growth rate is liable to fluctuate. Tumor growth rate is also known to be influenced by ionizing radiation and chemotherapy. Thus precise measurements of growth rates of human "solid" tumors have for these and other reasons[12] rarely been made. Indeed, even if data were available, they would be of dubious significance since they take no account of the considerable heterogeneity of human tumors. For example, tumor cell populations may be divided into three kinetic compartments: (1) cells that continuously move around the cell cycle (continuously proliferating or cycling cells), (2) cells that may leave the cycle but can be induced to re-enter by an appropriate stimulus (resting, G_o or nonproliferating cells), and (3) nondividing cells which have permanently left the cell cycle and will die without dividing again.[20-23] Therefore the growth of any population depends on at least three factors: the length of the cell cycle(s); the extent of cell loss due to death, exfoliation, or migration; and the proportion of resting or nonproliferating cells which can be brought back into cycle. Generally, attempts to measure these factors have met with limited success, as discussed earlier,[12,19] and in practice techniques allowing relevant estimates of the "proliferative parameters" of individual tumors remain to be developed.

It is important to realize that a reduction in the growth rate of a tumor, measured clinically, may be attributed to (1) an increased cell loss, (2) a reduction in number of proliferating cells and/or an increase in the percentage of resting cells, (3) an extension of cell cycle times, (4) selective killing of cells with shorter cell cycle times within the heterogeneous population, or (5) a combination of any or all of these factors. It is often difficult to distinguish between these alternatives in human tumors. Thus the need for more sensitive methods of tumor detection and of monitoring response to therapy remains, and tumor markers may be valuable in this respect. However, by applying our present knowledge to the optimal integration of various treatment modalities improved results may even now be achieved.

B. Proportion of Nonproliferating or Resting Cells in Normal and Malignant Cell Populations

The realization that proliferating cells were more sensitive to cytotoxic drugs led to the suggestion that tumors with a high "proliferative or growth fraction", and therefore few nonproliferating cells, such as transplantable animal tumors and leukemias, would be most easily destroyed by antitumor drugs. In contrast, in most "solid" tumors where the "growth fraction" is low, only a small percentage of the cells would be susceptible to chemotherapy.[12,24] Unfortunately, the use of this term in practice suffers from the major drawback that at present we are unable to distinguish accurately between nonproliferating and slowly or discontinuously proliferating cells.

Heterogeneity exists even among nonproliferating cells. Some are sterile or end cells, but others remain only temporarily at rest. For example, in "solid" tumors some resting cells held back by lack of nutrients or toxicity are destined to die, while others may recover when the supply of nutrients improves perhaps following partial destruction of the tumor by therapy. A partial depletion of the proliferative compartment, for example, by chemotherapy, also may trigger both normal and malignant resting cells back into cycle.[20,25,26] In addition, cells that are proceeding slowly through the cycle may speed up their traverse given the appropriate stimulus. In certain normal tissues, the resting or quiescent population represents an essential element in homeostasis, which may also be so in certain malignant tissues. Thus a knowledge of the size of all these subpopulations is of the utmost importance.

C. Stem Cells

Alterations in the "proliferative parameters" can also account, at least in part, for an increased growth rate or the regrowth of a tumor after damage by therapeutic agents. In this respect the existence of a small fraction of cells, the stem cells, is of paramount importance. It has been proposed that only these stem cells are responsible for maintaining the integrity and continued survival of any particular cell population.[10,27] Therefore, by definition, a stem cell is capable of an indefinite number of divisions, unlike the majority of cells which lack this unlimited capacity for proliferation. The existence of stem cells in normal tissues is well established with those in bone marrow and intestinal crypts being particularly well characterized[10,28] and evidence for malignant stem cells is gradually accruing.[9,29-32] Restraint, orderly proliferation, and differentiation distinguish stem cells of normal hematopoiesis from their equivalents in neoplastic tissue where responsiveness to regulation is greatly reduced or absent. However, definitive evidence of the presence of stem cells in human "solid" tumors has awaited the establishment of reliable assay procedures. Significant advances have been made with the development of in vitro agar colony-forming systems which support the growth of a variety of human tumor cells derived directly from patients' biopsy samples.[31,33,34]

These procedures allow us to start studying the biology of certain tumor "stem" cell populations, but the application of potential immense clinical value is that of drug-sensitivity testing (discussed in Section V). Preliminary clinical data from several centers in the U.S. provide evidence that these assays appear useful in predicting clinical response.[35-37]

Malignant stem cells are undoubtedly the most important cells in a tumor since they are capable of self-renewal and migration, so allowing growth of the primary and initiating distant metastases. Their growth properties must be characterized and their susceptibilities to drugs established. The object of chemotherapy is to eradicate the tumor stem cells with minimal damage to normal stem cells. Experimental studies which have demonstrated that antitumor drugs can be used to destroy selectively more malignant than normal stem cells are discussed in Section IV, together with their clinical relevance. An alternative approach has involved attempts to protect selectively normal stem cell populations. For example, by removal and storage of bone marrow from patients in remission for use as an autologous marrow rescue after chemotherapy.[38] This procedure, first used in treating acute leukemia,[39] is now being used to some advantage in certain human "solid" tumors.

D. Tumor and Normal Cell Repopulation

Stem cells are critical elements in the repopulation of both tumor and normal tissues. Successful therapy must allow normal stem cell renewal, preferably under conditions not favoring recovery of the tumor. Drug treatment is often limited by the amount of damage inflicted on the normal stem cells. The majority of drugs are most effective when given in full dose in intermittent schedules, repeated as soon as hematologic recovery has occurred with the number of marrow stem cells returned to the pretreatment level.[40] It should be remembered that two patterns of marrow recovery have been observed in mice and in man following the administration of different chemotherapeutic agents.[40] For most drugs recovery is complete within 17 to 21 days. However, following melphalan, BCNU, methyl CCNU, Myleran, and mitomycin C there is a delayed recovery, with the leukocyte count reaching the minimum value only at about the fourth week. In man recovery following these agents requires 6 to 8 weeks. Therefore their inclusion in a combination will require a minimal interval between courses of about 6 weeks, if cumulative toxicity to the normal marrow is to be avoided.[23] This fact is often ignored in protocols or only partly acknowledged by administering these drugs every 6 weeks but still including other drugs at three weekly intervals. The authors then reject the drugs because of severe and cumulative myelosuppression which they conclude prevents their successful use in drug combinations.[41] The rate of tumor regeneration between treatment courses must also be considered and may be a reason for excluding from combinations those agents which cause this delayed marrow recovery.

Recent studies by Hellman et al.[42] have suggested that damage to normal bone marrow caused by certain drugs for example, BCNU and Myleran, may never be completely restored. This may argue against their utilization in treating potentially "curable" malignancies.

Our knowledge of tumor cell repopulation is extremely limited. In experimental animal studies monitoring tumor mass behavior provides a poor estimation of the effects of treatment on the number of viable clonogenic tumor cells present, both in terms of response or tumor regrowth.[19,43] With the development of better techniques, it is essential to apply these specifically to malignant stem cell populations rather than to samples of heterogeneous collections of cells from "solid" tumor biopsies as has been done in the past.

Another crucial factor likely to influence tumor cell repopulation after chemotherapy is the selection/emergence and overgrowth of drug resistant populations. Whether drug resistant cells have altered "proliferative properties" remains to be established, but this may contribute to our failure to eradicate these tumors. Some generally accepted mechanisms of drug resistance are considered below.

III. BIOCHEMICAL FACTORS INFLUENCING DRUG RESISTANCE

Some tumor cells are more responsive than others to the cytotoxic effects of antitumor drugs. The numerous attempts to elucidate the precise mechanisms involved, however, have not met with unqualified success although they have implicated many different factors. Data from experimental studies need to be interpreted with caution since the ability to detect differences does not make them causal. Many experimentally induced drug-resistant tumors exhibit very high orders of resistance which have often been derived by repeated exposure to extremely high drug concentrations. These may not have their counterparts in human tumors. Factors of importance when resistance is of a lower order of magnitude may well be masked when a high degree of resistance develops involving alternative mechanisms. Therefore studies of the development of resistance may be most valuable. Experimental work with human cells showing low levels of resistance should be encouraged, since they may be of significance clinically, taking account of the fact that the dose and duration of chemotherapy in patients often may be limited.

Growth of resistant mutants is favored by certain conditions and the proportion of such mutants in any population will be influenced by kinetic and biochemical factors.

Resistance to antitumor drugs is generally associated with one or more of the following:

- Altered drug transport mechanisms
- Drug-induced metabolic alterations
- Cell cycle kinetic insensitivity
- Drug-induced modification of tumor cell antigenicity and modulation of the immune response
- Drug inaccessibility

These possibilities will be considered only briefly here since they have been discussed fully in several established reviews[44-47] and the Tables 1 to 5 provide summaries of some specific factors implicated for individual agents. Surprisingly little new data is available and few drugs have been studied in detail with repetitive emphasis on the "old favorites", particularly methotrexate. This may reflect our lack of knowledge of the *precise* mode of action in human tumors of most clinically useful antitumor drugs, which does not make the task of studying resistance any easier. However, since certain antitumor drugs are used effectively without this knowledge, perhaps resistance too can be circumvented and establishing precise mechanisms involved could become an academic problem.

A. Altered Drug Transport Mechanisms

Two main alterations known to occur in drug-resistant cells are impaired drug influx and/or enhanced efflux. These may result from changes in the passive permeability of the cell membrane to the drug or by modification of carrier transport systems. However, demonstration of an alteration in a transport parameter in a resistant cell does not necessarily mean that this change is the cause of resistance.[44] Furthermore, reduced drug accumulation is not always associated with resistance. For example, uptake of DDMP was reduced in methotrexate-resistant L5178Y cells but they were still killed by this drug as effectively or to a greater extent than the sensitive line.[48] Resistance to a specific drug may or may not be associated with a transport defect. Different results have been obtained not only with different cell types but also between independently derived resistant lines. For example: (1) in a series of seven methotrexate-resistant L1210 mutants established, only two demonstrated defective transport,[49] and (2) continued transplantation of a methotrexate-resistant L1210 subline with impaired drug uptake resulted in selection of a line with increased drug resistance characterized by elevated levels of the alleged "target" enzyme dihydrofolate reductase, but with a rate of drug transport similar to the parent drug-sensitive line.[40]

Table 1 provides examples of drugs whose antitumor effects are considered to be limited by alterations in drug permeability. Methotrexate, nitrogen mustard, actinomycin D, and daunomycin have been reviewed previously.[44] Some more recent studies, concentrating on adriamycin, the vinca alkaloids, and melphalan are summarized below.

Adriamycin — Cells resistant to adriamycin exhibit cross resistance to daunomycin, other anthracyclines and actinomycin D.[63,65,66] The primary resistance mechanisms seem to reflect decreased passage of the drug across cell membranes and decreased drug retention, as shown earlier with actinomycin D.[44] For various anthracyclines, influx has been shown to occur by passive facilitated diffusion,[62] while efflux is an active process.[63,67] The most common form of resistance is attributed to increased efflux.[68-71] However, transport studies with the anthracyclines are complicated by their binding to membranes, but the magnitude of this binding does not alter when resistance is induced.[67]

Table 1

BIOCHEMICAL FACTORS INFLUENCING DRUG RESISTANCE: ALTERED
DRUG TRANSPORT MECHANISMS

Impaired Drugs Influx	Examples
Altered cell membrane permeability	Act D[44,46], ADR[50], BLEO[51], DNR[46], HN2[44,46], L-PAM[52], VCR[53]
Modification of the carrier affinity	
Inactivation or deletion	MTX[44,54-56]
Alternative low affinity carrier	MTX[44,54-57], L-PAM[52]
Decreased nuclear drug accumulation	Act D[44], DNR[44], HN2[44], L-PAM[58]
Changes in membrane glycoprotein content	Act D[44,46,47], ADR[59] VLB[60]
Enhanced Drug Efflux	
Increased active outward drug transport	ADR[61,62], DNR[62,63], VCR[63,64], VDS[64]
Influence of change in calcium ion transport	DNR[63]

Vinca Alkaloids — Recent studies have shown that resistance to these drugs too is associated generally with a decreased capacity of the cells to retain the drug.[53,63,72,73] A sensitive line of Ehrlich ascites tumor cells accumulated six times more vincristine than the resistant line, but while cellular influx of vincristine was similar in both types, energy-dependent efflux differed.[73] Studies have shown that vincristine and the anthracyclines appear to be extruded by a common process,[63,72] perhaps explaining their cross-resistance, and enhanced efflux of vincristine and vinblastine was observed in adriamycin-resistant cells.[71] Enhanced efflux of vindesine in vindesine-resistant L5178Y cells has also been noted.[64]

Melphalan — Studies confirming the original observation of Goldenberg et al. that melphalan transport in cultured cells is carrier mediated have also provided further evidence for at least two distinct carrier systems.[52] In resistant L1210 cells with impaired melphalan transport, it is suggested that a specific mutation in the lower affinity system occurs rendering drug transport less efficient.[52] However, in human melanoma cells melphalan transport was not implicated in resistance since it was similar in both cell lines.[74]

Although the kinetics of drug transport have been carefully described for several agents in some normal tissues as well as tumor cells, many of the transport mechanisms have not been characterized biochemically and the molecular alteration(s) responsible for resistance have not been identified. Preliminary evidence suggests that methotrexate transport may be regulated by intracellular cAMP levels, perhaps through phosphorylation of the carrier protein.[75] Studies with the anthracyclines suggest that changes in such basic processes as ion transport may be involved since the active efflux mechanism appears to be influenced by calcium ion concentration.[63,76] Other work has centered on an examination of cell surface membranes, whose composition may affect drug penetration. Early studies showed marked differences in glycoprotein and glycolipid content in membranes prepared from sensitive mouse lymphoma cells, and an actinomycin D-resistant subline.[77] Further work by Ling and colleagues[78] with colchicine-resistant CHO cells has now shown that resistance is mediated via a particular component, the surface P-glycoprotein, decreasing drug accumulation into whole cells. Similarly studies investigating vinblastine resistance in human leukemic lymphoblasts have shown that high molecular weight (i.e., 170,000 - 190,000 daltons) membrane glycoproteins are present in increased amounts in resistant cells.[60] Although previously the P-glycoprotein has been observed to affect passively diffusing compounds, the possibility that interaction with certain actively transported compounds may also occur has recently been suggested involving melphalan,[58] adriamycin,[59] and perhaps the vinca alkaloids.[60] These data support the suggestion[77] that alterations in the cell membrane and in the biosynthesis and degradation of membrane constituents play a role in the development of resistance to these large, structurally complex molecules.

It is not suggested, however, that transport alterations represent the sole mechanisms of resistance for any of these drugs. For example, (1) an altered affinity of tubulin for the vinca alkaloids would be expected to confer resistance and this is being investigated,[76] (2) evidence that resistance to adriamycin[69] and daunomycin[63] may occur by other mechanisms has been provided, and (3) repair of drug-induced lesions has been implicated for melphalan (see below), and in CHO cell mutants resistance appears to be associated with a specific nuclear alteration,[58] as discussed in Chapter 1.

B. Drug-Induced Metabolic Alterations

Examples of these metabolic alterations are legion and Table 2 lists some of the most widely studied. It is clear that several factors are involved for the "antimetabolite" drugs such as methotrexate, 5-fluorouracil, cytosine arabinoside, 6-mercaptopurine, and thioguanine. This perhaps illustrates the numerous biochemical pathways with which these drugs may or may not interfere and the deviousness of tumor cells which so readily appear able to bypass these many insults.

Most of these studies were carried out prior to 1973 and were reviewed by Brockman,[46] so only a few recent reports will be mentioned here.

Methotrexate — The increases in dihydrofolate reductase in drug-resistant sarcoma 180 cells were shown to result solely from increased rates of enzyme synthesis.[101] This overproduction of enzyme was accompanied by a proportional increase in cellular dihydrofolate reductase mRNA content.[101] Most interestingly, however, in methotrexate-resistant L5178Y and CHO cell lines this overproduction was associated with amplification of genes coding for the enzyme,[86,102] as discussed in Chapter 1. A recent paper describes a method for exploiting this phenomenon and selectively killing resistant mutants.[103] Further evidence suggests that resistance may not be accounted for only by a simple increase in reductase, and a second species of enzyme has been detected in certain resistant cells. Resistant sublines of Chinese hamster cells were shown to overproduce one of two molecular weight forms of dihydrofolate reductase, only one of which was parenteral like. Each species was encoded by a different mRNA present in elevated amounts in resistant cells.[104] In another study,[89] in addition to the principle form of reductase, markedly sensitive to methotrexate, found in parent L5178Y cells, a methotrexate insensitive variant of folate reductase was found in two drug-resistant lines.

PALA — This is one of the newer pyrimidine antagonists undergoing clinical trials. An inverse relationship has been observed between aspartate transcarbamylase activity and sensitivity to PALA,[87,90] but other factors also contribute to resistance. For example, nucleoside kinase activities, necessary to allow utilization of salvage pyrimidines which would bypass the inhibited enzyme, were increased in some refractory tumors, but not all. Elevated activity of carbamyl phosphate synthetase II has been demonstrated in PALA-resistant variants of the Lewis lung carcinoma. Since carbamyl phosphate synthetase II exists as a complex with aspartate transcarbamylase, an augmented pool of carbamyl phosphate in the resistant variants may competitively displace PALA from aspartate transcarbamylase, diminish enzyme inhibition, and allow pyrimidine biosynthesis to proceed despite therapy. The role of these elevated synthetase activities as modulators of PALA resistance is reinforced by studies on the chemotherapeutic potentiation of PALA in these resistant tumors by the L-glutamine antagonist Acivicin.[95] While studies to identify other factors involved continue, it has already been shown that PALA is not preferentially detoxified by refractory tumor cells and that drug uptake was slow but comparable in all cell lines studied.[90-95]

Table 2

BIOCHEMICAL FACTORS INFLUENCING DRUG RESISTANCE: DRUG INDUCED METABOLIC ALTERATIONS

Specific effects and examples		Ref.
Increased drug degradation		
Elevated deoxycytidine deaminase	- Ara C	46
Elevated alkaline phosphohydrolase	- 6MP	46, 47
Increased drug-inactivating enzyme	- BLEO	79, 80
Inadequate drug activation		
Decreased uridine kinase	- 5AZA; 5FU	46; 47
Decreased adriamycin reductase	- ADR	81
Decreased deoxycytidine kinase	- Ara C	46
Decreased uridine phosphorylase	- 5AZA; 5FU	46
Decreased phosphoribosyltransferase	- 5FU; 6MP; 6TG	46, 47
Lacks detectable adenosine kinase	- 6MP; PYF	47; 82, 83
Deletion or inactivation of pyrimidine monophosphase kinase	- 5FU	84
Increased level of the "target" enzyme:		
Elevated levels of dihydrofolate reductase	- MTX	46, 85, 86
Elevated levels of aspartate transcarbamylase	- PALA	87
Elevated levels of orotidylate decarboxylase	- PYF	82
Change in the conformation of the "target" enzyme rendering it insensitive to drug action		
Altered dihydrofolate reductase with decreased drug affinity	- MTX	46, 88, 89
Altered PRPP amidotransferase less inhibited by drug	- 6MP; 6TG	46
Structural modification of thymidylate synthetase with decreased affinity for the active form of drug	- 5FU	47
Decreased requirement for a specific metabolic product:		
Reduced requirement for asparagine	- ASP	46
Enhanced levels of a normal substrate able to overcome the drug induced lesion or compete for tbe "target":		
Utilization of exogeneous thymidine	- 5FU; MTX	46; 47
Utilization of exogeneous uridine	- PALA	90
Elevated asparagine synthetic capacity	- ASP	46
Elevated levels of dCTP	- Ara C	91, 92
Increased concentration of thiol groups	- HN2	46
Development of an alternative biochemical pathway by-passing the drug induced block		
Increased dependence on the salvage pathway for DNA synthesis	- 5FU; MTX	46, 47; 93, 94
Increased synthesis of a competitive substrate, carbamyl phosphate	- PALA	95
Altered "repair" of drug induced lesions:		
Enhanced ability to repair DNA damage	- CYCLO; HN2; MeCCNU	46; 47; 96
Enhanced ability to excise or inactivate Pt-DNA mono-adducts	- Cis-Pt	97
Alteration in the assembly of new DNA chains	- HN2	98
Reduced ability to accumulate lethal cross linkages:		
Decreased platination of DNA with decreased sensitivity to that which does occur	- Cis-Pt	99
Decreased accessibility of DNA to the cross-linking effects of the drug	-Cis-Pt: L-PAM	100; 74, 100

Cis-platinum — Of the platinum complexes cis-platinum is the most commonly used clinically. It causes DNA inter- and intra-strand cross-links and DNA-protein cross-links.[97,100] Resistance mechanisms have recently been investigated, using a resistant L1210 subline; markedly reduced (25-fold) levels of cross-linking compared with the sensitive line were observed which correlated with the degree of resistance. However, it was suggested also that resistance may depend both on reduced platination of DNA and on different sensitivity to the platination which occurred.[99] A correlation between DNA cross-linking and tumor sensitivity was similarly claimed for cis-platinum in L1210 cells by Zelling et al.,[100] who also reported a reduction in DNA-protein cross-linking and attributed resistance to a reduced ability to transport the drug or an increased ability to inactivate it within the cell. A more recent report[97] from this group, comparing a normal human embryo cell strain with an SV-40 transformed line, also showed that cytotoxicity differences with cis-platinum correlated with differences in interstrand cross-linking. However, the presence of similar levels of DNA-protein cross-linking in the two lines excluded a difference in drug uptake or intracellular metabolic activation or inactivation prior to DNA interaction. In attempting to explain these data, Erikson et al.,[105] refer to the fact that DNA-interstrand cross-linking was found previously to correlate with differences in sensitivity among human cell strains treated with nitrosoureas. These differences were attributed to the presence or absence of a specific repair mechanism. However, the relative sensitivity of the two cell types studied was reversed: the transformed line was more sensitive to the nitrosoureas than the normal strain, while the reverse was true for cis-platinum. Therefore, in the case of cis-platinum they suggested that cells might differ in their ability to repair platinum-DNA monoadducts before they are converted to interstrand cross-links.[97] A similar mechanism was proposed for L1210 cells resistant to melphalan which also exhibited cross-resistance to cis-platinum.[106]

These results therefore indicate that differential cytotoxicity associated with interstrand cross-linking can be drug specific. Such observations further contribute to the growing body of evidence that wide differences in mechanisms of action exist even among the so-called "alkylating agents."[107-109] The corollary to this of course, is that mechanisms of resistance are likely to differ too.

C. Cell Cycle Kinetic Insensitivity

Responses of cells to treatment with drugs and radiation vary depending on their position in the cycle and whether they are proliferating or resting.[20,23] Cells within a population might therefore be considered resistant to certain drugs which exert lethality only at a specific phase of the cycle or which are ineffective against nonproliferating cells, if exposure time was limited.

Drugs exert two main effects on cells which may or may not be exerted at similar points in the cycle: (1) a lethal or cell killing effect, and (2) cell cycle progression delay and/or arrest. Cytotoxic effects may show no phase specificity or may be maximal in certain phase(s) of the cycle. Examples of truly phase specific drugs are few since current techniques show that for most agents several phases may be susceptible, although often to different degrees. Interpretation of effects caused by drugs on progression through the cycle are complicated by the fact that the drug concentration employed or the period of treatment may determine whether a drug exerts a lethal or a blocking effect, the latter being favored generally by lower drug concentrations and short exposure times. Such factors will also often influence whether the arrest is temporary and reversible or irreversible leading to cell death. In addition, a given single drug may by blocking progression at one point in the cycle, diminish its own effectiveness as a cytotoxic agent by protecting a proportion of the cells by preventing their reaching the phase where the lethal effect of the drug is exerted. These surviving cells could then reestablish the tumor posttreatment. This possibility was raised by work with AMSA which showed that cells initially in G_1 arrest during the period of drug exposure were most refractory to the cytotoxic effects of AMSA.[110] So this could be considered another expression of drug resistance and provides added argument in favor of well designed combination chemotherapy.

These cell cycle dependent effects have been established in vitro for most of the standard anticancer drugs and have been reviewed.[20,23] Table 3 summarizes data for the newer antitumor drugs currently being considered for clinical evaluation. With the advent of flow microfluorimetry more detailed information is becoming available concerning the kinetic effects of drugs on asynchronous nonperturbed population. These data however do not allow firm discrimination between dead or dying cells and those cells which retain viability, and hence need cautious interpretation. However, results and studies investigating possible phase specificity may also be unreliable since they are generally obtained after cell synchronization.

These recent data provide two main points for consideration: (1) several of these drugs show no evidence of phase specific cytotoxicity. Thus the problem of resistance due to kinetic insensitivity may be diminished and these drugs would therefore be good candidates for inclusion in combinations, and (2) many of these drugs result in an apparent G_2 block. However, after drug exposure in several cases, for example, with DHAQ, ellipticine, and AMSA an enrichment of cells with 4n DNA content has also been identified suggesting an interference with cytokinesis.[110,119,120] This aspect needs further careful evaluation and concurrent chromosome analyses with flow microfluorimetric studies may be valuable. From the therapeutic standpoint the presence of these drug-induced tetraploid cells may be encouraging since experimental studies suggested that they are among the first in a population to die.[130]

The differential sensitivity of resting, noncycling cells and cycling cells to chemotherapeutic agents has been extensively documented. In vitro studies comparing cells in the plateau or stationary growth phase with those growing exponentially have shown that most drugs exert selective toxicity for proliferating cells, as reviewed earlier.[20,131] Data for newer antitumor agents is provided in Table 4. Conflicting results continue to be reported for different drugs in various cell types. For example: with vindesine no cell kill of nonproliferating human neuroblastoma cells or Syrian hamster ovary cells was reported even following a 24 hr drug exposure,[64] contrasting with extensive kill observed after exposing LoVo cells for 1 hr to very high vindesine concentrations and these stationary phase cells proved significantly more sensitive than proliferating cells.[132] For vincristine, however, these groups both recorded negligible kill of resting cells. Drewinko et al.[132] also reported extensive but comparable kill of both exponential and stationary phase LoVo cells to Mitoxantrone, one of the anthracenedione derivatives, contrasting with data for an almost identical compound (NSC 279836) where enhanced cell kill (eightfold) was noted for proliferating rather than resting cells.[119] Such conflicting information has in the past been explained by variations in duration of exposure and conditions of culturing,[20] although it is also possible that drugs might exert different kinetic effects on different cell types, so perhaps explaining why certain tumors appear more responsive than others to cytotoxic drugs.

Another factor to be considered is that some of the cells which are out of cycle or slowly progressing through the cycle may be hypoxic. Within solid tumors these hypoxic cells are known to be relatively resistant to the cytotoxicity of ionizing radiation and are presumed also to be relatively resistant to cell cycle-specific chemotherapy.[136] The cytotoxicities of a number of drugs to oxygenated and hypoxic EMT6 mouse mammary tumor cells in vitro have recently been evaluated and the drugs were placed in three categories based on the relative sensitivity of cells (see Table 5). Some drugs preferentially killed cells under aerobic or hypoxic conditions and others exhibited no

Table 3
LETHAL AND CELL CYCLE KINETIC EFFECTS OF CERTAIN NEWER ANTITUMOR DRUGS

Drugs	Phase(s) of the cell cycle where:		
	Lethal effects predominate	Progression delay and/or arrest occurs	Ref.
Aclacinomycin	ns^a	$G_2 + M > G_1 + S$	111
AMSA	$G_2 >> G_1$	$S + G_2$	110
Anguidine	No phase specificity	$G_1/S + G_2/M$	112
ANT	No phase specificity	G_2/M	113
Chartreusin	S	$G_2 + M >> G_1/S$	114
DDMP	$S > G_1 >> G_2 + M$	$S >> G_2 + M$	115
Dibromodulcitol	$G_1 : G_1 + S$	G_1/S	116, 117
Dihydro-5-AZA	$S > M + G_1 > G_2$	S	118
DHAQ	ns	G_2	119
Ellipticine	early $G_1 + M >> S + G_2$	G_2	120
4'-Epiadriamycin	$S + $ early G_2	G_2	121
Formyl-leurosine	S	ns	117
Maytansine	$M + G_2 > S >> G_1$	M	122
Mitoxantrone	No phase specificity	$G_2 + M$	123, 124
Nogalamycin	S	ns	125
7-OMEN	Early $G_1 + S + G_2 >> $ mid $+$ late G_1	ns	125
Prospidine	ns	G_2	126
Pyrazofurin	$G_2 > S : G_1 + S$	$G_1/S \pm S$	127, 128
Spirogermanium	No phase specificity	None	129
Vindesine	S	M	64

preferential toxicity. Although again there are conflicting reports. For example, hypoxic CHO cells were found to be more resistant to adriamycin than their oxygenated counterparts,[137] while in another EMT6 line both oxic and hypoxic cells proved equally sensitive to the drug.[139] Further investigation is clearly warranted and in particular results from experimental in vivo studies would be of interest.

Selective proliferative toxicity of chemotherapeutic agents has also been observed in vivo. In mice an increased cytotoxicity against proliferating as opposed to resting hematopoietic colony-forming units has been noted for 19 standard agents.[15] These authors have however expressed caution in extrapolating these results to man since the distribution of resting and proliferating cells and their kinetic behavior may differ. A review of the effects of antitumor agents on normal hematopoietic precursors cells also concluded that most drugs are more effective against rapidly proliferating cells although Myleran proved the exception.[140] This survey prompted the optimistic proposal that results from such studies might allow prediction of the magnitude of human hematologic toxicity for new agents or combinations. This has been justified by recent studies with carminomycin, marcellomycin, and spirogermanium.[141] The in vitro assays accurately predicted for significant in vivo myelosuppression in man with carminoycin and marcellomycin and a lack of toxicity for spirogermanium, consistent with the reported absence of marrow toxicity in preclinical and clinical studies.

A knowledge of the effects of cytotoxic drugs on bone marrow and specifically on normal stem cell populations is vital for successful chemotherapy. This factor was first highlighted by Bruce and colleagues[9] when they demonstrated that there was a major kinetic difference between normal and malignant stem cells which could be exploited to increase the selectivity of anticancer drugs. These studies have provided a basis for safer cancer chemotherapy (discussed in Section IV).

Table 4
THE DIFFERENTIAL SENSITIVITIES OF RESTING (STATIONARY) AND CYCLING (EXPONENTIALLY GROWING) CELLS TO CERTAIN NEWER ANTITUMOR DRUGS

Drugs preferentially toxic to cycling cells	Drugs equally toxic to cycling and resting cells	Drugs preferentially toxic to resting cells
Aclacinomycin[a]	AD 32[b]	Cis-Platinum[c]
AMSA[c,d]	Anguidine[e]	
DDMP[f]	Mitomycin C[c]	
Dibromodulcitol[g]	Mitoxantrone[c]	
Dihydro-5-AZA[h]		
DHAQ[i]		
Formyl-leurosine[g]		
Maytansine[c]		
Nogalamycin[j]		
7-OMEN[j]		
Rubidazone[c]		
Spirogermanium[k]		
VP-16-213[c]		
[Vindesine][l]		[Vindesine][c]

[a]   Traganos, F., Staiano-Coico, L., Darynkiewicz, Z., and Melamed, M. R., *Cancer Res.,* 41, 2728, 1981.
[b]   Krishan, A., Dutt, K., Israel, M., and Ganapathi, R., *Cancer Res.,* 41, 2745, 1981.
[c]   Drewinko, B., Patchen, M., Yang, L-Y., and Barlogie, B., *Cancer Res.,* 41, 2328, 1981.
[d]   Wilson, W. R., Giesbrecht, J. L., Hill, R P., and Whitmore, G. F., *Cancer Res.,* 41, 2809, 1981.
[e]   Dosik, G. M., Barlogie, B., Johnston, D. A., Murphy, W. K., and Drewinko, B., *Cancer Res.,* 38, 3304, 1978.
[f]   Hill, B. T., *Eur. J. Cancer,* 16, 147, 1980.
[g]   Olah, E., Palyi, I., and Sugar, J., *Eur. J. Cancer,* 14, 895, 1978.
[h]   Traganos, F., Staiano-Coico, L., Darynkiewicz, Z., and Melamed, M. R., *Cancer Res.,* 41, 780, 1981.
[i]   Traganos, F., Evenson, D. P., Staiano-Coico, L., Darynkiewicz, Z., and Melamed, M. R., *Cancer Res.,* 40, 671, 1980.
[j]   Bhuyan, B. K., Blowers, C. L., Crampton, S. L., and Shugars, K. D., *Cancer Res.,* 41, 18, 1981.
[k]   Hill, B. T., Whatley, S. A., Bellamy, A. S., Jenkins, L. Y., and Whelan, R. D. H., *Cancer Res.,* in press, July, 1982.
[l]   Hill, B. T., Whelan, R. D. H., *J. Natl. Cancer Inst.,* 67, 437, 1981.

D. Drug-Induced Modification of Tumor Cell Antigenicity and/or Modulation of the Immune Response

Immunotherapy still has its foundations in theory rather than clinical observation.[142] As with all forms of therapy any hypothetical immunological cancer treatment will have its hypothetical hazards and perhaps the most worrying is immunological enhancement of tumor growth, a phenomenon observed in experimental animals.[143] It has also been postulated that since anticancer agents may cause selective immune imbalances, both immunosuppressing and immunoaugmenting, this may be another mechanism of resistance. Several reviews by Mihich[45] in the early 1970s discussed this possibility and little data to support or refute this proposal have since become available. However, one interesting aspect of recent studies is that treatment conditions, including the timing and duration of drug therapy, could determine whether immuno-

Table 5
THE DIFFERENTIAL SENSITIVITIES OF OXYGENATED
AND HYPOXIC TUMOR CELLS TO ANTITUMOR
DRUGS

Drugs preferentially toxic to oxygenated cells	Drugs equally toxic to oxygenated and hypoxic cells	Drugs preferentially toxic to hypoxic cells
Actinomycin D[9]	AMSA[b]	Metronidazole[a]
Bleomycin[a]	BCNU[a]	Misonidazole[a]
Procarbazine[a]	CCNU[a]	Mitomycin C[a]
Streptonigrin[a]	Cis-Platinum[a]	
Vincristine[a]	5-Fluorouracil[a]	
	Methotrexate[a]	
[Adriamycin][c]	[Adriamycin][d]	[Adriamycin][a]

[a] Teicher, B. A., Lazo, J. S., and Satorelli, A. C., *Cancer Res.,* 41, 73, 1981.
[b] Wilson, W. R., Whitmore, G. F., and Hill, R. P., *Cancer Res.,* 41, 2817, 1981.
[c] Smith, E., Stratford, I. J., and Adams, G. E., *Br. J. Cancer,* 41, 568, 1980.
[d] Harris, J. W. and Shrieve, D. C., *Int. J. Radiat. Oncol. Biol. Phys.,* 5, 1245, 1979.

suppression may be minimized or, in fact, whether immunoaugmentation may result.[144,146] Thus *if* this is a factor of importance in drug resistance it may be possible by deliberate pharmacological intervention to overcome this and lead to therapeutically advantageous imbalances of the immune response.

E. Drug Inaccessibility

Brain tumors represent the classic example of sites inaccessible to polar antitumor agents unable to penetrate the blood-brain barrier. Efforts to overcome this problem have centered on an exploitation of pharmacokinetic factors, for example the use of lipophylic drugs such as the nitrosoureas.

Drug penetration into solid tumors is also an area requiring investigation. A suitable model for quantitative evaluation of this parameter may be the multicellular spheroids recently introduced into laboratory studies[147] (discussed in Section V).

IV. EXPERIMENTAL STUDIES INDICATING HOW PROBLEMS OF DRUG RESISTANCE MAY BE MINIMIZED OR CIRCUMVENTED

A. The Fractional Cell Kill Hypothesis

A major contribution to the era of combination chemotherapy derives from experimental studies by Skipper and Schabel and colleagues.[13,148] They developed a better understanding of quantitative aspects of tumor growth and realized and stressed their importance in designing optimal drug schedules for drug-sensitive malignancies. They proposed that the ability to eradicate malignant cells with a drug depended not only on the dose used but also on the number of tumor cells present. Furthermore, cell destruction by drugs was said to follow "first order kinetics". This means that a given treatment destroys a constant fraction of cells, not a fixed number, i.e., a treatment reducing a tumor cell population from 1000,000 to 10 should reduce a population of 100,000 to 1 cell. It also means that there would be a 99.999% chance of eradicating the tumor if only 1 malignant cell were present. A simplified version of this concept is illustrated by the experimental results in Table 6. These data emphasize that drug treatment is most likely to be curative when a minimum number of malignant cells is pres-

Table 6
THE RELATIONSHIP BETWEEN "CURE-RATE" AND TUMOR CELL NUMBER

Effects of a Drug which Achieves a 6
Log Cell Kill (99.9999%)

Number of tumor cells in animals	Percentage of animals "cured"
10 thousand (10^4)	almost all
1 million (10^6)	40%
1 billion (10^9)	none

Effects of Different Therapeutic Strategies on Fractional Cell Kill in Solid Tumours with Different Growth Rates

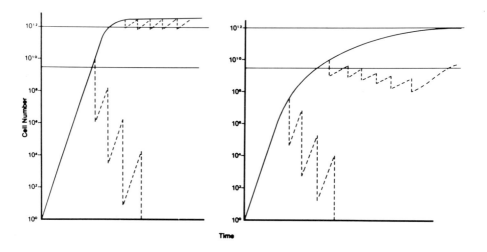

FIGURE 2.   Schematic representation of fractional cell kills in rapidly growing and slowly growing human tumors (reproduced from Shackney et al.[149] with the kind permission of the authors and the editor of *Annals of Internal Medicine*).

ent. This fractional cell kill hypothesis, indicating that effectiveness of drug treatment increases with decreasing volume of tumor cells was derived from the exponentially growing L1210 leukemia, although it has subsequently been validated in other animal tumors.[14,149] For Gompertzian growth, which may be the pattern in many human tumors, it can be seen in Figure 2 that the necessity for early treatment is even more vital if cure is to be achieved. This diagram illustrates that a form of therapy effective at the time of clinical detection for exponentially growing tumors, since fractional cell kills were large, would not result in cure if the tumor exhibited Gompertzian growth. Under these conditions, with small fractional cell kills, at best a shallow response would be followed by early recurrence. Only treatment of subclinical disease, producing larger fractional cell kills, may lead to cure.[150]

Skipper also emphasized that the interval between multiple drug treatments was critical for effective therapy.[13] Net tumor cell kill per treatment was shown to be the result of initial cell kill less the regrowth of the tumor population before the next treatment.

If enough time elapsed between treatments to allow regrowth to pretreatment levels or greater, the eventual outcome would be the death of the animal. The possibility of drug resistance developing between treatments must also be considered.[151] It is important to be able to anticipate when the nadir in tumor burden is likely to be achieved so that at or near this point, drugs may be switched to those still effective against these specifically drug-resistant tumor cells. If the initial treatment is continued long past its nadir, even though clinical relapse has not yet become apparent, the chance for cure or extended remission may well have been missed.[151] This importance of timing applies both to treatment of advanced disease and for effective adjuvant chemotherapy.[23]

The implications of the fractional cell kill hypothesis are, that to eradicate a tumor effectively by drug treatment it is necessary both to increase the dose of drug or drugs within limits tolerated by the host, and to start treatment when the number of tumor cells present is small enough to allow their eradication by a tolerated dose. These experimental studies have therefore provided the rationale for (1) drug combinations, attempting to overcome limits imposed on escalating doses of single agents because of toxicity to normal tissues, and (2) "adjuvant" chemotherapy combined with local therapy, attempting to increase the "cure" rate. An extension of these ideas and a new approach based on a mathematical analysis relating the drug sensitivity of tumors to their spontaneous mutation rate to drug resistance has been described[152] and is presented in Chapter 3.

The requirement for full dose intensive chemotherapy as an adjuvant has also been established beyond doubt experimentally.[14,38,153,154] Its importance is at last being appreciated clinically although often in the past a less intensive regimen has been selected in an effort to reduce acute toxicity. Unfortunately in many cases this conservative approach has failed to improve the disease-free interval and often a reduction of dosage or the use of single agents is not necessarily accompanied by lower toxicity. Recent clinical data support the critical role that dose rate plays in prolonging disease-free survival,[38,155-157] and so the need for reducing side-effects becomes increasingly important.

B. Selective Toxicity of Antitumor Drugs for Malignant Stem Cells

In 1966 Bruce and colleagues[9] assessed the sensitivity of normal hematopoietic and AKR lymphoma colony-forming cells to a number of antitumor drugs. They provided the first demonstration that kinetic differences existed between normal and malignant tissues, and indicated how these differences might be exploited so as to achieve increased selective toxicity against malignant stem cells.

Using the quantitative spleen colony-forming assay they showed that three distinct types of survival curve were obtained, and, for some agents, as much as 10,000-times greater cell kill of lymphoma over bone marrow stem cells could be achieved. These studies formed the basis for a Kinetic Classification of Antitumor Drugs. In Class I (see Figure 3) there was no difference in toxicity exerted against normal hematopoietic and lymphoma colony-forming cells. These agents (e.g., X-irradiation) were said to be "nonspecific", appearing equally toxic for both proliferating and resting stem cells. Class II agents were considerably more toxic to lymphoma than to normal stem cells, with increasing drug doses killing a greater number of cells until a plateau was reached, after which there was no further increase in cell kill. Class II agents were called "phase-specific" because proliferating cells were killed during a specific phase(s) of the cycle. Resting cells appeared to be unaffected by these agents, provided the exposure time was kept short (24 hr). For Class III drugs survival curves were exponential with dose, but there was a significant difference (× 6) in the slope for normal and lymphoma

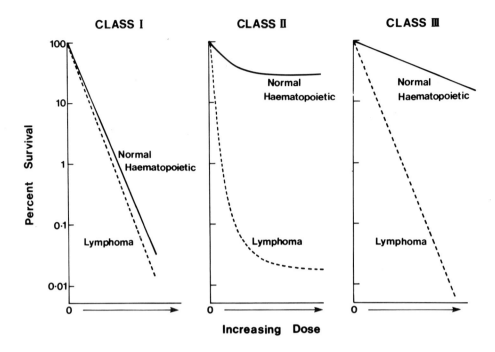

FIGURE 3.   The basis for a Kinetic Classification of Antitumor Drugs dose-survival curves for both normal hematopoietic and transplanted lymphoma colony-forming units. Normal or tumor-bearing mice were given a range of doses of a given drug and their femoral marrows were assayed 24 hours later for their content of colony-forming units. (After Bruce et al.[9])

colony-forming cells. These agents were termed "cycle-specific" since although they damaged both proliferating and resting stem cells, dividing cells were much more sensitive being killed throughout the cycle. This selectivity of Class II and Class III drugs appeared to be associated with the fact that in untreated animals most normal hematopoietic stem cells were resting, while nearly all detectable malignant cells appeared to be cycling.[29] Therefore, short courses (i.e., over 24 hr) of Class II and Class III agents, which preferentially kill cycling cells, would cause much greater kill of malignant as opposed to normal stem cells. If the time of exposure is prolonged, however, this kinetic difference between normal and malignant stem cells is abolished and increasing damage to bone marrow occurred.[25,26] Similarly, if mice were treated after previous injury to the marrow, when hematopoietic stem cells were being recruited to a proliferating state to repair damage, the selectivity of these drugs for malignant stem cells was lost, i.e., the kinetically exploitable difference between normal and malignant stem cells applies for only a limited exposure time (24 to 36 hr). These studies have been extended to include other agents, reviewed earlier[23] and results are summarized in Table 7.

A major implication of these studies is that they have provided a basis for safer cancer chemotherapy involving minimal toxicity to normal bone marrow without compromising antitumor effectiveness. Certain predictions of potential clinical relevance can therefore be made.[20,23]

1. Bone marrow toxicity will be less if drugs are given over approximately 24 hr in man.
2. A knowledge of the Kinetic Classification of Antitumor Drugs is essential if chemotherapy is to be given safely.

Table 7
THE KINETIC CLASSIFICATION OF
ANTITUMOR DRUGS

CLASS II	CLASS III
5-Azacytidine	Actinomycin D
Cytosine arabinoside	Adriamycin
Hydroxyurea	BCNU
ICRF 159	CCNU
6-Mercaptopurine	Chlorambucil
Methotrexate	Cis-Platinum
Procarbazine	Cyclophosphamide
Pyrazofurin	Daunomycin
6-Thioguanine	Dibromodulcitol
Vinblastine	DTIC
Vincristine	5-Fluorouracil
Vindesine	Melphalan
VM26	Methyl CCNU
VP-16-213	Nitrogen Mustard
	Thiotepa

Note: Adapted from Hill.[23]

3. Toxicity of Class II agents to normal stem cells (e.g., bone marrow) is not dose dependent. Class II drugs therefore may be added to combinations without reducing their dose, provided the total treatment time does not exceed 48 hr.
4. Class III agents in combination will be additively toxic to the marrow and doses should be reduced proportionately.
5. The practice of giving small daily doses of drugs from either Class should be avoided, since normal bone marrow stem cells will be drawn into the cycle and killed. This would increase toxicity to normal bone marrow and may reduce the number of malignant cells killed because treatment has to be postponed or interrupted.

Some potential clinical applications of this approach were suggested by Bergsagel.[40] However, the first clinical demonstration of the value of these principles came from a study showing that marrow toxicity of combination chemotherapy using cyclophosphamide, methotrexate, vincristine, and 5-fluorouracil in treating miscellaneous solid tumors could be significantly reduced if drugs were given over 24 hr only.[158] Subsequently, it has been established that scheduling drugs according to these principles reduces toxicity but not effectiveness of combination chemotherapy. For example: (1) with vinblastine, actinomycin D and methotrexate in advanced testicular teratomas,[159] (2) with adriamycin, 5-fluorouracil and methotrexate in advanced nonsquamous cell lung cancers,[160] (3) in advanced breast cancer a 24 hr protocol including cyclophosphamide, 5-fluorouracil, vincristine, and methotrexate produced a 63% response rate, comparable to the more conventional 5 day approach, but side effects were minimal,[161] and (4) improved results with markedly reduced toxicity have also been achieved by giving combination cancer chemotherapy over 24 hr in head and neck cancer.[162]

The prediction that toxicity of Class II agents to normal tissues is more related to duration of exposure than to dose was confirmed in 1969 by the demonstration that up to 20,000 mg of methotrexate (Class II agent) could be given safely over 24 hr, while usual doses of 5-100 mg could produce profound marrow depression if given in divided doses over 5 days.[163] This study also showed that the value of "high dose" methotrexate infusions in overcoming resistance was remarkably short-lived and so this group abandoned this approach in the early 1970s. Current studies have also demonstrated that very high doses of other Class II agents such as hydroxyurea and procarbazine can be given safely provided that the duration of treatment does not exceed 30 hr.[159,164] In addition it has been shown, as predicted, that agents in Class III would be less toxic if given over 24 hr or so rather than on a more prolonged schedule. For example, actinomycin D is known to produce severe side-effects when given as single intravenous injections over several days. However, a single injection of actinomycin D in the same total dose can be given without toxicity.[159]

The application of these principles has enabled combination chemotherapy to be given more safely clinically than in the past, provided of course, standard medical precautions are always observed.[159] This approach is now being used for treating other tumors. For example, recent feasibility studies have shown that it is possible (1) to redesign the conventional MOPP protocol for Hodgkin's disease according to these principles administering drugs on days 1 and 2 only and this resulted in significantly reduced toxicity,[164] and (2) to design 24-hr combination chemotherapy protocols for integration with radiation therapy for the treatment of squamous cell carcinoma of the cervix or bronchus.[159]

The impact of these kinetically designed protocols on survival is now being investigated. Encouraging data are provided from a study of advanced squamous cell carcinoma of the head and neck involving a combination of vincristine, bleomycin, methotrexate, hydrocortisone, and 5-fluorouracil given over 24 hr on days 1 and 14 prior to local "curative" therapy with radiation and/or surgery on day 28.[165] In the first 96 patients eligible for assessments overall 5 year survival is 43% compared with an expected 20%, with chemotherapy responders having the longest median duration of survival. Toxicity was minimal, there was 100% patient compliance and 80% of patients received full dose radiotherapy as planned without interruption.

Therefore conditions for minimizing or overcoming drug resistance, involving the use of drugs in full dosage, in combination protocols, administered at frequent intervals and integrated optimally with local therapies, can be met by this approach. It remains to be established in most common "solid" tumors in randomized prospective controlled clinical trials whether the addition of such effective cancer chemotherapy significantly improves overall survival compared with local therapy alone.

C. Cell Cycle Dependent Drug Cytotoxicities

Much of the promise that cell cycle information would prove valuable in designing optimal drug combinations has not been realized in clinical practice. In particular, attempts to exploit synchronization and recruitment, as discussed earlier,[23] to enhance tumor cell kill have failed generally. This has often contributed to disillusionment of several authors and the suggestion that cell kinetic information in general is of no clinical value.[5,7,8] The above discussions and data show that this conclusion is incorrect.

When selecting drugs for combination therapy it may also be valuable to choose at least one which (1) will be effective at killing cells in each phase of the cycle, perhaps favoring some newer drugs which showed no phase specific lethality, (2) will be preferentially cytotoxic to nonproliferating cells, provided care is taken to minimize damage to "resting" normal stem cells, for example, in the bone marrow, by limiting the exposure time to less than 48 hr (see above), and (3) will be preferentially cytotoxic to hypoxic cells, for example, mitomycin C or questionably adriamycin.

D. Patterns of Cross-Resistance and Collateral Sensitivity

A knowledge of patterns of cross-resistance between various drugs may be useful when making selections for combinations or sequential schedules. The inclusion of drugs to which certain resistant populations are collaterally sensitive also would be a positive approach to overcoming resistance.

The incidence of collateral sensitivity and cross-resistance in experimental animal tumors in vivo and in vitro has been reviewed recently,[109] and some data are summarized in Tables 8 to 10. In general, (1) cross-resistance appears frequent among vinca alkaloids, actinomycin D, and anthracyclines, perhaps associated with common membrane alterations implicated in resistance to these agents, (2) cross-resistance is *not* invariable among drugs with alkylating moieties, providing further evidence for marked differences both in the biological mechanism of action and selective toxicity for tumor cells in this group of agents, and (3) collateral sensitivity is most often seen between cells resistant to methotrexate, 5-fluorouracil, 6-mercaptopurine, or cytosine arabinoside. This suggests that alternative drugs are readily available when resistance to these develops. However, it also highlights the fact that alternatives may *not* be readily available for cell populations resistant to other widely used drugs such as cyclophosphamide, melphalan, the nitrosoureas, and cis-platinum.

It is emphasized that these results are not intended to imply that patterns of cross-resistance or lack of cross-resistance will hold for all tumors.[65] However, remarkably similar patterns of response were observed in the different tumor types selected,[109] in spite of the fact that the extent of resistance varied and may have been derived using different treatment schedules. There were of course a few exceptions. A comparison of in vitro and in vivo data also produced some similarities and a few differences.[109] These may be real discrepancies or may be associated with heterogeneous cell populations exhibiting a range of drug sensitivities, a factor even more relevant when considering human tumors. The clinical relevance of this experimental information is uncertain. However an encouraging recent development, discussed later in Section V, concerns the evaluation of drug sensitivity and cross-resistance in human tumors.

V. FUTURE PROSPECTS FOR OVERCOMING DRUG-RESISTANCE

A. Identification and Study of Human Tumor Stem Cell Populations

A therapeutic strategy based on exploitation of kinetic differences between normal and malignant murine stem cells, and its successful introduction into clinical practice has been described above. To extend these ideas it became essential to establish an assay for stem cells in human "solid" tumors. Pioneering work by Courtenay[33] in England and Salmon and his group[31] in the U.S. has provided methodology for successful cloning of cells from some types of human tumors. Although in several major centers in North America where over 1,000 biopsy specimens have been processed, a wide range of tumor types has been cultured successfully, using the Hamburger and Salmon[31] method, it must be emphasized that this remains an elaborate and time consuming procedure with plating efficiencies often of only 0.1 to 0.0001%. Results from smaller groups have generally been more disappointing, and our limited experience has shown that while colonies can be grown from ascitic tumors and metastatic deposits we have not been successful with primary tumors including melanomas, head and neck tumors, and colorectal carcinomas.[166,167] In addition, we have found plating efficiency and colony size to be significantly improved using the more involved Courtenay assay.

The controversy which rages over whether colonies grown under these conditions are representative of true "stem" cells or their clonogenic progeny is probably of little importance. The true value of this approach can only be decided when it can be shown (1) whether the in vitro sensitivity of these tumor "stem" cells to cytotoxic agents correlates with clinical response, and (2) whether treatments based on these predictive tests result in improved survival. The first preliminary evidence that this assay system

Table 8

PATTERNS OF CROSS-RESISTANCE AMONG
"ALKYLATING AGENTS", ESTABLISHED IN
EXPERIMENTAL ANIMAL TUMORS

	Tumor lines resistant to				
Drug tested	BCNU	CYCLO	HN2	MTC	L-PAM
Cis-Pt	S	S	ns	ns	CR
CCNU	CR	S	ns	ns	S
BCNU	—	CR	CR	ns	S
CYCLO	S	—	CR	ns	CR
HN2	ns	CR	—	CR	CR
MTC	ns	CR	CR	—	S
L-PAM	S	S	CR	ns	—
MYL	ns	CR	ns	ns	CR
ThioTEPA	CR	CR	ns	CR	CR

Note: S, sensitive; CR, cross-resistant; ns, not studied.
Adapted from Hill.[109]

Table 9

PATTERNS OF CROSS-RESISTANCE AMONG "MITOTIC
INHIBITORS" AND "ANTITUMOR ANTIBIOTICS" IN
EXPERIMENTAL ANIMAL TUMORS

	Tumor lines resistant to:					
Drug Tested	Act D	ADR	DNR	VLB	VCR	VDS
Act D	—	CR	CR	ns	CR	CR
ADR	CR	—	CR	CR	CR	CR
DNR	CR	CR	—	CR	CR	ns
VLB	CR	CR	CR	—	CR	CR
VCR	CR	CR	CR	CR	—	CR
VDS	ns	CR	CR	ns	CR	—

Note: CR, cross-resistant; ns, not studied.
Adapted from Hill.[109]

Table 10

PATTERNS OF COLLATERAL SENSITIVITY ESTABLISHED IN
EXPERIMENTAL ANIMAL TUMORS

	Tumor lines resistant to						
Drug Tested	ADR	AraC	ASP	5FU	6MP	MTX	VLB
Act D	CR	ns	ns	CS	S	CS	CS
ADR	—	ns	ns	CS	S	CS	CR
Ara C	CS	—	ns	ns	S	S	CS
ASP	ns	CS	—	ns	ns	CS	ns
BCNU	S	S	ns	ns	ns	ns	CS
CYCLO	S	S	S	S	CS	CS	ns
5FU	S	CS	ns	—	S	CS	ns
HN2	S	S	ns	S	CS	CS	ns
6MP	S	CS	ns	CS	—	CS	S
MTC	S	ns	ns	CS	ns	ns	ns

Table 10 (continued)
PATTERNS OF COLLATERAL SENSITIVITY ESTABLISHED IN
EXPERIMENTAL ANIMAL TUMORS

	Tumor lines resistant to						
Drug Tested	ADR	AraC	ASP	5FU	6MP	MTX	VLB
MTX	CS	S	CS	S	CS	—	S
L-PAM	S	ns	ns	CS	ns	CS	ns

Note: CR, cross-resistant; CS, collaterally sensitive; S, sensitive; ns, not studied.
Adapted from Hill.[109]

might prove useful for prediction of clinical response came in 1978[168] and further data now support the predictive clinical value for certain tumors, particularly ovarian carcinomas, where a plentiful supply of material is often available.[35-37,169] Furthermore a recent report has shown that in relapsing ovarian carcinoma when the chemotherapy was selected on the basis of the in vitro assay results this was associated with improved survival.[170] Major efforts to optimize the methodology and modify the assays for routine clinial use are now underway.

B. Elucidation of Patterns of Cross-Resistance in Human Tumors
Studies initiated with experimental tumors (discussed abve) may now be carried out directly on certain human tumor biopsy material. Recently Alberts et al.[171] evaluated drug sensitivities of ovarian tumor colony-forming units from patients with relapsing disease. These in vitro results showed that (1) vinblastine and cis-platinum were the most active of the second line drugs, (2) there was no evidence of collateral sensitivity between adriamycin and methotrexate, unlike that observed in some experimental systems, (3) cross-resistance between vindesine and vinblastine was complete, and (4) adriamycin was not cross-resistant with AMSA. These results were used to select agents for treatment of relapsed patients on an individual basis. The authors point out that a clinical study to identify active agents with a similar degree of accuracy would have required 450 evaluable patients, in contrast to the 32 examined here.

Further such work with other tumor types is clearly indicated. However, a large quantity of clinical material is needed for these studies and an alternative approach, adopted by my group, involves the use of established human tumor cell lines. We are attempting to (1) study the development of resistance following exposure to *clinically achievable* drug levels, and (2) checking patterns of cross-resistance or collateral sensitivity.

C. Methods for Preventing the Development of Drug-Resistance
Resistance to certain drugs develops more easily than others, either spontaneously or following specific drug exposure.[109,153,154] This is almost certainly reflected in the number of literature reports of various drug resistant cells lines. For example, numerous cell types resistant to methotrexate or 5-fluorouracil have been described but little data has been reported for mitomycin C or bleomycin resistance and none for the podophyllotoxins. Our laboratory experience confirms the ease of developing in vitro resistance to methotrexate and/or 5-fluorouracil, but we have been far less successful in establishing lines resistant to cis-platinum and some of the anthracyclines. Further studies of this type may help in deciding which agent(s) should be included in initial therapy and which could be used for second line treatment.

D. More Reliable Methods for Screening Potential "New" Drugs

The applications of the human tumor "stem" cell assay to new drug evaluation and screening are now accepted and some recent data is available.[172,173] Another possibility is the use of established human tumor cell lines. The few initial reports are sufficiently encouraging to hope that this approach will also be more widely pursued.[174,175] Studies with xenografted tumors are producing interesting preliminary data, some of which are conflicting, so again further work is indicated. In general a range of drug sensitivities is noted,[176,177] but it remains to be established whether these can be correlated with clinical responses.

E. New Model Systems for Studying Drug Resistance

Multicellular spheroids, first described by Sutherland et al.[147] provide a system of intermediate complexity between standard tissue culture systems and tumors in vivo. They may be useful for evaluating drug responses since they contain a heterogeneous population with regard to growth kinetics and because the penetration barriers which exist in poorly vascularized regions of tumors can be simulated in part. Initial results have indicated poor drug penetration to be a major factor in drug resistance for several agents includng adriamycin,[178,179] vinblastine,[180] and AMSA.[138] An exception was 5-fluorouracil, which seemed to penetrate efficiently, at least through glioma spheroids.[180] However, other factors such as altered metabolism, protection by intercellular communication and different cell kinetic parameters have also been implicated in the resistance observed in these models[181] and these aspects require further study.

The fact that certain drugs exert preferential cytotoxicity on internal vs. external cells in a spheroid has also been investigated. This approach should aid identification of agents effective against internal hypoxic cells, for example, the nitrofuran selected in a recent study.[182]

Development of resistance may also be monitored in spheroids, preferably following exposure to clinically achievable drug levels.

F. Optimal Scheduling of "Old" Drugs in Combinations

Although the search for new and more effective drugs continues there remains a major need to use the drugs already available more effectively. The fact that successful chemotherapy depends on the schedule and dose of drug employed is appreciated by many, but attempts to change the administration of drugs are often not accepted. For example, repeated doses of certain "alkylating agents" and several "antimetabolites" favor the emergence of drug-resistant cells experimentally.[153,154] Unfortunately, treatment with a low dose of these agents on a prolonged daily basis is still used in some clinical studies. For example, the standard method of clinical administration of procarbazine[183] and dibromodulcitol[184] is daily administration over 14 or 10-20 days respectively, yet these drugs can be administered in large doses over 2 days without loss of activity and for procarbazine this results in significantly reduced nausea, vomiting, and myelotoxicity.[164,185]

Experimental studies have shown that a full dose combination of cyclophosphamide and 6-mercaptopurine, which resulted in complete regression and cure after four courses in the Ridgeway osteogenic sarcoma, when given in lower doses to animals carrying similarly staged advanced tumors, still produced regression but allowed tumor regrowth during continued treatment and all the animals died. Similarly, growth of drug-resistant cells in a tumor is favored by continuing with initially effective single drugs or combinations until it is obvious that treatment is failing before instituting alternative therapy.[154] These problems may be overcome or circumvented and clinical evidence is already available showing how this may be achieved. For example, (1) in tumors responsive to drug treatment such as oat cell carcinoma of the lung and breast carcinoma full dose chemotherapy results in better response rates than when the dose is reduced even by a factor of as little as two or less,[38,155-157] (2) variability in dosage is a major factor in the differing response rates obtained with the same clinical protocol, any reduction compromising efficacy,[38] and (3) the use of two different, yet effective noncross-resistant sequential schedules *ab initio*, may reduce the likelihood of tumor regrowth during drug treatment, as now being tried in Hodgkin's disease alternating MOPP with ABVD.[186]

The more widespread practice of these principles is essential since chemotherapy is now often given with curative intent. This can only be encouraged by the demonstration that full dose intensive drug combinations can be administered more safely now than in the past.[187]

ACKNOWLEDGMENTS

I am extremely grateful to Drs. L. A. Price, J. R. W. Masters, and A. M. Creighton for their helpful advice and criticisms in the preparation of this manuscript. I am indebted to Drs. L. A. Price and D. Alberts for allowing me to include some of their current data being prepared for publication. The valuable assistance and patience particularly of Mrs. E. Simmons and of Miss G. Yiangou in typing drafts and the final manuscript have been greatly appreciated.

LIST OF ABBREVIATIONS USED FOR CERTAIN DRUGS

Act D	actinomycin D
AD 32	*N*-tri-fluoroacetyl-adriamycin
ADR	adriamycin
AMSA	9-acridinylamino-methanesulfon-m-anisidide
ANT	9,10-anthracenedione, 1,4[(2-[(2-hydroxyethyl)amino]-ethyl)amino]-diacetate (NSC 287513)
Ara C	cytosine arabinoside
ASP	L-asparaginase
5 AZA	5-azacytidine
BCNU	1,3-bis(2-chloroethyl)-1-nitrosourea
BLEO	bleomycin
CCNU	1-(2-chloroethyl)-3-nitrosoureido)-*cis*-cyclohexanecarboxylic acid
Cis-Pt	cis-diamminedichloroplatinum II
CYCLO	cyclophosphamide
DDMP	2,4-diamino-5-(3′,4′-dichlorophenyl)-6-methylpyrimidine
DHAD	1,4-dihydroxy-5,8-bis[2((2-hydroxyethyl)amino)-ethyl)amino]-9,10-anthracenedione dihydrochloride (NSC 301739)
DHAQ	1,4-dihydroxy-5,8-bis[2((2-hydroxyethyl)amino)-ethyl)amino]-9,10-anthracendedione (NSC 279836)
DNR	daunorubicin
DTIC	5-(3,3-dimethyl-1-triazeno)imidoazole-4-carboxamide

5FU	5-fluorouracil
HN2	nitrogen mustard
MeCCNU	*trans*-1-(2-chloroethyl)-3-(4-methylcyclohexyl)-1-nitrosourea
Mitoxantrone	see DHAD
6MP	6-mercaptopurine
MTC	mitomycin C
MTX	methotrexate
MYL	Myleran
7-OMEN	7-con-O-methylnogarol (NSC 269148)
PALA	N-phosphonoacetyl-L-aspartate
L-PAM	L-phenylalamine mustard or melphalan
PYF	pyrazofurin
6TG	6-thioguanine
VCR	vincristine
VDS	vindesine or desacetyl vinblastine amidesulfate
VLB	vinblastine
VM26	4'-demethyl-epipodophyllotoxin-9-(4,6-O-thenylidene-β-D-glucopyranoside)
VP-16-213	4'-demethyl-epipodophyllotoxin-9-(4,6-O-ethylidine-β-D-glucopyranoside)

REFERENCES

1. Zubrod, C. G., Historic milestones in curative chemotherapy, *Semin. Oncol.*, 6, 490, 1979.
2. Einhorn, L. H., Testicular cancer as a model for a curable neoplasm, *Cancer Res.*, 41, 3275, 1981.
3. Holland, J. F., Bruchner, H. W., Cohen, C. J., Wallace, R. C., Gusberg, S. B., Greenspan, E. M., and Goldberg, J., Cisplatin therapy of ovarian cancer, in *Cisplatin: Current Status and New Developments*, Prestayko, A. W., Crooke, S. T., and Carter, S. K., Eds., Academic Press, London, 1980, 383.
4. Livingston, R. B., Review: small cell carcinoma of the lung, *Blood*, 56, 575, 1980.
5. Van Putten, L. M., Are cell kinetic data relevant for the design of tumour chemotherapy schedules? *Cell Tissue Kinet.*, 7, 493, 1974.
6. Hart, J. S., Livingston, R. B., Murphy, W. K., Barlogie, B., Gehan, E. A., and Bodey, G. P., Neoplasia, kinetics and chemotherapy, *Semin Oncol.*, 3, 259, 1976.
7. Steel, G. C., *Growth Kinetics of Tumours*, Clarendon Press, Oxford, 1977, 1.
8. Tannock, I., Cell kinetics and chemotherapy: a critical review, *Cancer Treat. Rep.*, 62, 1117, 1978.
9. Bruce, W. R., Meeker, B. E., and Valeriote, F. A., Comparison of the sensitivity of normal hematopoietic and transplanted lymphoma colony-forming cells to chemotherapeutic agents administered *in vivo*, *J. Natl. Cancer Inst.*, 37, 233, 1966.
10. McCullough, E. A. and Till, J. E., Regulatory mechanisms acting on hematopoietic stem cells: some clinical implications, *Am. J. Pathol.*, 65, 601, 1971.
11. Tattersall, M. H N. and Tobias, J. S., How strong is the case for intensive cancer chemotherapy? *Lancet*, 1, 1071, 1976.
12. Hill, B. T., The management of human "solid" tumours: some observations on the irrelevance of traditional cell cycle kinetics and the value of certain recent concepts, *Cell Biol. Int. Rep.*, 2, 215, 1978.
13. Skipper, H. E., Schabel, F. M., Jr., and Wilcox, W. S., Experimental evaluation of potential anti-cancer drugs. XIV. Further study of certain basic concepts underlying chemotherapy of leukemia, *Cancer Chemother. Rep.*, 45, 5, 1965.

14. Schabel, F. M., Jr., Surgical adjuvant chemotherapy of metastatic murine tumours, *Cancer,* 40, 558, 1977.
15. Valeriote, F. and van Putten, L., Proliferation-dependent cytotoxicity of anticancer agents: a review, *Cancer Res.,* 35, 2619, 1975.
16. Carter, S. K., The strategy of cancer treatment: introduction, in *Recent Results in Cancer Research,* Vol. 62, Mathe, G., Ed., Springer-Verlag, Berlin, 1977, 51.
17. Fisher, B., Redmond, C., Brown, A., Wolmark, N., Wittliff, J., Fisher, E. R., Plotkin, D., Bowman, D., Sachs, S., Wolter, J., Frelick, R., Dresser, R., and other NSABP investigators, Treatment of primary breast cancer with chemotherapy and tamoxifen, *N. Engl. J. Med.,* 305, 1, 1981.
18. Rossi, A., Bonadonna, G., Valagussa, P., and Veronesi, V., Multimodal treatment in operable breast cancer: five year results of the CMF programme, *Br. Med. J.,* 282, 1427, 1981.
19. Hill, B. T., Principles of tumour growth, in *Scientific Foundations of Respiratory Medicine,* Scadding, J. G. and Cumming, G., Eds., Heinemann Medical, London, 1981, 592.
20. Hill, B. T. and Baserga, R., The cell cycle and its significance for cancer treatment, *Cancer Treat. Rev.,* 2, 159, 1975.
21. Hill, B. T., Biochemistry of the cell cycle, in *Scientific Foundations of Oncology,* Symington, T. S. and Carter, R. L., Eds., Heinemann Medical, London, 1976, 63.
22. Prescott, D. M., The cell cycle and the control of cellular reproduction, *Adv. Genet.,* 18, 99, 1976.
23. Hill, B. T., Cancer chemotherapy - the relevance of certain concepts of cell cycle kinetics, *Biochim. Biophys. Acta,* 516, 389, 1978.
24. Mendelsohn, M. L., The growth fraction: a new concept applied to tumours, *Science,* 132, 1496, 1960.
25. Valeriote, F. A. and Bruce, W. R., Comparison of the sensitivity of hematopoietic colony-forming cells in different proliferative states to vinblastine, *J. Natl. Cancer Inst.,* 38, 393, 1967.
26. Bruce, W. R. and Meeker, B. E., Comparison of the sensitivity of hematopoietic colony-forming cells in different proliferative states to 5-fluorouracil, *J. Natl. Cancer Inst.,* 38, 401, 1967.
27. Lajtha, L. G., Oliver, G. R., and Gurney, C. W., Kinetic model of a bone-marrow stem cell population, *Br. J. Haematol.,* 8, 442, 1962.
28. Carnie, A. B., Lala, P. K., and Osmond, D. G., in *Stem Cells of Renewing Cell Populations,* Academic Press, New York, 1976, 1.
29. Bruce, W. R. and Valeriote, F. A., Normal and malignant stem cells and chemotherapy, in *Proliferation and Spread of Neoplastic Cells, 21st Annual Symp. on Fundamental Cancer Research at M.D. Anderson Hospital and Tumour Institute at Houston, Texas,* Williams & Wilkins, Baltimore, 1968, 409.
30. Park, C. H., Bergsagel, D., and McCullough, E. A., Mouse myeloma tumor stem cells: a primary cell culture assay, *J. Natl. Cancer Inst.,* 46, 411, 1971.
31. Hamburger, A. W. and Salmon, S. E., Primary bioassay of human tumour stem cells, *Science,* 197, 461, 1977.
32. Buick, R. N., *In vitro* clonogenicity of primary human tumor cells: quantitation and relationship to tumor stem cells, in *Cloning of Human Tumor Stem Cells - Progress in Clinical and Biological Research,* Vol. 48, Salmon, S. E., Ed., Alan R. Liss, New York, 1980, 15.
33. Courtenay, V. D. and Mills, J., An *in vitro* colony assay for human tumours grown in immune-suppressed mice and treated *in vivo* with cytotoxic agents, *Br. J. Cancer,* 37, 261, 1978.
34. Jones, S. E., Hamburger, A. W., Kim, M. B., and Salmon, S. E., Development of a bioassay for putative human lymphoma stem cells, *Blood,* 53, 294, 1977.
35. Ozols, R. F., Willson, J. K. V., Weltz, M. D., Grotzinger, K. R., Myers, C. E., and Young, R. C., Inhibition of human ovarian cancer colony formation by adriamycin and its major metabolites, *Cancer Res.,* 40, 4109, 1980.
36. Salmon, S. E., Alberts, D. S., Meyskens, F. L., Jr., Durie, B. G. M., Jones, S. E., Soehnlen, B., Young, L., Chen, H-S. G., and Moon, T. E., Clinical correlations of in vitro drug sensitivity, in *Cloning of Human Tumor Stem Cells - Progress in Clinical and Biological Research,* Vol. 48, Salmon, S. E., Ed., Alan R. Liss, New York, 1980, 223.
37. Von Hoff, D. D., Harris, G. J., Johnson, G., and Glaubiger, D., Initial experience with the human tumor stem cell assay system: Potential and problems, in *Cloning of Human Tumor Stem Cells - Progress in Clinical and Biological Research,* Vol. 48, Salmon, S. E., Ed., Alan R. Liss, New York, 1980, 113.
38. Frei, E., III and Canellos, G. P., Dose: a critical factor in cancer chemotherapy, *Am. J. Med.,* 69, 585, 1980.
39. Thomas, E. D., Fluornoy, N., and Buckner, C. D., Cure of leukemia by marrow transplantation, *Leuk. Res.,* 1, 67, 1977.
40. Bergsagel, D. E., An assessment of massive-dose chemotherapy of malignant disease, *Can. Med. Assoc. J.,* 104, 31, 1971.

41. Legha, S. S., Buzdar, A. U., Hortobagyi, G. N., DiStefano, A., Wiseman, C. L., Yap, H-Y., Blumenschein, G. R., and Bodey, G. P., Phase II study of hexamethylmelamine alone and in combination with mitomycin C and vincristine in advanced breast carcinoma, *Cancer Treat Rep.*, 63, 2053, 1979.

42. Botnick, L. E., Hannon, E. C., Vigneulle, R., and Hellman, S., Diferential effects of cytotoxic agents on hematopoietic progenitors, *Cancer Res.*, 41, 2338, 1981.

43. Griswold, D. P., Jr., Simpson-Herren, L., and Schabel, F. M., Jr., Altered sensitivity of a hamster plasmacytoma to cytosine arabinoside (NSC-63878), *Cancer Chemother. Rep.*, 54, 337, 1970.

44. Goldman, I. D., Uptake of drugs and resistance, in *Drug Resistance and Selectivity - Biochemical and Cellular Basis*, Mihich, E., Ed., Academic Press, London, 1973, 299.

45. Mihich, E., Tumour immunogenicity in therapeutics, in *Drug Resistance and Selectivity - Biochemical and Cellular Basis*, Mihich, E., Ed., Academic Press, London, 1973, 391.

46. Brockman, R. W., Mechanisms of resistance, in *Antineoplastic and Immunosuppressive Agents*, Part I, Sartorelli, A. C., and Johns, D. G., Eds., Springer-Verlag, Berlin, 1975, 352.

47. Hall, T. C., Prediction of responses to therapy and mechanisms of resistance, *Semin. Oncol.*, 4, 193, 1977.

48. Hill, B. T., Price, L. A., and Goldie, J. H., Methotrexate resistance and uptake of DDMP by L5178Y cells - selective protection with folinic acid, *Eur. J. Cancer*, 11, 545, 1975.

49. Jackson, R. C., Niethammer, D., and Huennekens, F. M., Enzymic and transport mechanisms of amethopterin resistance in L1210 mouse leukemia cells, *Cancer Biochem. Biophys.*, 1, 151, 1975.

50. Inaba, M. and Johnson, R. K., Uptake and retention of adriamycin and daunorubicin by sensitive and anthracycline-resistant sublines of P388 leukemia, *Biochem. Pharmacol.*, 27, 2123, 1978.

51. Brabbs, S. and Warr, J. R., Isolation and characterization of bleomycin-resistant clones of CHO cells, *Genet. Res. Camb.*, 34, 269, 1979.

52. Redwood, W. R. and Colvin, M., Transport of melphalan by sensitive and resistant L1210 cells, *Cancer Res.*, 40, 1144, 1980.

53. Bleyer, W. A., Frisby, S. A., and Oliverio, V. T., Uptake and binding of vincristine by murine leukemia cells, *Biochem. Pharmacol.*, 24, 633, 1975.

54. Niethammer, D. and Jackson, R. C., Changes of molecular properties associated with the development of resistance against methotrexate in human lymphoblastoid cells, *Europ. J. Cancer*, 11, 845, 1975.

55. Sirotnak, F. M. and Donsbach, R. C., Kinetic correlates of methotrexate transport and therapeutic responsiveness in murine tumours, *Cancer Res.*, 36, 1151, 1976.

56. Warren, R. D., Nichols, A. P., and Bendet, R. A., Membrane transport of methotrexate in human lymphoblastoid cells, *Cancer Res.*, 38, 668, 1978.

57. Hill, B. T., Bailey, B. D., White, J. C., and Goldman, I. D., Characteristics of transport of 4-amino antifolates and folate compounds by two lines of L5178Y lymphoblasts, one with impaired transport of methotrexate, *Cancer Res.*, 39, 2440, 1979.

58. Elliott, E. M. and Ling, V., Selection and characterization of Chinese hamster ovary cell mutants resistant to melphalan (L-phenylalanine mustard), *Cancer Res.*, 41, 393, 1981.

59. Kessel, D., Enhanced glycosylation induced by adriamycin, *Molec. Pharmacol.*, 16, 306, 1979.

60. Beck, W. T., Mueller, T. J., and Tanzer, L. R., Altered surface membrane glycoproteins in vinca alkaloid-resistant human leukemic lymphoblasts, *Cancer Res.*, 39, 2070, 1979.

61. Inaba, M., Kobayashi, H., Sakurai, Y., and Johnson, R. K., Active efflux of daunorubicin and adriamycin in sensitive and resistant sublines of P388 leukemia, *Cancer Res.*, 39, 2200, 1979.

62. Skovsgaard, T., Carrier-mediated transport of daunorubicin, adriamycin and rubidazone in Ehrlich ascites tumour cells, *Biochem. Pharmacol.*, 27, 1221, 1978.

63. Dano, K., Experimentally developed cellular resistance to daunomycin, *Acta Pathol. Scand. Sect. A*, Suppl. 256, 11, 1976.

64. Hill, B. T. and Whelan, R. D. H., Comparative cell killing and kinetic effects of vincristine or vindesine in mammalian cell lines, *J. Natl. Cancer Inst.*, 67, in press, 1981.

65. Skipper, H. E., Hutchison, D. J., Schabel, F. M., Schmidt, L. H., Goldin, A., Brockman, R. W., Venditti, J. M., and Wodinsky, I., A quick reference chart on cross-resistance between anticancer agents, *Cancer Chemother. Rep.*, 56, 493, 1972.

66. Biedler, J. L., Riehm, H., Peterson, R. H. F., and Spengler, B. A., Membrane-mediated drug resistance and phenotypic reversion to normal growth behaviour of Chinese hamster cells, *J. Natl. Cancer Inst.*, 55, 671, 1975.

67. Skovsgaard, T., Mechanism of resistance to daunorubicin in Ehrlich ascites tumour cells, *Cancer Res.*, 38, 1785, 1978.

68. Casazza, A. M., Pratesi, G., Giuliani, F., Formelli, F., and DiMarco, A., Enhancement of the antitumour activity of adriamycin by Tween 80, *Tumori*, 64, 115, 1978.

69. Nishimura, T., Muto, K., and Tanaka, N., Drug sensitivity of an adriamycin resistant mutant subline of mouse lympho-blastoma L5178Y cells, *J. Antibiot.*, 31, 493, 1978.

70. Peterson, C. and Trouet, A., Transport and storage of daunomycin and doxorubicin in cultured fibroblasts, *Cancer Res.*, 38, 4645, 1978.

71. Inaba, M. and Sakurai, Y., Enhanced efflux of actinomycin D, vincristine and vinblastine in an adriamycin-resistant subline of P388 Leukemia, *Cancer Lett.*, 8, 111, 1979.

72. Inaba, M., Fujikura, R., and Sakurai, Y., Active efflux common to vincristine and daunorubicin in vincristine-resistant P388 leukemia, *Biochem. Pharmacol.*, 30, 1863, 1981.

73. Skovsgaard, T., Mechanism of cross-resistance between vincristine and daunorubicin in Ehrlich ascites tumor cells, *Cancer Res.*, 38, 4722, 1978.

74. Parsons, P. G., Carter, F. B., Morrison, L., and Mary, R., Sr., Mechanism of melphalan resistance developed *in vitro* in human melanoma cells, *Cancer Res.*, 41, 1525, 1981.

75. Henderson, G. B., Zevely, E. M., and Huennekens, F. M., Cyclic adenosine 3':5'-monophosphate and methotrexate transport in L1210 cells, *Cancer Res.*, 38, 859, 1978.

76. Brockman, R. W., Yagisawa, Y., Ling, V., Schabel, F. M., DiMarco, A., Harrap, K. R., and Holland, J. F., Modes of acquiring resistance to chemotherapeutic agents, in *Current Chemotherapy*, American Society for Microbiology, Washington, D.C., 1978, 97.

77. Bosmann, H. B., Mechanism of cellular drug resistance, *Nature (London)*, 233, 566, 1971.

78. Baker, R. M. and Ling, V., Membrane mutants of mammalian cells in culture, *Meth. Membrane Biol.*, 9, 337, 1978.

79. Mayaki, M., Ono, T., Hori, S., and Umezawa, H., Binding of bleomycin to DNA in bleomycin sensitive and resistant rat ascites hepatoma cells, *Cancer Res.*, 35, 2015, 1975.

80. Akiyama, S.-I., Ikezaki, K., Kuramochi, H., Takahashi, K., and Kuwano, M., Bleomycin-resistant cells contain increased bleomycin-hydrolase activities, *Biochem. Biophys. Res. Commun.*, 1, 55, 1981.

81. Meriwether, W. D. and Bachur, N. R., Inhibition of DNA and RNA metabolism by daunorubicin and adriamycin in L1210 mouse leukemia, *Cancer Res.*, 32, 1137, 1972.

82. Dix, D. E., Lehman, C. P., Jakubowski, A., Moyer, J. D., and Handschumacher, R. E., Pyrazofurin metabolism, enzyme inhibition, and resistance in L5178Y cells, *Cancer Res.*, 39, 4485, 1979.

83. Suttle, D. P., Harkrader, R. J., and Jackson, R. C., Pyrazofurin-resistant hepatoma cells deficient in adenosinekinase, *Eur. J. Cancer*, 17, 43, 1981.

84. Ardalan, B., Cooney, D. A., Jayaram, H. N., Carrico, C. K., Glazer, R. I., Macdonald, J., and Schein, P. S., Mechanisms of sensitivity and resistance of murine tumors to 5-fluorouracil, *Cancer Res.*, 40, 1431, 1980.

85. Kaufman, R. J., Brown, P. C., and Schimke, R. T., Amplified dihydrofolate reductase genes in unstably methotrexate-resistant cells are associated with double minute chromosomes, *Proc. Natl. Acad. Sci. USA*, 76, 5669, 1979.

86. Melera, P. W., Lewis, J. A., Biedler, J. L., and Hession, C., Antifolate-resistant Chinese hamster cells: evidence for dihydrofolate reductase gene amplification among independently derived sublines overproducing different dihydrofolate reductases, *J. Biol. Chem.*, 255, 7024, 1980.

87. Johnson, R. K., Swyryd, E. A., and Stark, G. R., Effects of N-(phosphonacetyl)-L-aspartate on murine tumours and normal tissues *in vivo* and *in vitro* and the relationship of sensitivity to rate of proliferation and level of aspartate transcarbamylase, *Cancer Res.*, 38, 371, 1978.

88. Jackson, R. C., Hart, L. I., and Harrap, K. R., Intrinsic resistance to methotrexate of cultured mammalian cells in relation to the inhibition-kinetics of their dihydrofolate reductase, *Cancer Res.*, 36, 1991, 1976.

89. Goldie, J. H., Krystal, G., Hartley, D., Gudauskas, G., and Dedhar, S., A methotrexate insensitive variant of folate reductase present in two lines of methotrexate-resistant L5178Y cells, *Eur. J. Cancer*, 16, 1539, 1980.

90. Jayaram, H. N., Cooney, D. A., Vistica, D. T., Kariya, S., and Johnson, R. K., Mechanisms of sensitivity or resistance of murine tumours to N-(phosphonacetyl)-L-aspartate (PALA), *Cancer Treat. Rep.*, 63, 1291, 1979.

91. Chou, T. C., Arlin, Z., Clarkson, B. D., and Philips, F. S., Metabolism of 1-β-D-arabinofuranosylcytosine in human leukemia cells, *Cancer Res.*, 37, 3561, 1977.

92. Robert de Saint Vincent, B. R. and Buttin, G., Studies on 1-β-D-arabinofuranosylcytosine-resistant mutants of Chinese hamster fibroblasts. IV. Altered regulation of CTP synthetase generates arabinosylcytosine and thymidine resistance, *Biochim. Biophys. Acta*, 610, 352, 1980.

93. Moran, R. G., Mulkins, M., and Heidelberger, C., Role of thymidylate synthetase activity in development of methotrexate cytotoxicity, *Proc. Natl. Acad. Sci. USA*, 72, 3683, 1979.

94. Ayusawa, D., Koyama, H., and Seno, T., Resistance to methotrexate in thymidylate synthetase-deficient mutants of cultured mouse mammary tumour FM3A cells, *Cancer Res.*, 41, 1497, 1981.

95. Kensler, T. W., Mutter, G., Hankerson, J. G., Reck, L. J., Harley, C., Han, N., Ardalan, B., Cysyk, R. L., Johnson, R. K., Jayaram, H. N., and Cooney, D. A., Mechanism of resistance of variants of the Lewis lung carcinoma to N-(phosphonacetyl)-L-aspartic acid, *Cancer Res.,* 41, 894, 1981.

96. Erickson, L. C., Osieka, R., and Kohn, K. W., Differential repair of 1-(2-chloroethyl)-3-(4-methyl-cyclohexyl)-1-nitrosourea-induced DNA damage in two human colon tumour cell lines, *Cancer Res.,* 38, 802, 1978.

97. Erickson, L. C., Zwelling, L. A., Ducore, J. M., Sharkey, N. A., and Kohn, K. W., Differential cytotoxicity and DNA cross-linking in normal and transformed human fibroblasts treated with cis-diamminedichloroplatinum (II), *Cancer Res.,* 41, 2791, 1981.

98. Yin, L., Chun, H. L., and Rutman, R. J., A comparison of the effects of alkylation on the DNA of sensitive and resistant Lettre-Ehrlich cells following *in vivo* exposure to nitrogen mustards, *Biochim. Biophys. Acta,* 324, 472, 1973.

99. Strandberg, M. C., Studies on the resistance of a murine leukemia L1210 cell line to cis-diammine-dichloroplatinum (II), *Proc. Am. Assoc. Cancer Res.,* 22, 202, 1981.

100. Zwelling, L. A., Michaels, S., Schwartz, H., Dobson, P. P., and Kohn, K. W., DNA cross-linking as an indicator of sensitivity and resistance of mouse L1210 leukemia to cis-diamminedichloroplatinum (II) and L-phenylalanine mustard, *Cancer Res.,* 41, 640, 1981.

101. Alt, F. W., Kellems, R. E., Bertino, J. R., and Schimke, R. T., Selective multiplication of dihydro-folate reductase genes in methotrexate-resistant variants of cultured murine cells, *J. Biol. Chem.,* 253, 1357, 1978.

102. Dolnick, B. J., Berenson, R. J., Bertino, J. R., Kaufman, R. J., Nunberg, J. H., and Schimke, R. T., Correlation of dihydrofolate reductase elevation with gene amplification in a homogeneously staining chromosomal region in L5178Y cells, *J. Cell Biol.,* 83, 394, 1979.

103. Urlaub, G., Landzberg, M., and Chasin, L. A., Selective killing of methotrexate-resistant cells carrying amplified dihydrofolate reductase genes, *Cancer Res.,* 41, 1594, 1981.

104. Melera, P. W., Wolgemuth, D., Biedler, J. L., and Hession, C., Antifolate-resistant Chinese hamster cells: evidence from independently derived sublines for two dihydrofolate reductases encoded by different mRNAs, *J. Biol. Chem.,* 255, 319, 1980.

105. Erickson, L. C., Bradley, M. O., Ducore, J. M., Ewig, R. A. G., and Kohn, K. W., DNA cross-linking and cytotoxicity in normal and transformed human cells treated with anti-tumor nitrosoureas, *Proc. Natl. Acad. Sci. USA,* 77, 467, 1980.

106. Micetich, K., Michaels, S., Jude, G., Kohn, K., and Zwelling, L., Mechanism of resistance to cis-dichlorodiammine-platinum (II) in a line of L1210 cells, *Proc. Am. Assoc. Cancer Res.,* 22, 252, 1981.

107. Schabel, F. M., Jr., Trader, M. W., Laster, W. R., Jr., Wheeler, G. P., and Witt, M. H., Patterns of resistance and therapeutic synergism among alkylating agents, in *Fundamentals in Cancer Chemotherapy, Antibiotics Chemother.,* Vol. 23, Schonfeld, H., Brockman, R. W., and Hahn, F. E., Eds., S. Karger, Basel, 1978, 200.

108. Schmid, F. A., Otter, G. M., and Stock, C. C., Resistance patterns of Walker carcinosarcoma 256 and other rodent tumours to cyclophosphamide and L-phenylalanine mustard, *Cancer Res.,* 40, 830, 1980.

109. Hill, B. T., Collateral sensitivity and cross-resistance, in *Antitumour Drug Resistance - Handbook of Experimental Pharmacology,* Fox, B. W. and Fox, M., Eds., Springer-Verlag, Berlin, 1982, in press.

110. Tobey, R. A., Deaven, L. L., and Oka, M. S., Kinetic response of cultured Chinese hamster cells to treatment with 4'-[(9-acridinyl)-amino]methanesulphon-m-anisidide-HCl, *J. Natl. Cancer Inst.,* 60, 1147, 1978.

111. Traganos, F., Stainano-Coico, L., Darynkiewicz, Z., and Melamed, M. R., Effects of aclacinomycin on cell survival and cell cycle progression of cultured mammalian cells, *Cancer Res.,* 41, 2728, 1981.

112. Dosik, G. M., Barlogie, B., Johnston, D. A., Murphy, W. K., and Drewinko, B., Lethal and cyto-kinetic effects of anguidine, *Cancer Res.,* 38, 3304, 1978.

113. Evenson, D. P., Darzynkiewicz, Z., Staiano-Coico, L., Traganos, F., and Melamed, M. R., Effects of 9,10-anthracenedione, 1,4[[2-[(2-hydroxyethyl)amino]-ethyl]amino]-diacetate on cell survival and cell cycle progression in cultured mammalian cells, *Cancer Res.,* 39, 2574, 1979.

114. Bhuyan, B. K., Robinson, M. I., Shugars, K. D., Bono, V. H., and Dion, R. L., Effects of chartreu-sin on cell survival and cell cycle progression, *Cancer Res.,* 38, 2734, 1978.

115. Hill, B. T., Lethal and kinetic effects of DDMP (2,4-diamino-5-(3',4'-dichlorophenyl)-6-methylpyr-imidine), *Eur. J. Cancer,* 16, 147, 1980.

116. Hidvegi, E. J., Sebestyn, J., Szabo, L. D., Koteles, G. J., and Institoris, L., The effect of dibromo-dulcitol, diepoxydulcitol and various new cytostatic hexitol derivatives on the metabolic activities of nucleic acids and proteins - II, *Biochem. Pharmacol.,* 25, 1705, 1976.

117. Olah, E., Palyi, I., and Sugar, J., Effects of cytostatics on proliferating and stationary cultures of mammalian cells, *Eur. J. Cancer*, 14, 895, 1978.

118. Traganos, F., Staiano-Coico, L., Darynkiewicz, Z., and Melamed, M. R., Effects of dihydro-5-azacytidine on cell survival and cell cycle progression of cultured mammalian cells, *Cancer Res.*, 41, 780, 1981.

119. Traganos, F., Evenson, D. P., Staiano-Coico, L., and Darynkiewicz, Z., and Melamed, M. R., Action of dihydro-anthraquinone on cell cycle progression and survival of a variety of cultured mammalian cells, *Cancer Res.*, 40, 671, 1980.

120. Traganos, F., Evenson, D. P., Staiano-Coico, L., Darynkiewicz, Z., and Melamed, M. R., Ellipticine-induced changes in cell growth and nuclear morphology, *J. Natl. Cancer Inst.*, 65, 1329, 1980.

121. Hill, B. T. and Whelan, R. D. H., A comparison of the lethal and kinetic effects of doxorubicin and 4′-epi-doxorubicin *in vitro*, *Tumori*, in press, 1982.

122. Rao, P. N., Freireich, E. J., Smith, M. L., and Loo, T. L., Cell cycle phase-specific cytotoxicity of the antitumour agent maytansine, *Cancer Res.*, 39, 3152, 1979.

123. Wallace, R. E., Murdock, K. C., Angier, R. B., and Durr, F. E., Activity of a novel anthracenedione, 1,4-dihydroxy-5,8-bis[[-2-[(2-hydroxyethyl)amino]ethyl]amino]-9,10-anthracenedione dihydrochloride, against experimental tumors in mice, *Cancer Res.*, 39, 1570, 1979.

124. Murray, E. F. and Wallace, R. E., CL 232,315 (NSC 301739) 1,4-dihydroxy-5,8-bis[[2-[(2-hydroxyethyl)amino]-ethyl]amino]9,10-anthracenedione dihydrochloride: a novel antitumour agent, in *Anthracyclines: Current status and new developments*, Crooke, S. T. and Reich, S. D., Eds., Academic Press, London, 1980, 397.

125. Bhuyan, B. K., Blowers, C. L., and Shugars, K. D., Lethality of nogalamycin, nogalamycin analogs, and adriamycin to cells in different cell cycle phases, *Cancer Res.*, 40, 3437, 1980.

126. Traganos, F., Staiano-Coico, L., Darynkiewicz, Z., and Melamed, M. R., Effects of prospidine on survival and growth of mammalian cells in culture, *J. Natl. Cancer Inst.*, 65, 993, 1980.

127. Hill, B. T. and Whelan, R. D. H., Antitumour activity and cell kinetic effects of pyrazofurin *in vitro*, *Eur. J. Cancer*, 16, 1633, 1980.

128. Olah, E., Lui, M. S., Tzeng, D. Y., and Weber, G., Phase and cell cycle specificity of pyrazofurin action, *Cancer Res.*, 40, 2869, 1980.

129. Hill, B. T., Whatley, S. A., Bellamy, A. S., Jenkins, L. Y., and Whelan, R. D. H., Cytotoxic effects and biological activity of spirogermanium *in vitro*, *Cancer Res.*, in press, 1982.

130. Tobey, R. A. and Crissman, H. A., Comparative effects of three nitrosourea derivatives on mammalian cell cycle progression, *Cancer Res.*, 35, 460, 1975.

131. Bhuyan, B. K., Fraser, T. J., and Day, K. J., Cell proliferation kinetics and drug sensitivity of exponential and stationary populations of cultured L1210 cells, *Cancer Res.*, 37, 1057, 1977.

132. Drewinko, B., Patchen, M., Yang, L-Y., and Barlogie, B., Differential killing efficacy of twenty antitumour drugs on proliferating and non-proliferating human tumour cells, *Cancer Res.*, 41, 2328, 1981.

133. Wilson, W. R., Giesbrecht, J. L., Hill, R. P., and Whitmore, G. F., Toxicity of 4′-(-Acridinylamino)methanesulfon-*m*-anisidide in exponential- and plateau-phase Chinese Hamster cell cultures, *Cancer Res.*, 41, 2809, 1981.

134. Bhuyan, B. K., Blowers, C. L., Crampton, S. L., and Shugars, K. D., Cell kill kinetics of several nogalamycin analogs and adriamycin for Chinese hamster ovary, L1210 leukemia and B16 melanoma cells in culture, *Cancer Res.*, 41, 18, 1981.

135. Krishan, A., Dutt, K., Israel, M., and Ganapathi, R., Comparative effects of adriamycin and N-trifluoroacetyl-adriamycin-14-valerate on cell kinetics, chromosomal damage, and macromolecular synthesis *in vitro*, *Cancer Res.*, 41, 2745, 1981.

136. Teicher, B. A., Lazo, J. S., and Sartorelli, A. C., Classification of antineoplastic agents by their selective toxicities toward oxygenated and hypoxic tumor cells, *Cancer Res.*, 41, 73, 1981.

137. Smith, E., Stratford, I. J., and Adams, G. E., Cytotoxicity of adriamycin on aerobic and hypoxic Chinese hamster V79 cells *in vitro*, *Br. J. Cancer*, 41, 568, 1980.

138. Wilson, W. R., Whitmore, G. F., and Hill, R. P., Activity of 4′-(9-acridinylamino)methane-sulfon-m-anisidide against Chinese hamster cells in multicellular spheroids, *Cancer Res.*, 41, 2817, 1981.

139. Harris, J. W. and Shrieve, D. C., Effects of adriamycin and X-rays on euoxic and hypoxic EMT6 cells *in vitro*, *Int. J. Radiat. Oncol. Biol. Phys.*, 5, 1245, 1979.

140. Marsh, J. C., The effects of cancer chemotherapeutic agents on normal hematopoietic precursor cells: a review, *Cancer Res.*, 36, 1853, 1976.

141. Marsh, J. C., Bone marrow colony forming cell sensitivity to carminomycin, marcellomycin and spirogermanium, *Proc. Am. Assoc. Cancer Res.*, 22, 241, 1981.

142. Currie, G., *Cancer and the Immune Response*, 2nd ed., Edward Arnold, London, 1980.

143. Kaliss, N., Immunological enhancement of tumour homografts in mice - a review, *Cancer Res.*, 18, 992, 1958.

144. Mihich, E., Chemotherapy and immunotherapy as a combined modality of cancer treatment, in *Advances in Tumour Prevention, Detection and Characterization*, Vol. 4, Davis, W. and Harrap, K. R., Eds., Excerpta Medica, Amsterdam, 1978, 113.

145. Mihich, E. and Ehrke, M. J., Selectivity of antitumour agents on immunity, in *Advances in Medical Oncology, Research and Education - Proc. 12th Int. Cancer Congress*, Volume V, Fox, B. W., Ed., Pergamon Press, Oxford, 1979, 131.

146. Braun, D. P. and Harris, J. E., Modulation of the immune response by chemotherapy, *Pharmacol. Ther.*, 14, 89, 1981.

147. Sutherland, R. M., McCredie, J. A., and Inch, W. R., Growth of multicell spheroids in tissue culture as a model of nodular carcinoma, *J. Natl. Cancer Inst.*, 46, 113, 1971.

148. Skipper, H. E., Kinetic considerations associated with therapy of solid tumours, in *The Proliferation and Spread of Neoplastic Cells, 21st Ann. Symp. on Fundamental Cancer Res. at M.D. Anderson Hospital and Tumor Institute at Houston, Texas*, Williams & Wilkins, Baltimore, 1968, 213.

149. Wilcox, W. S., Griswold, D. P., Laster, W. R., Jr., Schabel, F. M., Jr., and Skipper, H. E., Experimental evaluation of potential anticancer agents. XVII. Kinetics of growth and regression after treatment of certain solid tumours, *Cancer Chemother. Ref.*, 47, 27, 1965.

150. Shackney, S. E., McCormack, G. W., and Cuchural, G. J., Growth rate patterns of solid tumors and their relation to responsiveness to therapy, *Ann. Intern. Med.*, 89, 107, 1978.

151. Skipper, H. E., Schabel, F. M., Jr., and Lloyd, H. H., Dose-response and tumour cell repopulation rate in chemotherapeutic trials, in *Advances in Cancer Chemotherapy*, Vol. 1, Rosowsky, A., Ed., Marcel Dekker, New York, 1979, 205.

152. Goldie, J. H. and Coldman, A. J., A mathematical model for relating the drug sensitivity of tumours to their spontaneous mutation rate, *Cancer Treat. Rep.*, 63, 1727, 1979.

153. Skipper, H. E., Schabel, F. M., Jr., and LLoyd, H. H., Experimental therapeutics and kinetics: selection and overgrowth of specifically and permanently drug-resistant tumour cells, *Semin. Haematol.*, 15, 207, 1978.

154. Schabel, F. M., Jr., Skipper, H. E., Trader, M. W., Laster, W. R., Jr., Corbett, T. H., and Griswold, D. P., Jr., Concepts for controlling drug-resistant tumor cells, in *Breast Cancer. Experimental and Clinical Aspects*, Mouridsen, H. T. and Palshof, T., Eds., Pergamon Press, Oxford, 1980, 199.

155. Cohen, M. H., Creaven, P. J., Fossieck, J. R., Broder, L. E., Selawry, O. S., Johnston, A. V., Williams, C. L., and Minna, J. D., Intensive chemotherapy of small cell bronchogenic carcinoma, *Cancer Treat. Rep.*, 61, 349, 1977.

156. Salmon, S. E. and Jones, S. E., Studies of the combination of adriamycin and cyclophosphamide (alone or with other agents) for the treatment of breast cancer, *Oncology*, 36, 40, 1979.

157. Bonadonna, G. and Valagussa, P., Dose-response effect of adjuvant chemotherapy in breast cancer, *N. Engl. J. Med.*, 304, 10, 1981.

158. Price, L. A. and Goldie, J. H., Multiple drug therapy for disseminated malignant disease, *Br. Med. J.*, 4, 336, 1971.

159. Price, L. A. and Hill, B. T., Safer cancer chemotherapy using a kinetically-based approach: clinical implications, in *Safer Cancer Chemotherapy*, Price, L. A., Hill, B. T., and Ghilchick, M. W., Eds., Balliere Tindall, London, 1981, 9.

160. Anderson, G., Thomas, G., and Stewart-Jones, J., Treatment of advanced bronchogenic carcinoma with adriamycin, 5-fluorouracil and methotrexate, *Br. J. Dis. Chest.*, 71, 179, 1977.

161. Goldie, J. H. and Price, L. A., 20-hour combination chemotherapy in advanced breast cancer, *Br. Med. J.*, 2, 1064, 1977.

162. Price, L. A., Hill, B. T., Calvert, A. H., Dalley, V. M., Levine, A., Busby, E. R., Schachter, M., and Shaw, H. J., Improved results in combination chemotherapy of head and neck cancer using a kinetically-based approach: a randomized study with and without adriamycin, *Oncology*, 35, 26, 1978.

163. Goldie, J. H., Price, L. A., and Harrap, K. R., Methotrexate toxicity: correlation with duration of administration, plasma levels, dose and excretion pattern, *Eur. J. Cancer*, 8, 409, 1972.

164. Kitchen, G., Kinetically-designed 'short MOPP' therapy for Hodgkin's disease: a feasibility study, in *Safer Cancer Chemotherapy*, Price, L. A., Hill, B. T., and Ghilchick, M. W., Bailliere Tindall, London, 1981, 103.

165. Price, L. A. and Hill, B. T., Safe and effective induction chemotherapy without cisplatin for squamous cell carcinoma of the head and neck: impact on complete response rate and survival at five years, following local therapy, *Med. Ped. Oncol.*, in press, 1982.

166. Rupniak, H. T. and Hill, B. T., The poor cloning ability in agar of human tumour cells from biopsies of primary tumours, *Cell Biol. Int. Rep.*, 4, 479, 1980.

167. Rupniak, H. T., Marks, P., Watkins, S., Bourne, G., Slevin, M., Bancroft-Livingston, G. H., Simmons, C. A., and Hill, B. T., Studies on the drug sensitivities of human tumour cells obtained directly from biopsy material, in *Proc. 12th Int. Congress of Chemotherapy, Florence, Italy*, in press, 1981.

168. Salmon, S. E., Hamburger, A. W., Soehnlen, B. J., Durrie, B. G. M., Alberts, D. S., and Moon, T. E., Quantitation of differential sensitivity of human tumor stem cells to anticancer drugs, *N. Engl. J. Med.,* 298, 1321, 1978.

169. Alberts, D. S., Salmon, S. E., Chen, H. S. G., Surwit, E. A., Soehnlen, B., Young, L., and Moon, T. E., *In vitro* clonogenic assay for predicting response of ovarian cancer to chemotherapy, *Lancet,* 2, 340, 1980.

170. Alberts, D. S., Young, H. S. G., Moon, T. E., Leigh, S. A., Surwit, E. A., and Salmon, S. E., Improved survival for relapsing ovarian cancer patients using the human tumor stem cell assay to select chemotherapy, *Proc. Am. Soc. Clin. Oncol.,* 22, 462, 1981.

171. Alberts, D. S., Chen, H. S. G., Salmon, S. E., Surwit, E. A., Young, L., Moon, T. E., and Meyskens, F. L., Jr., Chemotherapy of ovarian cancer directed by the human tumor stem cell assay, *Cancer Chemother. Pharmacol.,* 6, 279, 1981.

172. Salmon, S. E., Meyskens, F. L., Jr., Alberts, D. S., Soehnlen, B., and Young, L., New drugs in ovarian cancer and malignant melanoma: in vitro Phase II screening with the human tumor stem cell assay, *Cancer Treat. Rep.,* 65, 1, 1981.

173. Von Hoff, D. D., Coltman, C. A., Jr., and Forseth, B., Activity of mitoxantrone in a human humor cloning system, *Cancer Res.,* 41, 1853, 1981.

174. Drewinko, B., Yang, L. Y., Ho, D. H. W., Benvenuto, J., Loo, T. L., and Freireich, E. J., Treatment of cultured human colon carcinoma cells with fluorinated pyrimidines, *Cancer,* 45, 1144, 1980.

175. Hill, B. T. and Whelan, R. D. H., Assessments of the sensitivities of cultured human neuroblastoma cells to antitumour drugs, *Pediat. Res.,* 15, 1117, 1981.

176. Bateman, A. E., Peckham, M. J., and Steel, G. G., Assays of drug sensitivity for cells from human tumours: In vitro and in vivo tests on a xenografted tumour, *Br. J. Cancer,* 40, 81, 1979.

177. Tveit, K. M., Fodstad, O., Olsnes, S., and Pihl, A., In vitro sensitivity of human melanoma xenografts to cytotoxic drugs. Correlation with *in vivo* sensitivity, *Int. J. Cancer,* 26, 717, 1980.

178. Sutherland, R. M., Eddy, H. A., Bareham, B., Reich, K., and Vanantwerp, D., Resistance to adriamycin in multicellular spheroids, *Int. J. Radiat. Oncol. Biol. Phys.,* 5, 1225, 1979.

179. Durand, R. E., Flow cytometry studies of intracellular adriamycin in multicell spheroids in vitro, *Cancer Res.,* 41, 3495, 1981.

180. Nederman, T., Carlsson, J., and Malmquist, M., Penetration of substances into tumour tissue - a methodological study on cellular spheroids, *In Vitro,* 17, 290, 1981.

181. Wibe, E., Resistance to vincristine of human cells grown as multicellular spheroids, *Br. J. Cancer,* 42, 937, 1980.

182. Olive, P. L., Different sensitivity to cytotoxic agents of internal and external cells of spheroids composed of thioguanine-resistant and sensitive cells, *Br. J. Cancer,* 43, 85, 1981.

183. Spivack, S. D., Procarbazine, *Ann. Intern. Med.,* 81, 795, 1974.

184. Mischler, N. E., Earhart, R. H., Carr, B., and Tormey, D. C., Dibromodulcitol, *Cancer Treat. Res.,* 6, 191, 1979.

185. Price, L. A., Unpublished data, 1981.

186. Santoro, A., Bonadonna, G., Bonfante, V., and Valagussa, P., Non cross resistant regimens (MOPP and ABVD) vs MOPP alone in stage IV Hodkin disease, *Proc. Am. Assoc. Clin. Oncol.,* 21, 470, 1980.

187. Price, L. A., Hill, B. T., and Ghilchick, M. W., Eds., *Safer Cancer Chemotherapy,* Balliere-Tindall, London, 1981, 1.

Chapter 3

A MATHEMATICAL MODEL OF DRUG RESISTANCE IN NEOPLASMS

Andrew J. Coldman and James H. Goldie

TABLE OF CONTENTS

I. INTRODUCTION

An essential requirement for effective cancer chemotherapy is that the drugs employed should be toxic to offending cells without causing unacceptable toxicity to the host. An increasing number of antineoplastic agents satisfy these conditions and chemotherapy has become one of the main cancer therapies available. Neoplasms, however, are not a homogeneous group and tumors show varying degrees of resistance to the whole range of chemotherapeutic agents.

It has been recognized for some years that drug insensitivity varies with both the histological type and the location of the tumor. These characters reflect, in part, inherent differences in the sensitivity of the cells from which the tumor originates and in the transport of the drug to the tumor site. Even allowing for such effects, there appear to be further differences present which affect the sensitivity of tumors to therapy. Such differences have variously been ascribed to systemic (host) factors which affect drug concentration and halflife, and to differences in the cellular material comprising the tumor. Both these general mechanisms have been found to exist and have been further subdivided into distinct processes.

In animal systems it has been shown that cell lines may be isolated which show variable amounts of resistance to given drugs.[1,2] It has also been demonstrated that the change to resistance is frequently stable and heritable, as discussed in Chapter 1. This would seem to indicate that some form of stable genetic alteration has occurred and thus, that this process may be viewed as being directly controlled by the genetic material.

Similar problems have been encountered previously in the resistance of various bacterial populations to viral infection. In their classic paper, Luria and Delbrück[3] showed that this process arose via random spontaneous mutations which occurred at a fixed frequency. The fluctuation test, as Luria and Delbrück called their experimental method, has been used extensively since to show that cellular resistance to a variety of chemotherapeutic agents in many different cellular populations arises in the same way. This was first demonstrated in mammalian tumor cells in the case of the origin of resistance to folic antagonists in L1210 leukemia.[4] This topic is dealt with in much greater detail in Chapter 1 and will not be addressed here. We will present a theory describing how resistance of neoplasms to chemotherapy can occur as a result of random mutations which are selected into prominence by the presence of the chemotherapeutic agent, and then explore the clinical implications of such a process.

II. A MODEL FOR A SINGLE CHEMOTHERAPEUTIC AGENT

A. Definitions and Assumptions

The defining postulate of this model will be that mutations occur at a fixed frequency α which confer resistance to a particular agent on the cell. This frequency will be referred to as the mutation rate and may be considered either as a rate per unit time or as a rate per cell division.[5] The distinction between these two definitions is of little importance when dealing with exponentially growing populations, as they are then equivalent.[5,6] In nonexponential populations they do not lead to identical quantitative conclusions and a choice must be made about the definition to use. Using a time dependent rate would imply that some uniform reference frame existed which was related to the origins and manifestations of the process independent of the cell cycle. Such a cause might well be cosmic rays, whose intensity is approximately uniform and which have been implicated as a possible initiator of mutations. Conversely, using a rate referenced to the cell cycle would imply that either the origins or manifestations of the process were regulated by the cell cycle and thus, would include mechanisms such as error of DNA transcription. We will choose to define the rate as cell-cycle dependent since this leads to greater mathematical simplicity when dealing with neoplasms displaying nonexponential growth. Either assumption will lead to qualitatively the same results although quantitatively they will differ.

Therefore, we will define α as follows:

1.   The mutation rate α is defined as the probability that a cell upon division will undergo a stable mutation which confers resistance immediately upon one of its progeny to a specific agent.

It must be kept in mind that we are interested in one property of tumor cells, i.e., resistance and that the mutation rate relates to the frequency of this event and not the frequency of any genetic change. No implication is made as to whether this change is single or multiple or that any one specific change exists. The essential postulate is that some heritable stochastic effect occurs at a constant frequency.

Cells selected to be resistant to a given dose of an agent may or may not be resistant to higher doses of the same agent. Examples exist where cells selected for low level resistance display resistance at much higher doses.[7] This situation is not universal and in referring to a mutation rate leading to resistance the dose of the agent must be considered. All further discussion of the mutation rate will relate to some fixed dosage level for the agent which will remain unspecified but may be taken as the clinical dosage.

2.   Let N be the number of cells present in the tumor which are sensitive to the agent in question.
3.   Let R(N) be the number of cells resistant to the given agent in the tumor when there are N sensitive cells present.

The size of the tumor, that is the total number of cells, is then $N + R(N)$.

A large number of models have been developed to explain the growth characteristics of neoplasms, (for example see Steel[8]). These have been developed from two distinct standpoints; one in which the processes are modeled upon a cellular level and combined to predict the gross growth characteristics of the tumor. The second involves fitting mathematical curves to empirical measurements of tumor growth. Of the latter type, the Gompertzian curve has enjoyed prominence.[9,10] In this section we will make no specific assumptions about tumor growth except that we will not allow the possibility of tumor regression or more precisely, cell loss, does not occur. This does not preclude the possibility of cellular differentiation and loss of proliferative capacity, extended periods in G_o or changes in cell cycle time. The assumption of no cell loss simplifies the derivation of the equations which follow. Its deletion would not substantially change the nature of the conclusions if relaxed. It is possible to replace N by either $N_o \exp\{\lambda t\}$ (an exponential model of growth), $N_o \exp\{A/B(1-e^{-Bt})\}$ (a Gompertzian model of growth) or any other nondecreasing functions of time and the equations derived will be identical to those derived using N (if all other assumptions are the same).

As another technical measure, we will also assume:

4.   Sensitive and resistant cells are dynamically identical (i.e., they replicate at the same rate).

There is abundant experimental evidence that for some drugs and experimental tumor lines this is true.[11] Situations have also been found where this is not the case[2] and in a consideration of a specific agent, this assumption could be modified accordingly.

In statistical terminology, the number of resistant cells in a tumor will be a random variable. Thus, if one takes 100 different tumors of the same size which have been grown from individual sensitive cells from the same line, the number of resistant cells will vary from tumor to tumor. As may be expected the average number of resistant cells present is not a good indicator of the resistant cell status of any particular tumor. (An essential finding of Luria and Delbrück when they first analysed this process was that the expected number of resistant cells is a remarkably poor indicator of the situation likely to be encountered.) Therefore, an approach utilizing the tools of probability theory is required for a complete solution to this problem. However, it is possible to obtain two interesting results using simple calculus which agree with those obtained from a more complete analysis. In order to do this we will further assume that N increases continuously and thus, that fractions of a cell are permitted. Although biological nonsense, this greatly simplifies the theoretical development and, again, it will not affect the conclusions.

B. Development and Discussion of Basic Relationships

Let $\mu(N)$ = expected number of resistant cells present where there are N sensitive cells present. Thus, $\mu(N)$ is the average value of R(N), and $\mu(N)$ is given by

$$\mu(N) = \alpha N \ln N \qquad (1)$$

where ln is the natural logarithm. Formula 1 is equivalent to the one previously obtained for this quantity,[12] however the meaning of N is somewhat different.

This function is plotted in Figure 1 for values of α ranging between $\alpha = 10^{-7}$ and 10^{-3}, which encompasses the range seen in experimental tumor systems. It can be seen from this that the number of resistant cells in the tumor increase at a faster rate than that of the total population. This is more obvious in Figure 2, where the fraction of cells resistant, F, is plotted against the total number of tumor cells.

$$\text{Thus, } F = \frac{\alpha N \ln N}{N + \alpha N \ln N} = \frac{\alpha \ln N}{1 + \alpha \ln N} \qquad (2)$$

$$\cong \alpha \ln N \qquad (\text{for } \alpha \ln N \ll 1) \qquad (3)$$

Figure 2 shows how the fraction of resistant cells increases as the tumor grows. This implies generally that tumor heterogeneity will be greater in larger tumors since this formula holds for all events caused by random mutation. For a tumor composed of 10^{10} cells and a mutation rate to resistance of 10^{-4}, we would expect that on average, one in every 500 cells would be resistant. If all sensitive cells are rapidly removed from the tumor, then in the order of 10^7 resistant cells will remain and remission may never be achieved although regression will be apparent.

Although the mean size of the resistant population does contain some information as to the general properties of the tumor during therapy, it does not give the whole picture. Another variable of interest is the probability, $P^o(N)$, that a tumor containing N cell has no resistant cells. This may also be obtained using calculus and is given by[12]

$$P^o(N) = \exp\{-\alpha(N-1)\} \qquad (4)$$

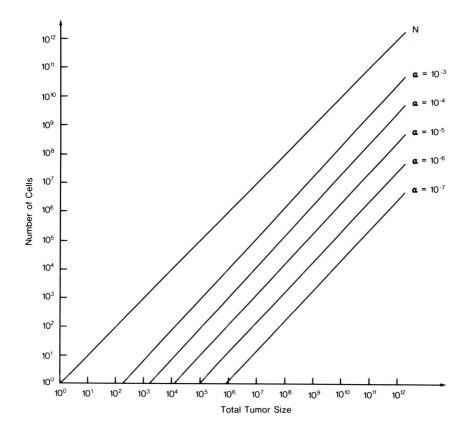

FIGURE 1.   Plot of the log of the expected number of mutant cells vs. the log of the total number of tumor cells for 4 values of the mutation rates (a). The straight line indicating the growth in total population is included as a reference. The lines for the resistant subpopulation are slightly curved and approach the total population line, illustrating that the mutant population increases at a greater rate than the total tumor population. This relationship will hold no matter what growth function is assumed for the tumor as a whole.

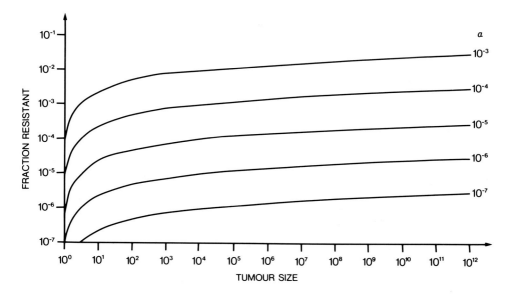

FIGURE 2.   This shows the increase in the proportion of resistant cells with the total number of tumor cells for several different values of the mutation rate α.

Usually N will be large and we may approximate (4) by:

$$P^O(N) \cong \exp\{-\alpha N\} \tag{5}$$

This function is plotted in Figure 3 for various values of the mutation rate α between 0^{-7} and 10^{-3}. From this it may be seen that the development of resistance ocurs at a random point in the history of the tumor and that when the size of the tumor exceeds $4/\alpha$, resistance is almost certain to be present. A very striking feature of this figure is that the shape of each curve is very similar, merely being shifted horizontally according to the value of the mutation rate. This property can be utilized by considering the increase in size required to change this probability from a high value to a low value for any value of the mutation rate α.

Let $P^o(N_2)$, $P^o(N_1)$ be the probability of no resistance at size N_2 and N_1 respectively. Equation 5 gives

$$P^O(N_2) = \exp\{-\alpha N_2\} \, ; \, P^O(N_1) = \exp\{-\alpha N_1\}$$

and we have:

$$\frac{\ln(P^O(N_2))}{\ln(P^O(N_1))} = \frac{-\alpha N_2}{-\alpha N_1} = \frac{N_2}{N_1} \tag{6}$$

For example, to go from a .95 ($= P^o(N_1)$) to a .05 ($= P^o(N_2)$) probability of no resistant cells requires a

$$\frac{(\ln(.05)}{(\ln(.95)} = \,)$$

60 fold increase in the size of the tumor which is independent of the value of the mutation rate. More precisely this says that there exists a period of 60-fold growth for any tumor line when the proportion of tumors with resistant cells will increase from 5% to 95%. For any individual tumor its transition from purely sensitive to one containing a resistant cell may be viewed as occurring instantaneously. Examination of the curves of $P^o(N)$ show that the rate of change of $P^o(N)$ varies with N. Using calculus it is easy to show that $P^o(N)$ may change by as much as 0.25 in one doubling period of the tumor. Once a resistant clone has emerged continuing therapy of that tumor with the agent cannot result in eradication of the tumor. If no such clone exists, then eradication is possible although other factors may well intervene to prevent this. We may regard the nonexistence of such a clone as a minimal condition for cure to be possible and that $P^o(N)$ represents the maximum probability of cure. The previous remarks may be reinterpreted as follows:

- The potential curability of a tumor line may change by as much as 95% to 5% in less than six doublings.
- The potential curability of a tumor line may change by as much as 25% in one doubling.

Generally, we would interpret this by saying that curability may change very rapidly in the lifetime of the tumor. This clearly can be important since the delay between diagnosis and the institution of chemotherapy is frequently of the order of 1 to 2 months. The doubling time of human cancers has been found to vary widely with

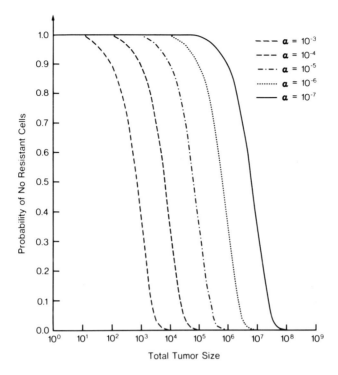

FIGURE 3.   Plot of Equation 3 which relates the probability of the existence of no resistant phenotypes to the mutation rate (α) and number of tumor cells. The almost identical profile of each curve reflects the independence of the changes required for a class of tumors to proceed from the state when only 5% have resistant phenotypes to that when 95% have such phenotypes.

doubling times of 40 days being common for breast carcinomas.[8,13] It is possible, therefore, that prompt treatment with chemotherapy may significantly affect survival. One adjuvant study of breast cancer found that the significant benefit associated with one course of cyclophosphamide was lost if administration was delayed for as little as 3 weeks.[14] Generally the relationship given in Equation 5 reflects the almost universal finding that chemotherapy is more effective for smaller tumor burdens. Furthermore it is also a statement of probability and thus only implies that this will be true on the average and not in every circumstance.

An alternative way to view the Relationship 5 is to fix N and examine how P° varies with α. This is displayed for $N = 10^6$ in Figure 4 and can be seen to be identical in shape to the previous curves. This clearly shows how measures to reduce the mutation rate will increase the likelihood that there are no resistant cells present. A very obvious example of such a measure would be the use of combinations of noncross-resistant agents, or perhaps, the administration of agents at higher doses.

In the language of probability, all information about the nature of a stochastic process is contained in its distribution function. This function is not easy to calculate although it is possible to calculate its Laplace transform.[6,15,16] From this the mean, variance and P°(N) may be simply calculated. These agree with the previous results for $\mu(N)$, P°(N) and we have for the variance:

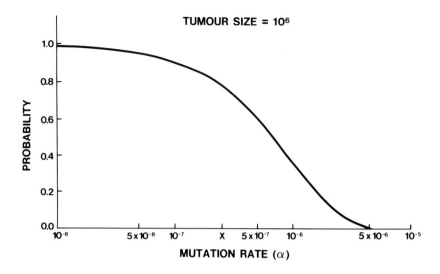

FIGURE 4.   The inverse relationship between mutation rate and the probability of no resistant cells for a tumor of size 10^6 cells.

$$\text{var}(R(N)) = 2\alpha N^2[1-N^{-1}(1+\tfrac{1}{2} \ln N)] \qquad (7)$$

and thus, the standard deviation is

$$SD(R(N)) = N\sqrt{2\alpha}\,[1-(1+\tfrac{1}{2}\ln N)/N]^{1/2} \qquad (8)$$

Examining the ratio:

$$\frac{\mu}{SD}(N) = \frac{\alpha}{\sqrt{2}}\ln N/[1-(1+\tfrac{1}{2}\ln N)/N]^{1/2}$$

we see that for α in the range 10^{-7} to 10^{-3} and N in the range 10^6 to 10^{12} this ratio is strictly less than one and the mean is substantially less than the standard deviation. This indicates that the process is very variable and that substantial variability in the number of resistant cells is to be expected. This relationship lies at the root of the Luria and Delbrück fluctuation test.

Using recursive relationships[16] it is possible to evaluate the distribution function of the number of resistant cells. Such a calculation is displayed in Figure 5 for $\alpha = 10^{-6}$, $N = 10^6$. This illustrates the very variable nature of the process, since $\mu(10^6) = 13.8$, $P_o(10^6) = 0.368$, mode of the distribution $= 0$, and the median $= 1$.

Another way of examining this variability is to consider the following quantity — given two tumors of the same size with the same mutation rate, what is the probability that one tumor will have a resistant subpopulation substantially larger than the other. In the example above the probability that in one tumor the resistant subpopulation is ten times that in the other is 0.26, i.e., there is a one in four chance that one resistant population will be at least 10 times larger than the other.

The magnitude of this relationship indicates substantial variability. However, this large value arises because the probability of there being zero resistant cells is large (i.e., $\exp\{-10^{-6}(10^6-1)\} = .37$). By the time two such tumors have grown to size 5×10^6, the probability of zero resistant cells diminishes from 0.37 to 0.007. The probability that one tumor will have a resistant subpopulation ten times as large as that of the other has then fallen to less than 0.09. From this we can see that despite the large variance

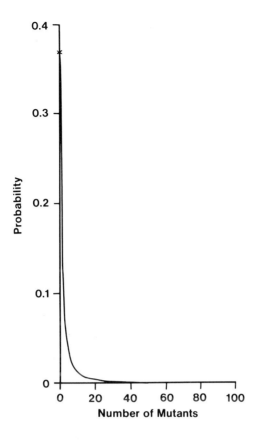

FIGURE 5. Probability distribution of the number of resistant cells for a mutation rate of $\alpha = 10^{-6}$, in a tumor containing 10^6 cells.

of the process, the probability that two otherwise identical tumors will have large multiplicative differences in the sizes of their resistant subpopulations is small.

III. A MODEL FOR TWO AGENTS

A. Introduction

When more than one agent is available it may be possible to use them in combination to increase the log-kill per cycle of each course. Combination chemotherapy is also desirable from a mutational point of view since it will have the result of decreasing the effective mutation rate to the combined regimen. In situations where some combinations of regimens are not possible and one agent (or combination) is clearly superior to the others available, then the more potent therapy would be used initially with other agents held in reserve in case of failure. There are some situations (i.e., Hodgkin's Disease)[17] where two almost equivalent therapies exist which cannot be given simultaneously and the question arises how they should be employed in general. This situation will now be examined from the view point of cellular resistance.

B. Definitions and Assumptions

There are now two agents, which we will call 1 and 2. An individual cell may be in one of four possible mutually exclusive states with respect to these agents:

1.　　　Sensitive to both agents　　　　　N

2.	Sensitive to 1 and resistant to 2	R_2
3.	Resistant to 1 and sensitive to 2	R_1
4.	Resistant to both 1 and 2	R_{12}

This is illustrated schematically in Figure 6. Each subpopulation is referred to by subscript 1 or referring to agents 1 and 2.

If resistance to Agent 1 implies resistance to Agent 2, then $R_1 = 0$ as no cells can be sensitive to 2 and resistant to 1. This example may be viewed as one extreme case of cross-resistance. The term cross-resistance can be used in a number of ways and requires definition here. We will define cross-resistance as the reduction of log-kill or increase in the spontaneous mutation rate to resistance to one agent in those cells which have been selected for resistance to another agent. Evidence from a variety of experimental tumor systems indicate that such cross-resistance exists for certain agents,[2] but that it is by no means universal. For the purposes of simplicity we will assume temporarily that no cross-resistance exists and that the various mechanisms which produce resistance to each agent work independently. We may refer to the two mutation rates to resistance as α_1 and α_2. We assume that the two therapies are equally effective and this implies that α_1 equals α_2. Cells in N can be eliminated by either agent, cells in R_1 by agent 2 and cells in R_2 by agent 1. However, cells in R_{12} cannot be eliminated by either therapy alone or in combination and thus, no regimen composed of these two agents will extinguish a tumor containing members of R_{12}. R_{12} now plays the same role that R did in the previous calculations, and we wish to find ways in which the probability that $R_{12} = 0$ is kept as high as possible.

Assumptions used previously will be extended to this case in the obvious way. We will also assume that simultaneous mutations to both agents do not occur, but that the double-resistant mutant arises from a two-step process.[18] Double mutations may well occur; however, no estimates for such rates are available. If one were to assume that such a rate was the product of the individual rates, then it is easy to show that this has a negligible quantitative effect on the model developed here. Thus, double resistance is assumed to arise by the appropriate mutation giving resistance to the second agent in a cell already resistant to the first agent or vice-versa. We will further assume that these mutations occur at the same rate as they would in a sensitive cell.

Every sensitive cell is not removed upon a single administraton of an agent but the probability of cell death is related to the dose of agent via a log-kill law[19] or modifications of it for phase specific agents. We will assume that each time an agent is given that it is given at the maximum tolerated dose and results in a constant log-kill among sensitive cells. The log-kills for each agent will be referred to as k_1 and k_2. After each administration, the log-kill will be assumed to take effect instantaneously and will then be followed by a period of regrowth which corresponds to the interval between subsequent courses of therapy. To calculate the regrowth which occurs in a calendar period, it is necessary to postulate some form of growth curve. Here, we will assume an exponential form which has the advantage of simplicity and does not require further assumptions about the nature and location of the tumor burden (i.e., the properties of the exponential model will be invariant when subjected to division into arbitrarily sized units).

C. Derivation and Statement of Relationships

The previous assumptions used to set up this model require that members of R_{12} arise by self replication and mutation from R_1 and R_2. The sizes of R_1 and R_2 are calculated using their expected values and by modifying Equation 1 to allow there to be $\mu(N_o)$ resistant cells present when the tumor is of size N_o. The equation becomes:[20]

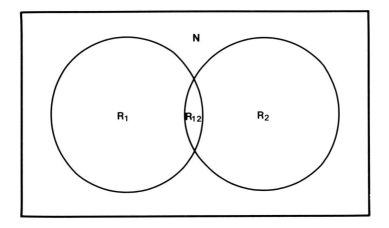

FIGURE 6. Schematic representation of the four compartments as defined by the therapies available. The relative sizes of these compartments are not in proportion to their true sizes.

$$\mu_1 (N) = \mu_1 (N)N/N_0 + \alpha_1 N \ln (N/N_0) \qquad (9)$$

and similarly, for $\mu_2(N)$ (where $\mu_1(N)$ is the expected value of $R_1 (N)$, etc.). Using this expression it is now possible to calculate the probability that $R_{12} = 0$ (hereafter referred to as $P_{12}(N)$) using the same method as was used for deriving Equation 9, but extending it slightly to cover the existence of two resistant compartments and approximating the size of the singly resistant compartments to be $\mu_1(N_o)$, $\mu_2(N_o)$ at N_o. We then obtain:

$$P_{12} (N) = \exp \{-\alpha_2 [\mu_1(N_2)-\mu_1(N_1)] - \alpha_1 [\mu_2(N_2)-\mu_2(N_1)]$$

$$+ 2\alpha_1 \alpha_2 (N_2-N_1)\} \qquad (10)$$

which, as might be expected, relates the probability to the increase in the number of singly resistant cells in each compartment in the same way as for the single compartment model.

D. Calculation and Discussion of Some Examples

The model described has been programed on a computer in order that the behavior of tumors with such properties could be explored. This requires that the following information be input at initiation of the program.

1. The size of the sensitive population, N (which is approximately equal to total tumor size)
2. The doubling time of the tumor, D
3. The mutation rate for each of the agents, α_1 and α_2
4. The log-kill for each of the agents, k_1 and k_2
5. The therapeutic interval for each therapy, l_1 and l_2 (That is the time between subsequent courses of therapy for each agent.)

In this idealization, we are assuming that the two agents are equivalent in that they have the same mutation rate, the same log-kill and the same therapeutic interval.

Therefore, *a priori*, these two agents are equally effective and (assuming one is not more toxic to normal tissue) either would be equally suitable for therapeutic use.

Figure 7 plots the tumor size for a regimen composed exclusively of 18 courses of Agent 1 (or equivalently, Agent 2). In this case, $N = 10^{10}$; $D = 40$ days; $\alpha_1 = \alpha_2 = 10^{-6}$; $k_1 = k_2 = 1$; $l_1 = l_2 = 21$ days. Initially, the tumor responds to the therapy and it regresses. Quickly this response is lost and the tumor begins to regrow. Table 1 gives a breakdown of the cellular composition of the tumor from which it may be seen that regrowth occurs as the tumor becomes increasingly composed of resistant cells and that thereafter continued therapy with this agent is ineffective.

It is clearly a suboptimal strategy to initiate therapy with the second agent when the tumor clinically recurs,[11] since we can see from the graph that therapy with agent 1 has failed for a long time. Figure 8 plots the tumor size for a regimen in which the second agent is instituted after tumor regression ceases. This regimen is seen to result in eradication of the tumor since all the cells resistant to the second therapy have been eliminated by the 1st therapy. This regimen can only truly result in eradication if both no doubly resistant cells have emerged and if no cells resistant to the second agent have emerged after therapy has commenced with this agent. The probability of there being zero doubly resistant cells present is displayed in Table 2 and is seen to be very low. When one further considers the probability that a clone resistant to 2 will have emerged, the likelihood that the regimen will have resulted in tumor eradication is small. We may view P_{12}, the probability that no such cells develop, as the maximal probability that the regimen will be successful. This probability is detailed in column 7 of Table 2. During therapy, this probability declines rapidly, and stabilizes when therapy with the second agent is instituted. It could thus be inferred that earlier institution of the second therapy may prove beneficial. Nevertheless, therapy with the first agent must be continued since the population resistant to the second therapy persists during the first 7 cycles of therapy.

One protocol achieving both these objectives is to alternate therapy at each course until eradication of the tumor is complete. Figure 9 plots tumor size for this protocol and it too is seen to result in eradication of the tumor. Furthermore, examination of Table 3 shows that this is achieved with less diminution of P_{12} than before and thus, this represents a protocol with a higher probability of success.

Although it is by no means obvious beforehand, this regimen has proven to be the most effective for a variety of mutation rates and tumor sizes which are likely to be encountered in clinical situations. Similar computations have been made using a Gompertzian model of tumor growth, and other models of chemotherapy kill.[9] Although quantitative differences naturally occur because of the different kinetics, qualitatively the same results were found. It seems reasonable to propose that any tumor growth models where cell growth or loss does not differ between the various resistant subtypes will lead to similar conclusions. It is also interesting to view sequential alternation of therapy from another perspective. The beginning or end of one cycle of therapy in a regimen is a matter of nomenclature used by the experimentalist or clinician. In many examples of combination chemotherapy different agents may be administered on different days during one cycle of therapy. This might then be viewed as alternation of therapy. Similarly, one could view a sequentially alternated therapy as being a regimen in which the two drugs (or combinations) are seen as a single combined therapy given over a longer period.

One major limitation to the development has been the use of expected values $\mu_1(N)$, $\mu_2(N)$ for the quantities $R_1(N)$, $R_2(N)$. This ignores the added complexity which results when $R_1(N)$ and $R_2(N)$ are substantially different in size due to the variable nature of the process. A rule of thumb would seem to be that this is unlikely to be a significant worry unless Z, the ratio of the sizes of the two resistant subpopulations ($= R_2(N)/$

Table 1

1 Treatment cycle	2 Treatment type	3 Prop. res. to 1	4 Prop. res. to 2	5 Tumor size	6 Interval prob.	7 Total prob.
0		2.303×10^{-5}	2.303×10^{-5}	1×10^{10}		0.6437
1	1	$2,306 \times 10^{-4}$	2.339×10^{-5}	2.439×10^{9}	0.8946	0.5759
2	1	2.301×10^{-3}	2.370×10^{-5}	2.075×10^{8}	0.8632	0.4971
3	1	0.0225	2.357×10^{-5}	3.048×10^{7}	0.8107	0.4030
4	1	0.1874	1.989×10^{-5}	5.276×10^{6}	0.7396	0.2980
5	1	0.6976	7.514×10^{-6}	2.040×20^{6}	0.6479	0.1931
6	1	0.9584	1.047×10^{-6}	2.136×10^{6}	0.5355	0.1034
7	1	0.9957	0	2.959×10^{6}	0.4071	0.0421
8	1	0.9996	0	4.241×10^{6}	0.2744	0.0115
9	1	1.0000	0	6.100×10^{6}	0.1555	0.0018
10	1	1.0000	0	8.778×10^{6}	0.0687	0.0001
11	1	1.0000	0	1.263×10^{7}	0.0212	0.0000
12	1	1.0000	0	1.817×10^{7}	0.0039	0.0000
13	1	1.0000	0	1.615×10^{7}	0.0003	0.0000
14	1	1.0000	0	3.763×10^{7}	0.0000	0.0000
15	1	1.0000	0	5.415×10^{7}	0.0000	0.0000
16	1	1.0000	0	7.792×10^{7}	0.0000	0.0000
17	1	1.0000	0	1.121×10^{8}	0.0000	0.0000
18	1	1.0000	0	1.613×10^{8}	0.0000	0.0000
19	1	1.0000	0	2.321×10^{8}	0.0000	0.0000
20	1	1.0000	0	3.340×10^{8}	0.0000	0.0000

Note: This table gives the detailed pattern of regrowth of a tumor treated continuously with agent 1. It can be seen from the third column that the tumor becomes increasingly resistant to that agent. The population resistant to the second agent exists initially, Column 4, but is gradually eradicated by the first agent. Column 5 shows that tumor regression occurs at first, but the effect is subsequently lost. Column 6 gives the probability that a doubly resistant clone will not emerge between treatments given that one has not emerged previously. This intertreatment probability is initially high but declines rapidly. Column 7 gives the probability that no doubly resistant clone has emerged prior to that treatment. It can be seen to decline through the therapeutic schedule and is calculated by taking the product of the interval probability (Column 6) and the previous entry in Column 7. The initial entry, 0.6437 in Column 7, represents the probability that no doubly resistant clone has emerged prior to therapy. Each value quoted relates to the instant of time immediately prior to the institution of the next course of therapy (or the time at which it would have occurred).

$R_1(N)$), or $1/Z$ exceeds the inverse of the fractional survival rate from either of the two therapies.

In this case, we are postulating that such a difference will not have too marked an effect since such differences would normally exist during the therapy schedule anyway. For the example we have discussed, the probability that one resistance compartment is 10 times larger than the other at the commencement of therapy is approximately 9%. Such an effect may be simulated by allowing one therapy to have a slightly higher mutation rate, i.e., ten times the other. If we assume, as we have done before, that we have no knowledge as to the size of the resistant compartments, then alternation is again superior to all other fixed protocols. This may be illustrated by using the previous example and allowing the mutation rate to single resistance to be 6.5×10^{-8} for the first treatment and 6.5×10^{-7} for the second. These values were chosen since one is ten times the other and they accord with percentiles of the distribution of $R(N)$ so that the probability that $R_1(N) < \alpha_1 N \ln N$ equals the probability that $R_2(N) > \alpha_2 N \ln N$. The mutation rates to double resistance from single resistance are both 10^{-6}. As both single

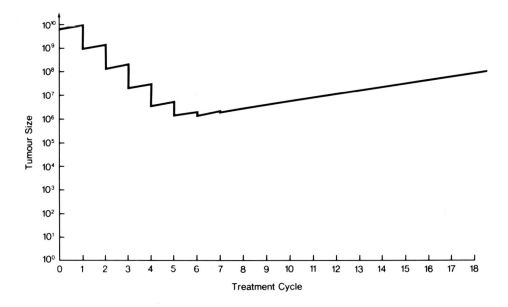

FIGURE 7.   Idealized plot of mean tumor size for a tumor treated continuously with one agent. Clearly this protocol is ineffective after 7 courses of therapy.

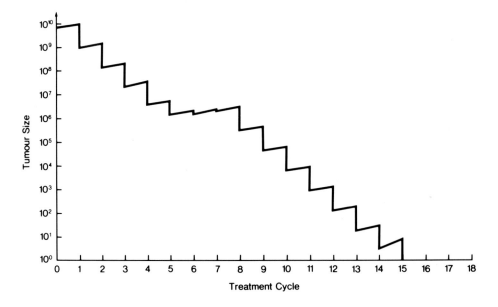

FIGURE 8.   Idealized plot of mean tumor size for a tumor where one therapy is given for 7 courses and is then changed. If no doubly resistant mutants emerge, this therapy will be successful.

Table 2

1 Treatment cycle	2 Treatment type	3 Prop. res. to 1	4 Prop. res. to 2	5 Tumor size	6 Interval prob.	7 Total prob.
0		2.303×10^{-5}	2.303×10^{-5}	1×10^{10}		0.6437
1	1	$2,306 \times 10^{-4}$	2.339×10^{-5}	2.439×10^{9}	0.8946	0.5759
2	1	$2,301 \times 10^{-3}$	2.370×10^{-5}	2.075×10^{8}	0.8632	0.4971
3	1	0.0225	2.357×10^{-5}	3.048×10^{7}	0.8107	0.4030
4	1	0.1874	1.989×10^{-5}	5.276×10^{-6}	0.7396	0.2980
5	1	0.6976	7.514×10^{-6}	2.040×20^{6}	0.6479	0.1931
6	1	0.9584	1.047×10^{-6}	2.136×10^{6}	0.5355	0.1034
7	1	0.9957	0	2.959×10^{6}	0.4071	0.0421
8	2	0.9957	0	4.258×10^{5}	0.8787	0.0370
9	2	0.9957	0	6.127×10^{4}	0.9816	0.0363
10	2	0.9956	0	8816	0.9973	0.0362
11	2	0.9955	0	1268	0.9996	0.0362
12	2	1.0000	0	180	1.000	0.0362
13	2	1.0000	0	26	1.0000	0.0362
14	2	1.0000	0	4	1.0000	0.0362
15	2	1.0000	0	1	1.0000	0.0362
16	2	1.0000	0	0	1.0000	0.0362

Note: This table gives values for the treatment protocol where the therapy is switched to agent 2, after 7 courses with agent 1. Explanation of each column is given in the caption to Table 1.

mutation rates have been chosen to be less than the value previously used (10^{-6}), the probability that there are no doubly resistant cells at presentation has increased to 0.854 from 0.643. The probability that either of the singly resistant compartments have no cells is effectively 0 and so continued therapy with either agent alone cannot be curative. Using seven courses of therapy 1 followed by continued therapy with 2, results in a 0.704 probability for the nonemergence of doubly resistant cells. This would thus appear to be quite a successful regimen. It must be considered, however, that we are trying to simulate a random process and that $R_1(N)$ may be ten times larger than $R_2(N)$ rather than vice-versa. To account for this, consider the protocol where seven courses of therapy 2 are followed by continuous therapy with 1. The probability that no doubly resistant clones develop during this protocol is 0.132. These two values are quite divergent and since either eventuality is equally likely it seems reasonable to combine them into one value by taking their average, i.e., 0.418. Simulations with various treatment strategies again show alternation to be the best with probabilities of 0.829 (1 first), 0.775 (2 first), and an average of 0.802. The most effective protocol for this situation was found to be sequential alternation where the agent given first was the one with the smaller number of cells resistant to it.

Even in the circumstance where random variation has led to one population being ten times larger than the other, alternation still appears superior to other fixed strate-

Table 3

1 Treatment Cycle	2 Treatment type	3 Prop. res. to 1	4 Prop. res. to 2	5 Tumor size	6 Interval prob.	7 Total prob.
0		2.303×10^{-5}	2.303×10^{-5}	1×10^{10}		0.6437
1	1	2.306×10^{-4}	2.338×10^{-5}	1.439×10^{9}	0.8946	0.5759
2	2	2.3089×10^{-4}	2.342×10^{-4}	2.071×10^{8}	0.9711	0.5592
3	1	2.304×10^{-3}	2.340×10^{-4}	2.987×10^{7}	0.9771	0.5464
4	2	2.300×10^{-3}	2.336×10^{-3}	4.307×10^{6}	0.9939	0.5431
5	1	0.0225	2.288×10^{-3}	6.326×10^{5}	0.9952	0.5405
6	2	0.0221	0.0224	9.290×10^{4}	0.9987	0.5348
7	1	0.1842	0.0187	1.602×10^{4}	0.9990	0.5393
8	2	0.1576	0.1601	1.693×10^{3}	0.9997	0.5392
9	1	0.6518	0.0662	938	0.9998	0.5390
10	2	0.4084	0.4148	215	0.9999	0.5390
11	1	0.8735	0.887	145	1.0000	0.5390
12	2	0.4857	0.4933	37	1.0000	0.5390
13	1	0.9042	0.0918	19	1.0000	0.5390
14	2	0.5000	0.5000	8	1.0000	0.5390
15	1	1.0000	0	6	1.0000	0.5390
16	2	1.0000	0	1	1.0000	0.5390
17	1	1.0000		1	1.0000	0.5390
18	2			0	1.0000	0.5390

Note: This table gives results for a protocol in which therapy is altered after each cycle.

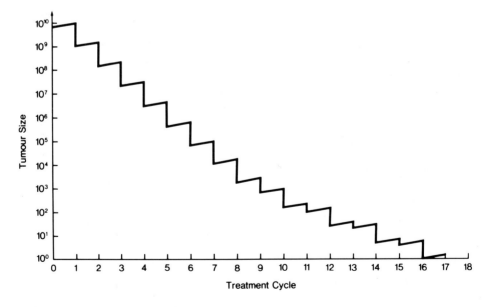

FIGURE 9.   Idealized plot of tumor size when therapy is switched after each course. This protocol is found to be most effective in eliminating the tumor and maximizing the probability that no doubly resistant clones will emerge.

gies. If alternation were not superior to other fixed strategies for differences greater than tenfold it would nevertheless be best overall. This is true because the mean gain in the probability of extinction (i.e., cure) exceeds the probability that the magnitude of the difference is greater than tenfold.

The relative sizes of the resistant subpopulations are unlikely to be known in advance of the institution of therapy, and therefore in giving this regime to a large number of patients there will be several individuals who have received a regimen which is not optimal for them. Although not ideal, this problem must be viewed as inevitable since a process whose nature is basically stochastic is unlikely to be amenable to a single fixed solution. Nevertheless, it should be noted that these strategies are still superior to those where a single agent is continued until some predetermined time or recurrence intervenes and then the second agent started. One clearly negative aspect of alternation is that if one agent is effective, while the other is not, for a particular individual, this fact will tend to be obscured so that it may no longer be apparent. Cessation of use of an ineffective agent, which is necessary no matter what protocol is being followed, may be delayed and thus, lead to undesirable prolongation of a partially ineffective therapy.

A question which arises from the previous example is the use of mutation rates of 6.5×10^{-7} and 6.5×10^{-8} to simulate fluctuations in the resistance process where the true rate is 10^{-6}. One would intuitively expect that one would choose rates, one of which is higher and one lower than 10^{-6}. This does not occur because of the extremely skewed nature of the distribution of R(N). In the single resistance case, the probability that $R(N) < \mu(N)$ for $\alpha = 10^{-6}$ is greater than 0.91. This clearly raises the question as to whether our simulations based on the expected values is likely to reflect the true situation. In the single agent case, we found that the predictions were based on the shape of the curve of $P^o(N)$ and not on any particular value of α. Similarly we would expect that the deductions we have made would also be true as long as the true shape of the curve of $P_{12}(N)$ is the same as that which has been used (Formula 10). More accurate calculations using Laplace transforms show that this is indeed the case as illustrated in Figure 10.

The rationale which emerges from these considerations is that prolonged therapy with a single agent (or combination) which allows subpopulations resistant to it to grow unimpeded will increase the probability that subtypes will develop which are resistant to all therapies available. Changing agents early in the therapeutic regimen will act to reduce this likelihood and thus, increase the effectiveness of such therapies. This approach is idealized when all active agents may be given simultaneously and by cyclical application for equally effective agents which may not be administered together.

The log-kill law implies that high concentrations of drug will lead to increased log-kill of sensitive cells and faster tumor regression. Also, we have suggested that higher drug concentrations may have a lower mutation rate and, thus, there may be fewer cells resistant at the higher concentration. When using a two drug alternating regime, as previously described, higher concentrations will also lead to more rapid depletion of the singly resistant compartments and thus, will lead to a higher probability of cure.

This can be modeled in the computer program by increasing the log-kills of each therapy while keeping the values of the mutation rates constant. This is portrayed in Figure 11 for the example previously examined using an alternating strategy, where k_1 and k_2 are increased to 2. The mutation rates are left unchanged. From this it may be seen, as expected, that the tumor is exterminated in fewer courses of therapy than were required previously. Table 4 shows that the probability P_{12} is larger than before and thus, this strategy is more successful. The rise is not great, and this illustrates that large increases in the log-kill of various therapies may not result in large gains in cur-

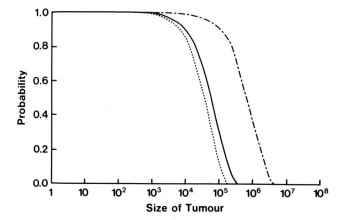

FIGURE 10. Plot of the probability that no doubly resistant clones emerge using three different methods of calculation —·—·—·plots where the mutation rate to double resistance is taken to be the product of the single resistance mutation rates, ———— represents a best calculation based upon the Laplace transform, ······ plots the values used in the computer model simulations. The abcissa is a log scale of the total number of tumor cells.

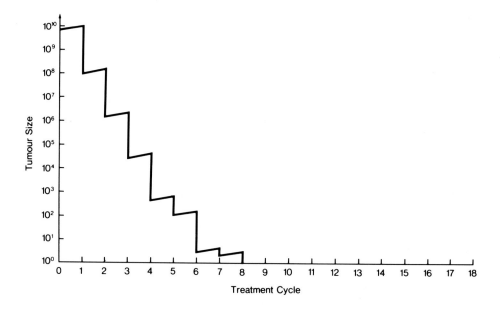

FIGURE 11. Plot of tumor size for an alternating therapeutic schedule where the log-kill factors have been doubled from the example previously used. As can be seen this brings about a rapid elimination of the tumor for small loss in the probability that no doubly resistant clones will emerge.

ability when mutation to resistance is a limiting factor. In situations where drugs are able to remove sensitive cells considerably faster than they can be replaced, the curability of the tumor is more sensitive to decreases in the mutation rate than increases in the log-kill. From this it is clear that for tumors where resistance is an important limiting factor attention must be paid to selecting agents with low mutation rates as well as high log-kills. We have postulated here that higher concentration of a drug will be

Table 4

1 Treatment cycle	2 Treatment type	3 Prop. res. to 1	4 Prop. res. to 2	5 Tumor size	6 Interval prob.	7 Total prob.
0		2.303×10^{-5}	2.303×10^{-5}	1×10^{10}		0.6437
1	1	2.298×10^{-3}	2.333×10^{-5}	1.442×10^{8}	0.9029	0.5812
2	2	2.293×10^{-3}	2.329×10^{-3}	2.080×10^{6}	0.9971	0.5795
	1	0.1869	1.898×10^{-3}	3.672×10^{4}	0.9979	0.5783
4	2	0.1573	0.1598	628	0.9999	0.5783
5	1	0.9492	0.64×10^{-3}	150	1.0000	0.5782
6	2	0.5000	0.5000	4	1.0000	0.5782
7	1	1.0000	0	3	1.0000	0.5782
8	2			0	1.0000	0.5782

Note: This table gives results for a one course alternating protocol in which the log-kill of each agent is doubled to simulate the use of agents with greater log-kills.

associated with lower mutation rates. However, one drug with a high log-kill may well have a higher mutation rate than another with a lower log-kill and thus, not be as suitable as the latter. In situations where the mutation rate is very high, the experimental kills achieved will be low since resistance will intercede to reduce the effectiveness. This will act to reduce the likelihood that drugs with high mutation rates will be selected as potential agents for chemotherapy. At lower values this will not be a problem although experimentally measuring the mutation rate is not an easy matter.

Consideration of the nature of the processes involved in resistance suggests that the maintenance of maximum tolerable dose chemotherapy may not be necessary throughout the treatment program and that high doses are more important at the beginning of the regimen. This follows since after a few courses in therapy the resistant compartments have been reduced sufficiently in size so that, as long as they are not permitted to regrow substantially, the probability of a doubly resistant clone emerging is comparatively small. This can be modeled using our example by reducing the log-kills of the therapies from 2 to 1 after 2 courses of therapy. This is illustrated in Figure 12 where the tumor is seen to be extinguished in somewhat more courses than required previously. Table 5 shows that the probability of cure has diminished very slightly even though the dosage has been considerably reduced overall.

It is clear from the viewpoint of resistance that achieving maximum tolerated dose is important at the commencement of chemotherapy but less important later in the therapy protocol. This may not always be the case because of the kinetic characteristics of the tumor (i.e., because of rapid regrowth) however, it is clear that 'front-end loading' is to be preferred if possible from the viewpoint of resistance.

We have assumed from the start that the two agents being used do not show cross-resistance and by this we have implied:

1. That cells resistant to one agent show the same chemosensitivity to the second agent as purely sensitive cells.
2. That cells sensitive to one agent show the same mutation rate to resistance for the second agent as purely sensitive cells.

These assumptions would make it very difficult to find agents which may be used in an alternating regimen. Fortunately, such requirements are over restrictive and may be relaxed considerably. The essential quality required for alternation to prove superior

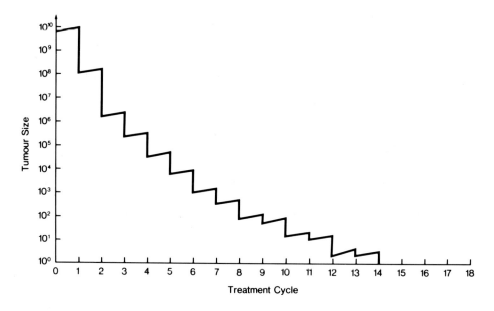

FIGURE 12.   Plots tumor size for which the reduced log-kill is reinstated after 2 cycles of therapy. This extends the treatment period considerably but does not greatly affect the probability that no doubly resistant cells emerge.

Table 5

1 Treatment cycle	2 Treatment type	3 Prop. res. to 1	4 Prop. res. to 2	5 Tumor size	6 Interval prob.	7 Total prob.
0		2.303×10^{-5}	2.303×10^{-5}	1×10^{10}		0.6437
1	1	2.298×10^{-3}	2.333×10^{-5}	1.442×10^{8}	0.9029	0.5812
2	2	2.293×10^{-3}	2.329×10^{-3}	2.080×10^{6}	0.9971	0.5795
3	1	0.0225	2.282×10^{-3}	3.055×10^{5}	0.9977	0.5782
4	2	0.0220	0.0224	4.486×10^{4}	0.9994	0.5778
5	1	0.1837	0.0187	7.733×10^{3}	0.9995	0.5775
6	2	0.2573	0.1598	1.300×10^{3}	0.9999	0.5775
7	1	0.6512	0.0662	452	0.9999	0.5774
8	2	0.4082	0.4146	104	1.0000	0.5774
9	1	0.8734	0.0887	70	1.0000	0.5774
10	2	0.4856	0.4933	18	1.0000	0.5774
11	1	0.9042	0.0919	14	1.0000	0.5774
12	2	0.50000	0.50000	4	1.0000	0.5774
13	1	1.0000	0.0000	3	1.0000	0.5774
14	2			8	1.0000	0.5774

Note: This table tabulates results for a regime where the log-kill of each agent is halved after 2 courses of the protocol. Comparison of these results with those from table 4, indicates how reductions in dose later in the course of therapy do not cause great reductions in the likelihood of no doubly resistant mutants, although prolonging the required treatment period. Comparison of this table with Table 3 indicates the possible advantages of "front-end loading".

is that the two agents should be symmetric with respect to their other properties. For example, agent 1 has 50% of the log-kill on cells resistant to agent 2 compared to that for sensitive cells then the equivalent situation must hold for agent 2. If cells resistant to agent 1 have double the mutation rate to agent 2 of sensitive cells, then again the equivalent condition must hold for agent 2. The following example may put these ideas on a more intuitive level. Two investigators, 1 and 2, have developed protocols for the therapy of a certain tumor based on the agents A, B, and C. Agents A and B may not be given simultaneously but A and C may, as may B and C. Their protocols are as follows:

1. A and B alternated at each cycle until 5 courses of each have been given, i.e., (A) (B) (A) (B) (A) (B) (A) (B) (A) (B).
2. 10 cycles of C, i.e., (C) (C) (C) (C) (C) (C) (C) (C) (C) (C).

We will assume that each drug is administered over the same cycle time. A third investigator believes both regimens to be effective but notes that since both are mutually compatible they may be given simultaneously as follows:

$$(A + C) (B + C) (A + C) (B + C) (A + C) (B + C) (A + C) (B + C) (A + C) (B + C)$$

However we are now dealing with an alternating regimen in which the two components exhibit cross-resistance to one another, i.e., cells resistance to $(A + C)$ will not be as sensitive to $(B + C)$ as purely sensitive cells and vice-versa. We have assumed that there is no cross-resistance between A and C or between B and C and thus the cross-resistance between the two components of the new regimen arises totally from them having one drug in common. Ignoring any toxicity, we would expect that this combination of drugs would be more effective than either of the original protocols. Clearly noncross-resistance is not essential for designing alternating protocols and this allows a more flexible development of effective drug combinations. However as the amount of cross-resistance increases the magnitude of improvement attained by using these drugs in an alternating strategy will diminish.

IV. CORRELATION BETWEEN PREDICTIONS AND EVIDENCE

Multiple agent chemotherapy has been unable to produce a significant number of cures in advanced breast cancer whereas apparent significant improvements in disease free survival using adjuvant chemotherapy have been reported for minimal disease burden.

Multiple agent therapy of limited small cell carcinoma of the lung has achieved cures where none were seen with single agents. Advanced stage Hodgkin's and non-Hodgkin's lymphoma have cure rates in the range of 30-50% because of multiple agent chemotherapy. Various strategies which utilize alternation to some degree have been found beneficial in both Hodgkins disease[21] and in oat-cell lung cancer.[22] The familiarity of the observation that small tumors are more curable than larger histologically similar tumors should be emphasized as being in perfect agreement with the considerations presented here. The lack of specificity of test observations in general do not permit a rigorous test of this model, but none of the general predictions contradict the empirical evidence available to date.

Variable response to chemotherapy is a common clinical experience and is explicitly predicted by this model due to the variable nature of the resistance process. Variability of response may be subclassified into two distinct types:

1. The distribution of cures
2. The distribution of remission and its length

In the first category, one would predict that given a therapy which could potentially eradicate the tumor (in the absence of resistance) then the variability would totally be due to the resistance phenomena. In the second category, variability of response would be due to a variety of factors of which cellular resistance would be only one. In this category, the largest source of variability would probably be the differing growth rates of tumors. Growth times for tumors which have originated from a very small number of cells have shown great variability, even in systems which otherwise show great regularity of growth.[23]

The greater wealth of detailed measurements available for experimental tumors permit more accurate comparisons of the model with empirical data. The phenomena of drug resistance at the cellular level has been recognized for over three decades, and is a known source of therapeutic failure. As the construction of this model was based on such observations they do not provide a true test of the validity of the model but do confirm its acceptability. Interpretation of the probability of no resistant cells as the maximal probability of cure allows a partial test of the model. Skipper[24] has fitted the vast amount of survival data he and his co-workers have collected on experimental leukemia against cures of P_0 generated for various values of α. The agreement appears good, although curves similar in shape to P_0 would be generated by any process which follows a poisson distribution. However no other process presently described has the additional property, which is well recognized, that the surviving tumors would then be resistant to further therapy with the same agent.

Another source of evidence comes from information collected upon treatment of experimental tumor lines with various agents consecutively.

For sufficiently large tumor burdens, experimental tumors such as L1210 leukemia, may not be cured with 100% probability with single agent therapy using either Ara-C or cyclophosphamide. Extensive empirical data collected by Skipper and his colleagues have allowed the calculation of the log-kill parameters and mutation rates for both these drugs. Also, the growth curve of the tumor is very nearly exponential and has a doubling time of 8 hr. Using this data it was possible to simulate therapy of the tumor with these two drugs and arrive at predictions of optimal scheduling. The parameters used were log-kills of 5.5, 4.5, and mutation rates of 5×10^{-8}, 10^{-7} for Ara-C and cyclophosphamide, respectively.[24]

The first course of therapy was given when the tumor was of size 6.3×10^7 and each course of therapy was given 3 days apart. It can be seen that these drugs cannot be considered as being equally effective with Ara-C having both a higher log-kill and a lower mutation rate than cyclophosphamide and is thus more effective. A number of simulations showed that one course of Ara-C followed by three courses of cyclophosphamide eradicated the tumor with maximum probability. One course of Ara-C only was needed as this removed all cells resistant to cyclophosphamide and left the tumor composed largely of Ara-C resistant cells. It then required three courses of cyclophosphamide to eliminate the remaining cells because of the very rapid regrowth of this tumor. This treatment plan coincides with the "treatment to nadir" protocol developed for the treatment of such tumors.[18] This agreement is not unexpected as these authors have developed their treatment strategies on the premise of eliminating the drug-resistant variants, however, it is reassuring that the model produces protocols which are similar to those derived experimentally.

V. CONCLUSIONS

The role of drug resistance in the chemotherapy of human tumors remains to be fully elucidated, though the behavior of many clinical tumors in the face of drug treatment strongly suggests that acquired resistance is occurring. Tumors which show initial sensitivity to chemotherapy can lose this property and exhibit regrowth in the face of therapy. Drug-resistant variants have been isolated in a number of experimental tumor lines and this characteristic has been shown to be stable and heritable. Evidence of genetic change in these variants has also been clearly demonstrated. In experimental tumor lines it has been shown that this process arises by random mutations which are then selected into prominence. Identical phenomena have been seen previously in bacterial populations and have been found to be due to random mutation occurring at a constant frequency. Observations on experimental tumor lines are totally consistent with such a process.

In the absence of other factors, the effect of this process on cancer chemotherapy was explored. The random nature of the process led to the isolation of two factors as the principal indicators of the resistance status of the tumor:

1. The expected number of resistant cells
2. The probability that no resistant cells are present

It was shown that the number and proportion of resistant cells will increase during the lifetime of the tumor and that advanced tumors will contain substantial proportions of such cells.

The probability that there were no resistant cells was shown to be inversely proportional to both tumor size and mutation rate. The rate of change of this quantity was shown to be small during the majority of the tumor's history. The period during which it changed rapidly was found to occupy about 5 to 6 doubling times for the tumor. This probability was identified as the maximal likelihood of cure and strategies were developed to maximize its value. Early treatment implies that the tumor size is smaller and thus, has a greater likelihood for potential cure. Combination chemotherapy will have the effect of reducing the mutation rate making the therapy more effective.

The same question was addressed for the case in which two agents or combinations were available, but could not be used simultaneously. Using the same reasoning, the doubly resistant mutant was identified as being a critical determinant of the success of therapy. Assuming that each agent was of equal efficacy, it was found that strategies for their utilization did not depend upon the values of their mutation rates or cell kills. Alternation after each course proved to be most effective in minimizing the probability of double resistance and was also effective in eliminating each singly resistant cell.

The magnitude of the role played by cellular resistance in (the therapy of) human tumors is difficult to fully assess with existing techniques; however, there is considerable evidence to suggest that it exists. Although the phenomenon is random, steps may be taken to both diminish its likelihood and minimize its effects when present. Although providing no new solutions to the basic problems of cancer chemotherapy this model suggests ways in which agents may be optimally used and how the effectiveness of agents, both old and new, should be evaluated. A more detailed review of the implications of this model in the therapy of human tumors is given in Volume II, Chapter 5.

ACKNOWLEDGMENT

We would like to thank Patricia Lambert, Barbara Williams, and Linda Wood for the hard work they did in typing and organizing this manuscript.

REFERENCES

1. Skipper, H. E., Schabel, F. M., Jr., and Lloyd, M. M., Selection and overgrowth of specifically and permanently drug-resistant tumor cells, *Exp. Ther. Kinetics,* 15, 207, 1978.
2. Ling, V., Genetic basis of drug resistance in mammalian cells, in *Drug and Hormone Resistance in Deoplasia, Volume I: Basic Concepts,* Bruchovsky, N. and Goldie, J. H., Eds., CRC Press, Boca Raton, Fla., 1983, 1.
3. Luria, S. E. and Delbruck, M., Mutations of Bacteria from virus sensitivity to virus resistance, *Genetics,* 28, 491, 1943.
4. Law, L. W., Origin of the resistance of leukemic cells to folic acid antagonists, *Nature (London),* 169, 628, 1952.
5. Kondo, S., A theoretical study on spontaneous mutation rate, *Mutat. Res.,* 14, 365, 1972.
6. Armitage, P., The statistical theory of bacterial populations subject to mutation, *J. R. Stat. Soc.,* 14, 1, 1952.
7. Stanley, P. and Siminovitch, L., Selection and characterisation of chinese hamster ovary cells resistant to the cytotoxicity of lectins, *In Vitro,* 12, 208, 1976.
8. Steel, G. C., *Growth Kinetics of Tumors,* Clarendon Press, Oxford, 1977.
9. Norton, L. and Simon, R., Tumor size, sensitivity to therapy, and design of treatment schedules, *Cancer Treat. Rep.,* 61, 1307, 1977.
10. Laird, A. K., Dynamics of tumor growth, in *Br. J. Cancer,* 18, 490, 1964.
11. Schabel, F. M., Jr., Skipper, M. E., Trader, M. W., Laster, W. R., Jr., Corbett, T. M., and Griswold, D. P., Concepts for controlling drug resistant tumor cells, in, *Breast Cancer-Experimental and Clinical Aspects,* Mourisden, M. T. and Palshof, T., Eds., Pergamon Press, Oxford, 1980, 199.
12. Goldie, J. H. and Coldman, A. J., A mathematical model formulating the drug sensitivity of tumors to their spontaneous mutation rate, *Cancer Treat. Rep.,* 63, 1727, 1979.
13. Philippe, E. and LeGal, Y., Growth of seventy-eight recurrent mammary cancers, *Cancer,* 21, 461, 1968.
14. Nisser-Meyer, R., Kjellgren, K., Malmio, K., Mansson, B., and Norin, T., Surgical adjuvant chemotherapy, *Cancer,* 41, 2088, 1978.
15. Parzen, E., *Stochastic Processes,* Holden Day, San Francisco, 1962, 144.
16. Crump, K. S. and Hoel, D. E., Mathematical models for estimating mutation rates in cell populations, *Biometrika,* 61, 237, 1974.
17. Bonnadonna, G., Monfordini, S., and Viller E., Non-cross resistant combinations in stage IV non-Hodgkins lymphomas, *Cancer Treat. Rep.,* 61, 1117, 1977.
18. Brockman, R. W., Circumvention of resistance, in, *The Pharmacological Basis of Cancer Chemotherapy,* Williams & Wilkins, Baltimore, 1975, 691.
19. Skipper, H. E., Schabel, F. M., Jr., and Wilcox, W. S., Exerimental evaluation of potential anticancer drugs XIV, further study of certain basic concepts underlying chemotherapy of leukemia, *Cancer Chemother. Rep.,* 45, 5, 1965.
20. Goldie, J. H., Coldman, A. J., and Gudauskas, G. A., A rationale for the use of alternating non-cross resistant chemotherapy, *Cancer Treat. Rep.,* 66, 439, 1982.
21. Santoro, A., Bonnadonna, G., Bonforte, V., and Valagussa, P., Non-cross resistant reginers (MOPP and ABVD) vs. MOPP alone in stage IV hodgkins disease, *Proc. Amer. Assoc. Clin. Oncol.,* 21, 595, 1980.
22. Sikic, B. I., Daniels, J. R., Chak, L., Alexander, M., Kohler, M., and Carter, S. K., Pocc versus Pocc/Vam therapy for small cell anaplastic (oat cell) lung cancer, in, *Nitrosoureas Current Status and New Developments,* Prestayko, A. W., Baker, L. H., Crooke, S. T., Carter, S. K. and Schein, P. S., Eds., Academic Press, New York, 1981, 221.
23. Skipper, H. E., Schabel, F. M., and Lloyd, M. M., Dose response and tumor cell repopulation rate in chemotherapeutic trials, in, *Advances in Cancer Chemotherapy, Vol. 1,* Rozownky, A., Ed., Marcel Dekkar, New York, 1979, 205.
24. Skipper, H., Some thoughts regarding a recent publication by Goldie & Coldman, entitled "A mathematical model for relating the drug sensitivity of tumors to their spontaneous mutation rate" Booklet # 9, Southern Research Institute, Birmingham, Ala., June, 1980.

Chapter 4

GLUCOCORTICOID RESISTANCE IN LYMPHOID CELL LINES

Marianne Huet-Minkowski, Judith C. Gasson, and Suzanne Bourgeois

TABLE OF CONTENTS

I. INTRODUCTION

The cytotoxic effects of glucocorticoids on lymphoid cells are the basis for the use of these hormones in the treatment of lymphoproliferative diseases and as immunosuppressants. Like other responses to steroid hormones, these effects are mediated by cytoplasmic receptors which, after binding of the steroid, undergo activation and translocation to the nucleus. The nature of the interaction of receptor-steroid complexes with the nucleus, and the molecular mechanism of steroid-mediated responses are not fully understood. However, since receptor-steroid complexes have the capacity to bind DNA, the current working hypothesis is that they affect gene expression by binding specific sites of the genome.

The growth-inhibitory and lethal effects of glucocorticoids have been studied for three decades, using lymphocytes and thymocytes in vitro or transplantable animal tumors such as the mouse lymphosarcoma P1798. In recent years glucocorticoid-sensitive cell lines derived from lymphoid tumors have been established in tissue culture and cloned. These cloned cell lines offer the possibility to analyze the mechanism of the cytolytic response — and of acquisition of resistance — by somatic cell genetics because these lines represent a genetically homogeneous population of cells which are killed in the presence of glucocorticoids. Therefore, rare unresponsive variants can easily be selected on the basis of their resistance, and their defects characterized.

Two murine cell lines have been used extensively for such studies: the S49 line[1] derived from a mineral oil induced T-lymphoma, and the WEHI-7 (W7) line[2] cloned from a thymoma which arose after X-ray irradiation. A cloned line recently derived from the P1798 mouse lymphosarcoma[3] was found to undergo reversible growth arrest in the presence of glucocorticoids, without loss of viability. One human leukemic line, CEM-C7, which is killed by glucocorticoids, has been cloned[4] from CCRF-CEM cells, a thymus derived line established from the blood of a patient with acute lymphoblastic leukemia. Most human lymphoid cell lines are resistant to the cytotoxic effects of glucocorticoids, e.g., among 20 human lymphoid lines recently examined,[5] only 4 were sensitive to pharmacological concentrations of glucocorticoids and, of these, the CEM-C7 line was by far the most sensitive.

Although somatic cell genetics is a powerful tool, problems can arise from the use of somatic cells maintained in tissue culture. It is important to remember that somatic cell lines commonly have abnormal karyotypes. Chromosome aberrations and aneuploidy are a feature, in particular, of certain leukemias and lymphomas. For example, karyotypic analysis of the 20 human lymphoid lines mentioned above[5] revealed that all these lines, including the CEM-C7, had multiple chromosome rearrangements. While some lines may display an abnormal karyotype from the onset, some lymphoid cell lines have been shown to undergo substantial chromosome rearrangements and aneuploidy during prolonged cultivation in vitro.[6] The two murine cell lines used in studies of lymphocytolysis, S49 and W7, appear quasidiploid with 40 acrocentric chromosomes, but no chromosome banding analysis has been carried out to examine the possibility of chromosome rearrangements. In fact, as will be discussed below, the pseudodiploid S49 line displays some functional hemizygosity. Moreover, pseudotetraploid derivatives appear spontaneously in S49 populations.[7]

Other types of variations can occur as well in vitro, e.g., mutations or epigenetic events. Although such events may be rare, prolonged cultivation could enrich for the resulting variants. Obviously, cells grown in the artificial conditions of tissue culture medium must be under strong selective pressures different from those exerted in vivo. Whatever their origin, variants that can better withstand the tissue culture conditions will have a selective advantage. Such variants could, for example, have developed a reduced dependency on a growth factor present only in limiting amount or resistance to a toxic substance or to a hormone present in the serum commonly used in tissue culture media.

One of the most useful methodologies of somatic cell genetics is the construction of cell hybrids to establish dominance relationships or complementation, and to examine gene dosage effects. Thanks to the introduction of appropriate markers and to improvements in cell fusion techniques, hybrids between a variety of cell types can conveniently be isolated. However, cell hybrids undergo segregation-like events predominantly involving chromosome loss but also chromosome rearrangements. Although the most rapid loss of chromosomes appears to occur in hybrids between cells of different species, especially man-mouse hybrids, extensive segregation also takes place in intraspecific hybrids, even in those produced from two very similar cells.[8] Such instability obviously calls for great caution in interpreting the results obtained with hybrids. This problem will be illustrated below in the case of S49 and W7 cell hybrids.

II. GENETIC NATURE OF GLUCOCORTICOID RESISTANCE

A. Spontaneous Resistance to High Doses of Glucocorticoids

S49 variants resistant to glucocorticoid-induced killing retain their resistant phenotype in the absence of steroid and arise spontaneously at a frequency on the order of 10^{-5}, which is surprisingly high for a genetic event in a pseudodiploid cell.[9] The development of resistance is stochastic, occurring at a rate of 3.5×10^{-6}/cell/generation, which is increased by classical mutagens.[7] However, this high frequency appeared to be independent of ploidy in that it was observed in a pseudotetraploid S49 line as well as in pseudodiploids.[7,9] These observations raised the possibility that the appearance of resistance involved a heritable phenotypic change not involving a genetic alteration, i.e., an epigenetic event. Therefore, we turned to another glucocorticoid-sensitive line, the thymoma W7.[2] As shown in Table 1, in contrast to the high frequency observed in S49, the frequency of spontaneous appearance of glucocorticoid-resistant variants of the W7 line is $< 1.2 \times 10^{-10}$, i.e., no resistant variant was found when a population of 8.1×10^9 cells was examined.[10,11]

These results prompted us to compare other relevant properties of the S49 and W7 lines. Figure 1 illustrates the effect of dexamethasone on the growth of these cells. Both lines have a doubling time of approximately 15 hr in the absence of steroid, and are equally sensitive to 10^{-6} M dexamethasone. As described by Harris,[12] in the presence of the hormone these cells become pycnotic, smaller, unable to exclude dye and eventually lyse. A difference in sensitivity of these two cell lines becomes apparent, however, at lower concentrations of dexamethasone: at 1.2×10^{-8} M dexamethasone, for example, the number of living cells in the S49 culture has remained essentially constant after 72 hr (Figure 1a), while the number of living W7 cells has decreased drastically (Figure 1b). Moreover, the S49 line is relatively resistant to the low concentration of 6×10^{-9} M dexamethasone (Figure 1a), at which the number of living W7 cells is considerably reduced as compared to the control (Figure 1b). In addition, dead cells and cell debris accumulate in the W7 culture containing 6×10^{-9} M dexamethasone. The W7 line appears, then, considerably more sensitive to the cytolytic effect of glucocorticoids than the S49 line.

The glucocorticoid receptor content of these lines was measured by binding of $[^3H]$-dexamethasone to whole cells.[13] This assay, which gives very reproducible results, gave an estimate of $15,000 \pm 1,500$ dexamethasone binding sites per cell in the S49 line.[10] This value is considerably higher than the value of only 2,400 sites per S49 cell which can be calculated from the previously reported data of Sibley and Tomkins.[14] This discrepancy is most likely due to the fact that these investigators used a cell-free bind-

Table 1

FREQUENCIES OF SPONTANEOUS DEXAMETHASONE-
RESISTANT VARIANTS

Cell line	Receptor sites per cell ± SE	Dexamethasone concentration M	Frequency	Ref.
S49	15,000 ± 1,500	10^{-5}	3.0×10^{-5}	7, 9, 10
W7	30,000 ± 3,000	10^{-5}	$< 1.2 \times 10^{-10}$	10, 11
W7	30,000 ± 3,000	5×10^{-9}	3.3×10^{-7}	10
W7-MS1	15,000 ± 1,500	10^{-6}	4.1×10^{-6}	10

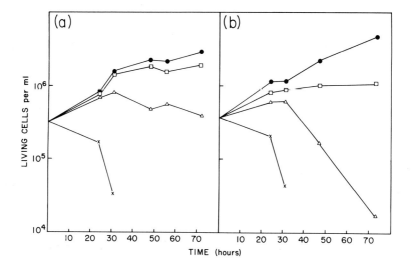

FIGURE 1.   Growth curves of the S49 and W7 lines in the presence of dexamethasone. Growth conditions and measurements of the number of living cells by trypan
blue exclusion are described elsewhere.[10] (a) S49 line; (b) W7 line. The symbols
represent the following dexamethasone concentrations: (X-X) 10^{-6} M; (Δ-Δ) 1.2 ×
10^{-8} M; (□-□) 6 × 10^{-9} M; (● — ●) control without dexamethasone.

ing assay in which some inactivation of receptor occurred. As listed in Table 1, measurements by the whole cell assay of the glucocorticoid receptor content of the W7
line revealed 30,000 ± 3,000 binding sites per cell. The receptors of both cell lines have
the same affinity for dexamethasone, $K_a = 1.3 \pm 0.3 \times 10^8 M^{-1}$.

The presence of twice as much receptor in the W7 line as in the S49 line is striking,
and led to the hypothesis that the S49 line is functionally hemizygous for the gene (r⁺)
encoding the glucocorticoid receptor. The intracellular receptor content would, then,
result from a gene dosage effect and reflect the presence of two active alleles in the
W7 line (r⁺/r⁺) and of only one allele in S49 (r⁺/r⁻). This interpretation would also
account for the much lower frequency of glucocorticoid-resistant variants arising from
the W7 line, and might explain the difference in glucocorticoid sensitivity between the
two lines.

B. Stepwise Acquisition of Resistance

The results described above suggest that acquisition of glucocorticoid resistance in
the W7 line could proceed in two steps:

$$r^+/r^+ \rightarrow r^+/r^- \rightarrow r^-/r^-$$

Each step, corresponding to the inactivation of one functional r^+ allele encoding the glucocorticoid receptor, would occur at a frequency on the order of 10^{-6} to 10^{-5}. Therefore, the frequency of resistant variants in the W7 line would be expected to be in the range of 10^{-12} to 10^{-10}, as observed (see Table 1). The S49 line behaves as having, accidentally, undergone the first step: this resulted in a twofold reduction in receptor content and a 10^5 to 10^6 times increased frequency of appearance of resistant variants. This interpretation is, however, based on the comparison of two different cell lines, a T-lymphoma (S49) and a thymoma (W7). While both cell lines originated in Balb/c mice and are thymus derived, they have been isolated independently. The S49 tumor appeared in a lymph node after injection of mineral oil, while the W7 tumor arose in the thymus after X-irradiation. To support the two-step model of acquisition of resistance, hemizygous derivatives (r^+/r^-) of the W7 line similar to the S49 line, had to be isolated.

The selection for such putative W7 (r^+/r^-) hemizygotes was achieved on the basis of the observation that the S49 line exhibits considerable resistance to dexamethasone in the range of 10^{-9} to 10^{-8} M (see Figure 1a). If this partial resistance is due to the reduced receptor content of this line, then selection for resistance to such low concentrations of dexamethasone should yield the desired W7 (r^+/r^-) hemizygotes. Table 1, line 3, shows that, if a population of W7 cells is exposed to 5×10^{-9} M dexamethasone, variants resistant to that concentration of the steroid appear at a frequency of 3.3×10^{-7}. Several of these partially resistant variants were analyzed,[10] and the results obtained for one such clone, W7-MS1, are shown in Table 1 (line 4) and Figure 2. Like S49 cells, the W7-MS1 variant contains $15,000 \pm 1,500$ dexamethasone binding sites per cell, and gives rise to fully resistant variants (selected in the presence of 10^{-6} M dexamethasone) at a high frequency of 10^{-6}. Moreover, as shown in Figure 2, clone W7-MS1 displays the same level of resistance as the S49 line. The fact that the phenotype of clone W7-MS1 (and other similar clones) is identical with that of S49 strongly supports the idea that these clones are, indeed, hemizygous for the receptor locus and represent intermediates in a two-step genetic mechanism of acquisition of resistance to glucocorticoids.

Similar studies carried out with the human leukemic line CEM-C7 established that glucocorticoid resistance arises in that line, like in S49 cells, as a random and stable event occurring at the high rate of 2 to 3×10^{-5}/cell/generation increased by mutagens.[15,16] It is likely, therefore, that resistance in the CEM-C7 line is acquired in a single step by mutation in a haploid or functionally hemizygous locus which, in this case as well as in S49, appears to be a gene encoding the glucocorticoid receptor.

III. INDUCTION OF GLUCOCORTICOID RESISTANCE

A. Induction by Classical Mutagens

Various classical mutagens have been shown to increase the frequency of glucocorticoid-resistant variants in all three cell lines examined. The alkylating agent N-methyl-N'-nitro-N'nitrosoguanidine (MNNG) raised this frequency 50- to 100-fold in the S49 line[7,17] and approximately 8-fold in the CEM-C7 line.[16] Two frame-shift mutagens have been used: 9-aminoacridine which increased the frequency of S49 variants up to 20-fold,[7] and ICR 191 which produced a 35-fold increase in the CEM-C7 line.[16] In addition, γ-irradiation also appeared effective on the S49 line.[7] In the case of the W7 line, the efficiency of mutagens is difficult to estimate quantitatively because the frequency of spontaneous mutations, $< 1.2 \times 10^{-10}$, is too low for a precise estimate. As shown in Table 2, three classical mutagens have been shown to be effective in the W7 line: two alkylating agents, MNNG and ethyl methanesulfonate (EMS), and UV irradiation.[18] These mutagens increase the frequency of W7 glucocorticoid-resistant variants to values ranging from 5×10^{-8} to 5×10^{-7}.

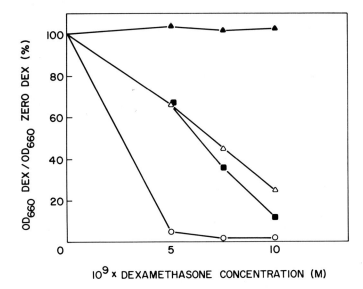

FIGURE 2.   Sensitivity to dexamethasone of the S49 and W7 lines, and of W7 variants. The cellular material present in the culture after eight doublings in the control culture without steroid, was monitored by turbidity at 660 nm.[10] The results obtained for the culture with dexamethasone are expressed as percentage of the OD_{660} reached in the control. The symbols represent the following cell lines: (O-O) W7; (■ — ■) S49; (△-△) W7-MS1; (▲ — ▲) a fully resistant derivative of W7-MS1 selected at 10^{-5} *M* dexamethasone. (From Bourgeois, S.; *Steroid Receptors and the Management of Cancer, Vol. II,* Thompson, E. B. and Lippman, M. E., Eds., CRC Press, Inc., Boca Raton, Florida, 1979, 99.

Table 2
INDUCTION OF W7 DEXAMETHASONE-RESISTANT VARIANTS BY VARIOUS MUTAGENS

Mutagen	Dose μg/mℓ	Time of treatment hr	Survival %	Frequency	Receptor negative[a] %	Ref.
MNNG	1.25	2	5 to 10[b]	5.2×10^{-7}	80	18
EMS	530	18	5 to 10[b]	2.5×10^{-7}	75	18
UV	—	—	10 to 40[b]	5.0×10^{-8}	87	18
Mitomycin C	0.5 or 1[c]	1	5	1.0×10^{-7}	95	11
Mitomycin C[d]	0.5 or 1[c]	1	5	7.2×10^{-8}	30	11
Bleomycin	47	22	10 to 15[b]	3.5×10^{-9}	35	11
Streptonigrin	0.1	5	2	1.2×10^{-8}	100	11
BD40	0.03	2	3 to 10[b]	1.8×10^{-9}	100	11
Colcemid	0.01	22	40	1.0×10^{-9}	75	11

[a]   Variants containing < 25% of the parental amount of receptor.

[b]   Range of percentage survival observed in several independent experiments.

[c]   Concentrations of 0.5 or 1 μg/mℓ mitomycin C were used in different experiments. In all cases, cells were incubated for 24 hr in the presence of 200 μg/mℓ caffeine, following mitomycin C treatment.

[d]   The 1 hr mutagenic treatment with mitomycin C was performed, in this case, in the presence of 10^{-6} *M* dexamethasone.

B. Induction by Various Cytotoxic Drugs
1. Mutagenicity of Various Cytotoxic Drugs

As will be described below (Section IIIC), all glucocorticoid-resistant variants isolated after treatment with classical mutagens resulted from receptor defects. To increase the probability of inactivating another, as yet unknown, function involved in the cytolytic response, we have recently turned to treatments by antitumor drugs known to induce large deletions and chromosome rearrangements or elimination.[11] This approach also is of intrinsic interest because it involves testing the mutagenicity of such drugs in animal cells and, in particular, their capacity to induce glucocorticoid-resistant lymphoid cell variants.

As listed in Table 2, five drugs used in cancer chemotherapy were shown to increase the frequency of glucocorticoid-resistant variants of the W7 line. Some of these drugs are known to interfere with DNA synthesis through covalent or noncovalent binding to DNA (mitomycin C and streptonigrin), removal of bases from DNA (bleomycin) or intercalation (ellipticines such as BD40), producing single- or double-strand breakage. On the other hand, colcemid at low concentration was shown to induce the elimination of one or two chromosomes, without chromosome breaks or rearrangements.[19] Of these five drugs, only mitomycin C was known to induce transmissible alterations in the genome of mammalian cells,[20] and caffeine was shown in some cases to potentiate this mutagenic activity.[21] Since little was known about the effect of the other four drugs on animal cells in culture, it was necessary to determine their toxicity for the W7 line. In preliminary experiments (not shown) these drugs were tested over a range of doses and for a variety of incubation periods.[11] The conditions used for mutagenesis, listed in Table 2, were chosen because they yield a substantial percentage of surviving cells, ranging from 2% to 40% of the population, among which the glucocorticoid-resistant variants were selected by plating in the presence of 10^{-5} M dexamethasone.

As shown in Table 2, the treatment by the alkylating agent mitomycin C (followed by caffeine) is as efficient as MNNG or EMS, inducing glucocorticoid-resistant variants at a frequency on the order of 10^{-7}. The other drugs are weaker mutagens, yielding variants at frequencies of 10^{-9} to 10^{-8}. All the resistant variants induced by these antitumor drugs turned out to be of the same type as those induced by classical mutagens, namely defective in the glucocorticoid receptor function, although the nature of the receptor defects varies with the mutagenic treatment (see below). These results raise the possibility that, in combination therapies involving cytotoxic drugs and a glucocorticoid, this type of steroid resistant lymphoid cell variant could be induced by the drug and selected by the presence of the hormone.

2. Absence of Cross-Resistance between Drugs and Glucocorticoids

The problem of drug resistance in mammalian cells, and the patterns of cross-resistance and collateral sensitivity, are discussed in detail in Chapters 1 and 2 and will only be mentioned briefly here. Since glucocorticoid resistant W7 variants were selected among populations of cells which had survived mutagenic treatments with highly toxic antitumor drugs, the question of a possible cross-resistance between the hormone and the drug used as mutagen had to be raised. The basis for drug resistance in cultured cells has been studied, in particular, in Chinese hamster ovary (CHO) cell mutants that are resistant to colchicine and display extensive cross-resistance to a number of apparently unrelated compounds[22] (see Chapter 1). This complex phenotype appears, however, to be the result of a single alteration in membrane permeability[23] affecting, in a pleiotropic fashion, the diffusion of various drugs. Membrane alteration is also the likely cause for bleomycin resistance in some CHO variants.[24] Tumor resistance to drugs is commonly observed clinically as well as in animal systems: in particular, the development of resistance to mitomycin C, one of the mutagens we have extensively used with the W7 line, has been described in a rat sarcoma.[25] Therefore, we tested the possibility of cross-resistance between dexamethasone and either bleomycin or mitomycin C in two variants induced by one or the other of these drugs.

Figure 3, panel a, illustrates that the parental W7 line is highly sensitive to all three compounds: dexamethasone, bleomycin, and mitomycin C. The variant B20 (panel b) is resistant to dexamethasone but has retained its sensitivity to 47 μg/mℓ bleomycin, the concentration of that drug used to induce this variant. Similarly, variant C23 (panel c) induced by treatment with 1 μg/mℓ mitomycin C has retained its sensitivity to that drug while developing resistance to dexamethasone.

These results are no surprise since, as will be described below, dexamethasone resistance in these variants results from glucocorticoid receptor defects which are not expected to affect sensitivity to bleomycin or mitomycin C. Moreover, all variants induced by antitumor drugs were selected for resistance to 10^{-5} M dexamethasone; changes in membrane permeability would probably not confer resistance to such a high concentration of glucocorticoids. Therefore, possible variants with membrane permeability alterations that could lead to cross-resistance would not be selected in those conditions. It is conceivable, however, that some changes in membrane permeability could result in resistance to much lower concentrations of dexamethasone. Selection for resistance to concentrations in the range of 10^{-9} to 10^{-8} M dexamethasone could possibly yield variants with altered membrane permeability, resulting in cross-resistance between glucocorticoids and antitumor drugs. Such variants, unlike the S49 or W7 (r^+/r^-) hemizygotes described earlier (see Section IIB), would have retained the parental amount of glucocorticoid receptor. We are currently screening a collection of W7 variants selected at low concentrations of dexamethasone to examine that possibility.

C. Types of Glucocorticoid-Resistant Variants

All S49 glucocorticoid-resistant variants isolated by Sibley and Tomkins[7] were selected in the presence of 5×10^{-7} M dexamethasone; in contrast, S49 variants obtained in our laboratory[17] were selected at 10^{-5} M dexamethasone. This difference in dexamethasone concentration used in the selection will be relevant to our discussion of the types of S49 variants obtained. Another significant difference between the two collections of S49 variants is that some of the variants isolated by Sibley and Tomkins[7] and characterized later in detail[14,26] were derived from a pseudotetraploid S49 line, while only variants derived from the pseudodiploid S49 line were studied in our laboratory.[17,27]

Various tests were used to characterize the variants obtained. All variants were screened qualitatively for binding of dexamethasone to whole cells. The amount of glucocorticoid receptor was assayed in some variants by Scatchard analysis of binding data performed over a range of dexamethasone concentrations using either cell extracts[14] or whole cells.[13,17] Because of inactivation of receptor in cell-free extracts, the whole cell assay is more reliable,[10] giving higher and more reproducible values. Variants which displayed dexamethasone binding were further characterized with respect to their ability to translocate the receptor-steroid complex to the nucleus. The conditions of the nuclear transfer assay described by Sibley and Tomkins[14] yield 50% of the radioactivity localized in the nuclear pellet, while the assay used in our laboratory[13] results in 70% of the radioactivity translocated to the nuclear fraction of wild-type S49 cells. Salt elution patterns of receptor-steroid complexes from DNA-cellulose[26] or from the nuclear fraction[13,17] were additional tests used to characterize glucocorticoid-resistant S49 variants. Representative variants were also analyzed genetically by cell hybridization.[26,27]

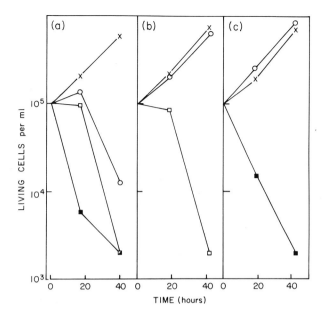

FIGURE 3. Tests of cross-resistance between dexamethasone and cytoxic drugs. Growth conditions and measurements of the number of living cells by trypan blue were as described elsewhere.[10] (a) Glucocorticoid-sensitive parental W7 line; (b) glucocorticoid resistant W7 variant B20, induced by bleomycin; (c) glucocorticoid resistant W7 variant C23, induced by mitomycin C. Symbols represent the following growth conditions: (X-X) controls without hormone or drug; (O-O) 10^{-6} *M* dexamethasone; ($\square$-$\square$) 47 $\mu g/m\ell$ bleomycin; ($\blacksquare$ — $\blacksquare$) 1 $\mu g/m\ell$ mitomycin C.

Approximately 200 glucocorticoid-resistant variants were isolated from the S49 line and examined in each laboratory. The results of the two groups concur in that the vast majority of the variants, derived either spontaneously or after mutagenesis, display greatly reduced glucocorticoid-binding activity: 75 to 90% of the variants either show no detectable glucocorticoid receptor or display less than 25% of the binding observed in wild-type S49 cells. These variants have been designated r⁻ for "receptorless" or "receptor deficient". The majority of the remaining variants contain levels of glucocorticoid receptor activity that are usually lower than in wild-type S49 cells, but can also be equal to or even higher than the activity of parental cells. However, these variants translocate receptor-steroid complex to the nucleus with a decreased efficiency and have, therefore, been designated nt⁻ for "nuclear transfer deficient". The receptors of these nt⁻ variants can also be distinguished from wild-type and from each other by the salt sensitivity of their interaction with DNA-cellulose or with the nuclear fraction.

Sibley and Tomkins[14] described a few resistant variants belonging to a third class, designated d⁻ for "deathless", in which hormone binding and nuclear transfer appeared normal. This class of variants, which was not observed in our laboratory, deserves close scrutiny because glucocorticoid-resistant variants with *bona fide* normal receptor must result from a defect in another function involved in the response, and would provide an important tool to analyze the as yet unknown steps in the lytic response. Upon close examination of the S49 variants originally classified as "deathless", most of them turned out to have an *increased* capacity to translocate the receptor-steroid complex to the nucleus.[26] This subclass of variants was redefined as "nuclear transfer increased" and designated nt^i, to distinguish them from the nt$^-$ variants mentioned above which have decreased nuclear transfer capacity. Interestingly, all nt^i variants have a receptor of considerably lower molecular weight than wild-type receptor.[26]

Two variants remained classified as "deathless" because they still had a receptor indistinguishable from the wild-type by all tests used. The phenotype of these two putative "deathless" variants has been interpreted as resulting either from a subtle alteration in the receptor or from a defect in another function. In retrospect, there is a much simpler, and more likely explanation for the nature of these "variants". It is important to point out that both these clones were derived from a tetraploid S49 line, and selected at 5×10^{-7} M dexamethasone. In view of the functional hemizygosity of the S49 line at the receptor locus, the tetraploid S49 parent contained only two active r$^+$ alleles. Moreover, such tetraploid lines are unstable and segregate chromosomes at high frequency. As will be discussed below (see Section IV), the loss of one r$^+$ allele from a tetraploid line occurs at a frequency on the order of 10^{-3}. Therefore, the two so-called "deathless variants" are most likely segregants, having lost one r$^+$ allele and retained a single copy of the r$^+$ gene. This would result in a tetraploid segregant containing a single dose of approximately 15,000 receptors per cell. These receptors would, obviously, be wild-type but the presence of only 15,000 receptors in a tetraploid cell results in considerable resistance to low concentrations of glucocorticoids (see Section IV). It is, therefore, likely that at the concentration of 5×10^{-7} M dexamethasone used by Sibley and Tomkins in the selection for variants, such segregants would yield colonies, although these colonies may be smaller and appear at a lower plating efficiency than would be the case for fully resistant variants. No data have been reported in the literature about the level of resistance of these two putative "deathless variants" compared to variants resulting from receptor defects. Moreover, their precise receptor content has not been measured since, unfortunately, the two "deathless" clones in which Sibley and Tomkins[14] measured dexamethasone binding quantitatively turned out later to belong to the nt^i class.[26]

Genetic complementation and dominance tests in cell hybrids were carried out for representative variants of each class.[26,27] All hybrids between wild-type cells and either r$^-$, nt$^-$ or nt^i variants were glucocorticoid sensitive, indicating that the wild-type phenotype is dominant. All tested combinations of variant x variant fusions yielded resistant hybrids, i.e., no complementation was observed which would have resulted in recovery of the sensitive phenotype. Complementation could have been expected if the defects resulted from mutations in different alleles such as, e.g., genes encoding several nonidentical receptor subunits or a locus necessary to modify the receptor protein into its active form. The absence of complementation is consistent with the idea that all defects result from mutations in the same allele, r, encoding a single receptor polypeptide. No complementation tests of the two putative "deathless variants" were carried out because these clones are already tetraploid.

Approximately 300 glucocorticoid-resistant variants were isolated in one step after mutagenesis of the W7 line and characterized.[11,18] A wide variety of mutagenic treatments were used on this line, as discussed earlier (section III) and listed in Table 2. Again, all variants resulted from defects in the receptor and only two types of defects were observed, receptor negative (r$^-$) and nuclear transfer defective (nt$^-$). As shown in Table 2 (column 6), the vast majority (75 to 100%) of the variants induced by most mutagenic treatments were receptor negative. There are, however, two striking exceptions: only 30 to 35% of the variants induced by mitomycin C (in the presence of dexamethasone) or by bleomycin were of the r$^-$ type, while most variants were nt$^-$ in those cases. While r$^-$ defects can result from deletions as well as point mutations, the nt$^-$ phenotype probably results from point mutations since nt$^-$ receptors are only altered in their nuclear transfer capacity but retain high dexamethasone binding activity. The reason for this high incidence of nt⁻ defects is unclear. Since mostly r⁻ variants were induced by mitomycin C in the absence of dexamethasone (Table 2, line 4), it appears that dexamethasone might affect transcription of the r⁺ gene. The hormone might modulate the synthesis of its receptor and/or change the conformation of the r⁺ gene in a fashion that renders it more sensitive to point mutations, resulting in the nt⁻ phenotype. The high incidence of point mutations (nt⁻ phenotype) induced by bleomycin indicates that this compound acts differently from the other mutagenic treatments used. This result is surprising because bleomycin is known to induce chromosome breaks resulting in deletions and extensive rearrangements that would be expected to inactivate the r⁺ gene and result mostly in r⁻ defects. The high proportion of nt⁻ variants obtained suggests that such extensive DNA damage is usually lethal and that the only events detected as receptor defects would be mutations resulting from error-prone repair of DNA breaks. This observation makes bleomycin the mutagen of choice to induce receptor alterations observed rarely with classical mutagens.

Over 100 glucocorticoid-resistant variants of the human leukemic line CEM-C7 were isolated, by selection in the presence of 10^{-6} *M* dexamethasone, and characterized.[16] Approximately 50 clones arose spontaneously and 60 clones were induced by mutagens. Again, all CEM-C7 variants result from defects in the glucocorticoid receptor. Among the spontaneous variants, no clone was entirely devoid of receptor, but the majority of these variants contained 10 to 30% of the parental receptor activity of 20,000 dexamethasone binding sites per cell. This distribution is somewhat different from that observed with the S49 line where most spontaneous variants lack detectable receptor activity. The majority of the CEM-C7 variants induced by classical mutagens, ICR 191 and MNNG, had < 10% of the parental receptor level. One glucocorticoid-resistant CEM-C7 clone, containing approximately 30% of the parental level of receptor, exhibited a phenotype not previously observed among the murine cell line variants, namely a complete absence of nuclear translocation.[28] Further characterization of this variant revealed that its receptor cannot form stable activated receptor-steroid complexes, and this defect was designated "receptor activation-labile". The stability of the altered receptors of nt⁻ variants of the S49 or W7 lines has not been examined. It is likely that some of the murine nt⁻ receptors also have increased lability, either in their activated or nonactivated form. This would account for the observation that most of the nt⁻ variants contain a reduced amount of glucocorticoid-binding activity.

The fact that all of > 400 S49 variants and > 100 CEM-C7 variants examined result from defects in the glucocorticoid receptor is reasonable in view of the evidence (see section II) for functional hemizygosity at the r locus. One would, however, have anticipated obtaining defects in another function in the case of the W7 line which is likely to be diploid for the r allele. The absence of W7 variants containing normal receptor amongst the > 300 variants induced by a variety of mutagenic treatments is highly significant and deserves comment. The lymphocytolytic response is relatively slow (see Figure 1) and certainly complex: it is, therefore, unlikely that the receptor is the only function involved. Mutations in a relevant locus other than r would have to be at least 300 times less frequent than in the r⁺ gene to explain the result obtained. It is conceivable that alterations in the other functions involved are lethal. Glucocorticoids could also induce more than one independent pathway leading to cell death; simultaneous mutations in several genes would then be required to block the process. This point remains to be clarified.

IV. CORRELATION BETWEEN GLUCORTICOID RECEPTOR AND CYTOLYTIC RESPONSE IN CELL HYBRIDS

A. Characteristics of Hybrids

The question of the correlation between glucocorticoid receptor content and cytolytic response of lymphoid cells is of great interest: a positive correlation would support the idea that receptor measurements in human leukemic lymphocytes and lymphomas might be useful in predicting the outcome of glucocorticoid therapy. The W7 thymoma line and its derivatives offer the possibility to examine quantitatively this controversial issue in a murine model system.

Three types of W7 clones containing different levels of glucocorticoid receptors are available: the homozygous (r^+/r^+) parental line, the hemizygous (r^+/r^-) derivatives selected for resistance to 5×10^{-9} M dexamethasone (Table 1), and the receptor deficient (r^-/r^-) lines resistant to 10^{-5} M dexamethasone (Table 2). Clones of each type exist which are resistant either to thioguanine or to 5-bromodeoxyuridine. The presence of these markers allows the selection of cell hybrids in hypoxanthine-aminopterin-thymidine medium, without imposing any selective pressure for full or partial resistance to glucocorticoids. The hybrid clones described below were never exposed to glucocorticoids before receptor assays or tests for sensitivity to dexamethasone were performed.

As shown in Table 3, hybrids were constructed which contained one, two, three or four r^+ alleles per tetraploid cell.[29] The receptor content of these hybrids reflects the number of copies of the r^+ allele: the number of dexamethasone binding sites per cell was approximately 15,000, 32,000, 43,000, and 57,000. All these hybrids are sensitive to glucocorticoids (see below) but, when plated in the presence of 10^{-5} M dexamethasone, they give rise to resistant clones at frequencies orders of magnitude higher than expected on the basis of the ploidy of the r^+ allele. Table 3 shows that glucocorticoid-resistant clones arise at a frequency of 1.6×10^{-3} from the clone containing a single copy of the r^+ allele, i.e., three orders of magnitude higher than in the case of a diploid hemizygous (r^+/r^-) cell. Similarly, the hybrid containing two r^+ alleles gives rise to resistant clones at a frequency of 7.6×10^{-6}, at least 4 orders of magnitude higher than the frequency of $< 1.2 \times 10^{-10}$ observed for diploid W7 (r^+/r^+) cells, which also contain two r^+ alleles (see Table 1).

These results suggested that, in the case of tetraploid cells, resistance can be acquired not only by mutation but also by chromosome segregation, involving loss or rearrangement. The karyotype of a $r^+/r^+ \times r^-/r^-$ hybrid clone was analyzed and revealed that these cells contained a modal number of 80 chromosomes,[30] while a glucocorticoid-resistant derivative of that hybrid contained only 78 chromosomes.[30] This indicated that two chromosomes were lost during the selection for glucocorticoid resistance. Giemsa banding of the chromosomes of a hybrid between S49 cells (r^+/r^-) and EL4 cells (which appear to be nt^-/nt^-) showed that glucocorticoid-resistant derivatives consistently lose one of the two chromosomes 18 of S49 origin.[31] This result assigns the gene encoding the glucocorticoid receptor to chromosome 18 of the mouse, and confirms that the S49 line is functionally hemizygous at that locus. This instability of tetraploid cells accounts for the high frequency of glucocorticoid-resistant variants derived from a tetraploid S49 cell line by Sibley and Tomkins;[7] indeed, because of segregation-like events, the frequency of mutations to dexamethasone-resistance behaves as if it were independent of ploidy when diploid cells containing a single r^+ allele, such as S49 or W7 (r^+/r^-) are compared with tetraploid cells containing two r^+ alleles (see Table 3, lines 2 and 6).

B. Sensitivity of Hybrids

Figure 4 illustrates the sensitivity to dexamethasone of the four hybrid lines listed in Table 3. The effect of 10^{-5} M dexamethasone on the growth of these hybrids is

Table 3
CHARACTERISTICS OF HYBRID CLONES

Receptor alleles	Number of r⁺ alleles per cell	Receptor sites per cell ± S.E.	Frequency of Dex^r
r^+/r^+	2	$30,000 \pm 3,000$	$< 1.2 \times 10^{-10}$
r^+/r^-	1	$15,000 \pm 1,500$	9.6×10^{-6}
r^-/r^-	0	< 100	1
$r^+/r^+ \times r^+/r^+$	4	$57,500 \pm 3,900$	$< 2.5 \times 10^{-8}$
$r^+/r^+ \times r^+/r^-$	3	$42,800 \pm 1,800$	$< 7.1 \times 10^{-9}$
$r^+/r^- \times r^+/r^-$ or $r^+/r^+ \times r^-/r^-$	2	$32,500 \pm 1,500$	7.6×10^{-6}
$r^+/r^- \times r^-/r^-$	1	$12,700 \pm 1,500$	1.6×10^{-3}

From Bourgeois, S., *J. Supramolecular Structure*, 13, 401, 1980. With permission.

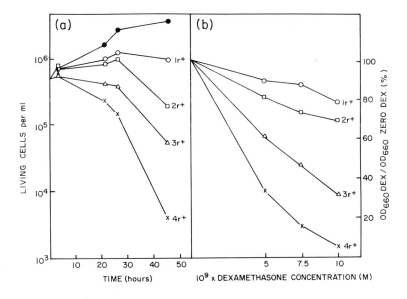

FIGURE 4.   Correlation between glucocorticoid receptor content and sensitivity of cell hybrids. Growth conditions were as described elsewhere.[10] (a) Number of living cells measured by trypan blue exclusion as a function of time; (b) Cellular material, present after eight doublings in the control culture without steroid, monitored by turbidity at 660 nm, and expressed as percentage of OD_{660} reached in the control as function of dexamethasone concentrations. The closed circles (●—●) in panel (a) represent the growth in the control cultures without dexamethasone: the control growth rates were very similar for all hybrids and are represented as a single symbol for simplicity. All other symbols represent cultures in the presence of 10^{-5} *M* dexamethasone (panel a) or of the indicated concentrations of dexamethasone (panel b) of the following hybrids: (X-X) W7TB (r^+/r^+) × W7TG (r^+/r^+); (△-△) MS1 (r^+/r^-) × W7TG (r^+/r^+); (□-□) W7TB (r^+/r^+) × SL3 (r^-/r^-); (O-O) MS1 (r^+/r^-) × SL3 (r^-/r^-). The number of functional r^+ alleles present in each hybrid cell line is indicated on each curve. Panel (A) is reproduced from Bourgeois, S. and Newby, R. F., *First International Congress on Hormones and Cancer,* Iacobelli, S., King, R. J. B., Linder, H. R., and Lippman, M. E., Eds., Raven Press, Rome, 1980, 67. With permission.

shown in Figure 4a. The rate of the cytolytic response is highly correlated with the receptor content, and the sensitivity of the hybrids increases with the number of receptor sites per cell. The hybrid containing a single dose of receptor (1 r⁺) is the most resistant, the number of living cells increasing for 30 hr, although lysis will eventually occur at later times. Figure 4b illustrates the sensitivity of these hybrids at lower dexamethasone concentrations. Again, there is a good correlation between their level of sensitivity and their receptor content. The hybrid containing a single receptor allele (1 r⁺) is the most resistant and, even at concentrations of dexamethasone of 5×10^{-8} M or above (data not shown), at which all receptor sites are saturated, this hybrid fails to show complete sensitivity. As mentioned earlier (see section IIIC), the considerable level of resistance of this hybrid could account for the selection of segregants from tetraploid S49 cells containing a single r⁺ allele, and which would be classified as "deathless" on the basis of their wild type receptor.

These results indicate that, in this model system, both the rate and extent of the cytolytic response depends on the steroid concentration and on the number of intracellular receptors: the concentration of receptor-steroid complexes limits this biological response. However, the lymphocytolytic response in mice, a glucocorticoid-sensitive species, may not be directly comparable to the inhibitory effects of glucocorticoids in humans, and the therapeutic benefits of glucocorticoids could involve other effects as well.

V. CONCLUDING REMARKS

The evidence is overwhelming that the acquisition of glucocorticoid resistance observed in vitro in three different T-lymphoid cell lines has a genetic basis. Although early studies in the S49 line were complicated by unsuspected functional hemizygosity and chromosome segregation events, these phenomena have now been recognized. Glucocorticoid resistance occurs at low frequencies that are dependent on cell ploidy and can be increased by various mutagens, including antitumor drugs. The resistant phenotype is associated with defects or alterations in the properties of a specific protein, the glucocorticoid receptor. Resistance, which is inheritable and stable in the absence of selection, can arise not only by mutations but also by chromosome segregation: this observation allowed the assignment of a gene encoding the glucocorticoid receptor to a specific chromosome of the mouse. Obviously, caution should be used in generalizing to humans the observations made with cells derived from the mouse, a glucocorticoid-sensitive species. However, the similarity between the results obtained in the human leukemic CEM-C7 line and in two murine lines, S49 and W7, is certainly striking.

The fact that glucocorticoid resistance can be acquired in two steps could have important clinical implications, because the r⁺/r⁻ hemizygous intermediates are resistant to low concentrations of glucocorticoids. Since such hemizygotes arise spontaneously at relatively high frequency, they are probably always present in vivo among the sensitive T-cell population. The presence of physiological concentrations of glucocorticoids would selectively enrich the population for these partially resistant cells. Fully resistant variants, arising spontaneously from such hemizygotes at a frequency on the order of 10^{-5}, could then be selected by pharmacological doses of glucocorticoids. This frequency could, possibly, be further increased if mutagenic antitumor drugs are used in combination therapies.

The absence of resistant variants resulting from defects in function(s) other than the glucocorticoid receptor is puzzling and as yet unexplained. Some possible interpretations of this observation have been mentioned in Section IIIC. The fact that receptor defects account for the resistance of all variants selected in vitro, together with the tight correlation observed in murine cell hybrids between receptor content and gluco-corticoid sensitivity, raises hopes that such a correlation might be uncovered in some lymphoproliferative diseases. However, acquisition of resistance by genetic events at the level of a locus encoding the receptor is certainly not the only mechanism playing a role in vivo: resistance is also acquired by epigenetic events taking place during the natural process of differentiation. Recent evidence from our laboratory indicates that resistance in a murine thymic lymphoma line, SAK8, appears to have an epigenetic origin and to be due to a defect in a function other than the receptor, since the gluco-corticoid receptor of SAK8 cells is functional and complements receptor defects in W7 (r^-/r^-) variants.[32]

ACKNOWLEDGMENTS

This work was supported by Grant GM20868 from the National Institutes of General Medical Sciences and by a grant from the Whitehall Foundation to Suzanne Bourgeois. Marianne Huet-Minkowski was an Exchange Scientist under the Hormone Regulation and Cancer Program Area of the U.S.-France (NCI-INSERM) Cancer Program, and Judith C. Gasson is recipient of fellowship AM06179 from the National Institute of Arthritis, Metabolic and Digestive Diseases.

REFERENCES

1. **Horibata, K. and Harris, A.W.**, Mouse myelomas and lymphomas in culture, *Exp. Cell Res.*, 60, 61, 1970.
2. **Harris, A. W., Bankhurst, A. D., Mason, S., and Warner, N. L.**, Differentiated functions expressed by cultured mouse lymphoma cells. II. θ antigen, surface immunoglobulin and a receptor for antibody on cells of a thymoma cell line, *J. Immunol.*, 110, 431, 1973.
3. **Thompson, E. A., Jr.**, Properties of cell culture line derived from lymphosarcoma P1798, *Molec. Cell. Endocrinol.*, 17, 95, 1980.
4. **Norman, M. R. and Thompson, E. B.**, Characterization of a glucocorticoid-sensitive human lymphoid cell line, *Cancer Res.*, 37, 3785, 1977.
5. **Burrow, H. M., Bird, C. C., Warren, J. V., Steel, C. M., Barrett, I. D., and Panesar, N. S.**, Human lymphoid cell lines and glucocorticoids: I. Characterization and cytolethal responses of lymphoblastoid, leukaemia and lymphoma lines, *Diagn. Histopathology*, 4, 175, 1981.
6. **Steel, C. M., Woodward, M. A., Davidson, C., Philipson, J., and Arthur, E.**, Non-random chromosome gains in human lymphoblastoid cell lines, *Nature (London)*, 270, 349, 1977.
7. **Sibley, C. H. and Tomkins, G. M.**, Isolation of lymphoma cell variants resistant to killing by glucocorticoids, *Cell*, 2, 213, 1974.
8. **Engel, E., McGee, B. J., and Harris, H.**, Recombination and segregation in somatic cell hybrids, *Nature (London)*, 223, 152, 1969.
9. **Harris, A. W. and Cohn, M.**, Physiology and genetics of some lymphoid cell functions, in *Developmental Aspects of Antibody Formation and Structure*, Sterzl, J. and Riha, I., Eds., Academia Publishing House of the Czechoslovak Academy of Sciences, Prague, 1970, 275.
10. **Bourgeois, S. and Newby, R.**, Diploid and haploid states of the glucocorticoid receptor gene of mouse lymphoid cell lines, *Cell*, 11, 423, 1977.
11. **Huet-Minkowski, M., Gasson, J. C., and Bourgeois, S.**, Induction of glucocorticoid resistant variants in a murine thymoma line by antitumor drugs, *Cancer Res.*, 41, 4540, 1981.
12. **Harris, A. W.**, Differentiated functions expressed by cultured mouse lymphoma cells, *Exp. Cell Res.*, 60, 341, 1970.
13. **Pfahl, M., Sandros, T., and Bourgeois, S.**, Interaction of glucocorticoid receptors from lymphoid cell lines with their nuclear acceptor sites, *Molec. Cell. Endocrinol.*, 10, 175, 1978.
14. **Sibley, C. H. and Tomkins, G. M.**, Mechanisms of steroid resistance, *Cell*, 2, 221, 1974.

15. Harmon, J., Norman, M., and Thompson, E. B., Human leukaemic cells in culture - A model system for the study of glucocorticoid-induced lymphocytolysis, in *Steroid Receptors and the Management of Cancer,* Thompson, E. B. and Lippman, M. E., Eds., CRC Press Inc., Boca Raton, Florida, 1979, 113.

16. Harmon, J. M. and Thompson, E. B., Isolation and characterization of dexamethasone-resistant mutants from human lymphoid cell line CEM-C7, *Molec. Cell. Biol.,* 1, 512, 1981.

17. Pfahl, M., Kelleher, R. J., and Bourgeois, S., General features of steroid resistance in lymphoid cell lines, *Molec. Cell. Endocrinol.,* 10, 193, 1978.

18. Bourgeois, S., Newby, R. F., and Huet, M., Glucocorticoid-resistance in murine lymphoma and thymoma lines, *Cancer Res.,* 38, 4279, 1978.

19. Cox, D. M., Birnie, S., and Tucker, D. N., The in vitro isolation and characterization of monosomic sublines derived from a colcemid-treated Chinese hamster cell population, *Cytogenet. Cell Genet.,* 17, 18, 1976.

20. Vig, B. K., Mutagenic effects of some anticancer antibiotics, *Cancer Chemother. Pharmacol.,* 3, 143, 1979.

21. Roberts, J. J., Sturrock, J. E., and Ward, K. N., The enhancement by caffeine of alkylation induced cell death, mutations and chromosome aberrations in Chinese hamster cells as a result of inhibition of post-replication DNA repair, *Mutation Res.,* 26, 129, 1974.

22. Bech-Hansen, N. T., Till, J. E., and Ling, V., Pleiotropic phenotype of colchicine-resistant CHO cells: Cross-resistance and collateral sensitivity, *J. Cell. Physiol.,* 88, 23, 1976.

23. Lalande, M. E., Ling, V., and Miller, R. G., Hoechst 33342 dye uptake as a probe of membrane permeability changes in mammalian cells, *Proc. Natl. Acad. Sci. USA,* 78, 363, 1981.

24. Brabbs, S. and Warr, J. R., Isolation and characterization of bleomycin-resistant clones of CHO cells, *Genet. Res. Camb.,* 34, 269, 1979.

25. Usubuchi, I., Sato, T. and Kudo, H., Mechanism of the development of resistance to mitomycin C in Hirosaki sarcoma, *Tohoku J. Exp. Med.,* 132, 237, 1980.

26. Yamamoto, K. R., Gehring, U., Stampfer, M. R., and Sibley, C. H., Genetic approaches to steroid hormone action, in *Recent Progress in Hormone Research,* Greep, R. O., Ed., Vol. 32, Academic Press, New York, 1976, 3.

27. Pfahl, M. and Bourgeois, S., Analysis of steroid resistance in lymphoid cell hybrids, *Somat. Cell Genet.,* 6, 63, 1980.

28. Schmidt, T. J., Harmon, J. M., and Thompson, E. B., "Activation labile" glucocorticoid receptor complexes of a steroid resistant variant of CEM-C7 human lymphoid cells, *Nature (London),* 286, 507, 1980.

29. Bourgeois, S. and Newby, R. F., Correlation between glucocorticoid receptor and cytolytic response of murine lymphoid cell lines, *Cancer Res.,* 39, 4749, 1979.

30. Bourgeois, S. and Newby, R. F., Genetic analysis of glucocorticoid action on lyphoid cell lines, in *First International Congress on Hormones and Cancer,* Iacobelli, S., King, R. J. B., Linder, H. R., and Lippman, M. E., Eds., Raven Press, Rome, 1980, 67.

31. Francke, U. and Gehring, U., Chromosome assignment of a murine glucocorticoid receptor gene (Grl-1) using intraspecies somatic cell hybrids, *Cell,* 22, 657, 1980.

32. Gasson, J. C. and Bourgeois, S., Genetic evidence for a function other than the receptor involved in the cytolytic response to dexamethasone, *J. Cell Biol.,* 91, 210a, 1981.

Chapter 5

BIOCHEMICAL ASPECTS OF ANDROGEN RESISTANCE

Paul S. Rennie

TABLE OF CONTENTS

I. INTRODUCTION

The role of endocrine therapy in the management of prostatic carcinoma is to inhibit the growth of androgen-dependent tumor cells through a reduction of the tissue levels of androgenic hormones. The success of this approach is determined first, by the degree to which the tumor cells require androgens for viability and growth, and second, by the effectiveness of the surgical or medical procedures used to lower the tissue concentration of androgens. The latter is generally achieved either by castration or by the administration of pharmacological doses of estrogens which reduces testicular androgen production primarily through the suppression of the circulating levels of luteinizing hormone. Additional endocrine manipulations which are occasionally used include adrenalectomy, pituitary ablation, or treatment with antiandrogens, such as cyproterone acetate.[1,2]

Most patients with advanced prostatic carcinoma are symptomatically improved after hormonal therapy. The response rate in unselected patients is between 60 to 80%,[3,4] although in only about one third of these cases is there objective evidence of tumor regression (i.e., a 50% reduction in the size of observed tumors). Furthermore, the duration over which tumor activity is controlled by these means is usually just two or three years.[1] Hence, while endocrine therapy is of definite palliative value in the treatment of prostatic cancer, its effect upon the length of patient survival is less certain.

The apparent failure of hormonal therapy to eradicate all prostatic tumor cells in a patient is largely due to the presence or emergence of androgen-resistant cells. In this context, androgen resistance is defined as the loss or decrease in sensitivity of cells, derived from an androgen-dependent organ, to respond to the growth modulating effects of androgens. While the primary etiological factors responsible for the development of the androgen-resistant phenotype have not been fully determined, there are several reports describing the characteristics associated with androgen resistance both at the cellular and molecular level. The purpose of this chapter is to discuss observations and theories relating to androgen resistance with the goal of providing an overview of the subject, as well as insight into the biochemical deletions or alterations most likely to cause androgen resistance in tumors.

II. A CELLULAR BASIS FOR ANDROGEN RESISTANCE

A. Tumor Progression

1. Tumor Progression and Androgen Resistance

The tendency of neoplastic cells to escape the regulating signals which are operational in the adult progenitor cells is termed tumor progression. The concept of tumor progression as originally formulated by Furth[5] and by Foulds[6,7] implies that an increased capacity to invade locally and metastasize, an increased growth rate, and a general reversion toward immaturity are phenotypic characteristics commonly acquired by malignancies.[8] As applied specifically to endocrine tumors, tumor progression refers to the transition from hormone sensitive to hormone-resistant growth.[7]

The development of hormone resistance may be an early event in the progression of individual tumors, although in many instances it appears to arise in association with either hormonal withdrawal therapy or tumor regression.[9] Noble has investigated the possible link between hormonal manipulations and tumor progression in studies with estrogen-dependent tumors of both the mammary gland[9] and the dorsal prostate gland[10] of Nb rats. In these experiments, the effects of complete estrogen withdrawal and fractional estrogen replacement on tumor progression to hormone resistance were compared. As anticipated tumor regression was observed after estrogen withdrawal but eventually the tumors regrew and were estrogen resistant. In those hosts which received low doses of estrogen, both tumor regression and tumor progression were reduced. Within this latter treatment group, a stationary growth pattern was achieved in some animals; none of these tumors progressed to estrogen resistance.

Recently, Noble[11,12] has extended these observations showing that estrogen-dependent prostatic tumors regress or cease to grow after treatment with the antiestrogen, tamoxifen, in the presence of estrogen. After prolonged administration of tamoxifen the tumors regrew but remained estrogen-dependent when transplanted. Together these results suggest first, that tumor regression per se does not accelerate tumor progression; second, that fractional hormone-replacement in many instances will block tumor progression; and third, that titration of the optimal dose necessary to prevent both tumor growth and tumor progression may potentially be best achieved by the combined administration of both hormone and antihormone.

2. Mechanisms for Tumor Progression

Although androgen resistance is a consequence of tumor progression, it is not clear whether the androgen resistance of a tumor represents the emergence of a particular clone in a heterogenous population of tumor cells or simply an adaptational response of a single clone to alterations in the cellular environment.

a. Clonal Selection

On the basis of cytogenetic, biochemical, and immunological studies, it is generally believed that most primary tumors originate from a single cell or clone.[13] However, despite an apparent unicellular origin, tumor heterogeneity has been noted with respect to growth and invasiveness,[14,15] drug resistance,[16] and a variety of other biochemical and molecular properties.[17-19] To account for tumor progression and tumor heterogeneity it has been postulated that irreversible mutations occur in the genomes of tumor cells, leading to the continual production and evolution of new, stable clones which successively predominate as a result of selective pressures in their cellular environment. According to this theory the rate of tumor progression is tied directly to the mutational rate, which in turn is a function of the genetic lability of the particular neoplasm. Since there is a strong correlation between chromosomal changes and tumor progression, and since many tumors have abnormal karyotypes, inherent genetic instability of neoplastic cells may account for their apparent rapid adjustment to environmental challenges.[13,20]

Another theory for tumor progression which is also based on clonal selection is that malignant transformation occurs simultaneously in more than one cell and as a result produces several unique tumor clones. As with the genetic mutational theory, environmental pressures and the properties of the individual clones will determine which clone predominates although the selection of phenotypes will be restricted since new clones are not being continually produced.

In support of at least limited tumor heterogeneity, kinetic studies with the Dunning rat tumor model have indicated that the R-3327-H tumor variant is composed of 80% androgen-sensitive and 20% androgen-resistant cells.[21,22] Progression to hormonal autonomy in this instance is due to the continuous, unhindered growth of the androgen-resistant clone. However, despite the attractiveness of clonal selection theories, they do not provide an adequate explanation of the observation made by Noble[9,10] that progression to hormone resistance can be delayed or prevented by the fractional replacement of hormones: a finding which is contrary to the inexorable progression to hormonal autonomy that would be predicted by clonal selection theories. Furthermore, it is not obvious what selective advantage favors, in rare instances, the clonal dominance of androgen-dependent tumor cells over those neoplastic cells which do not require androgens for growth.[23,24]

b. Epigenetic or Adaptive Changes

An alternative explanation to account for tumor progression proposes that environmental pressures induce changes in the morphological and functional properties of a tumor cell population through alterations in gene expression rather than through clonal selection. In instances where these adaptive changes are heritable and yet do not represent a permanent change in the genetic integrity of the cell, they are termed epigenetic changes.[25,26] Since this process implies stable but reversible changes in the malignant phenotype, there is the prospect of regulating or directing the state of differentiation of tumors. Examples of spontaneous or induced reversion of the malignant phenotype although infrequent, include the spontaneous differentiation of metastatic neuroblastomas into nonmalignant ganglion cells;[25] the induction of differentiation in teratocarcinomas in mice;[26] and the reversion of malignancy in myeloid leukaemia through the induction of normal cell differentiation by macrophage and granulocyte inducer.[27] Although less dramatic, the blocking of hormone resistance by fractional hormone replacement therapy is also consistent with an epigenetic or adaptive mechanism.

Uriel[8] has postulated that the increasingly malignant and autonomous character assumed by most cancer cells is achieved by unbalanced retrodifferentiation. Retrodifferentiation, defined as the reversion of cells toward stationary states with reduced complexity of structure and function, is a common adaptive process associated with normal cell regeneration and tissue repair. Uriel argues that in normal tissue, retrodifferentiation is followed by restoration to the original differentiated phenotype, whereas in neoplasia, the latter process does not occur; rather, the cells continue to divide and retain the adaptability conferred by the state of retrodifferentiation. As a result of sensitivity to the microenvironment the phenotypic expression of this adaptability may manifest itself in a degree of heterogeneity obscuring the monoclonal nature of a tumor.

As yet no judgment can be made as to whether hormone resistance evolves as a consequence of successive clonal selection or adaptive changes in a single clone. However, the distinction is important for future therapeutic considerations. If as a result of genetic instability or polycentric origins, a clone of hormone-resistant cells is present, then it is unlikely that endocrine therapy alone will prevent or alter tumor progression. On the other hand, if the tumor population is derived from a single clone of highly adaptable cells, then endocrine therapy can theoretically, at least, induce the expression of desirable, growth constraint mechanisms.

B. Homeostatic Constraint Mechanisms
1. Normal Constraint Mechanisms

On the basis of observations of the growth patterns of hormone sensitive cells, Bruchovsky and associates[28,29] have proposed a model in which the hormonal control of growth in a target tissue is ascribed to the expression of intrinsic cellular mechanisms. The three phases of growth, each of which are regulated by a separate homeostatic constraint mechanism, are termed initiation, negative feedback and autophagia. As shown in Figure 1, the growth responses of rat prostate to changes in the androgenic status of the animal are governed by these mechanisms. When the number of epithelial cells in the prostate is below normal, as is the case after a period of androgen withdrawal, administration of androgen will result in the initiation of DNA synthesis and cell proliferation. After restoration to the normal complement of cells in the organ,

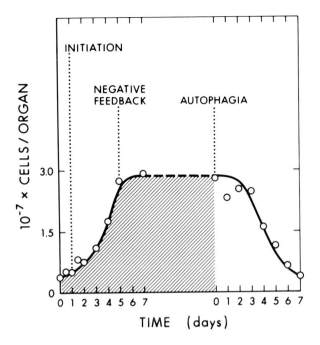

FIGURE 1. Basic responses of a hormone-sensitive organ. Groups of three to seven rats castrated 7 days previously were treated with daily doses of 400 μg of dihydrotestosterone/100 g body weight, and at various times the number of cells per prostate was determined by measuring the number of nuclei in glandular tissue. The shaded area under the curve indicates the period of hormonal treatment. (From Bruchovsky, N. and Lesser, B., *Adv. Sex Horm. Res.*, 2, 1, 1976. With permission.)

cell proliferation is curtailed by the activation of the negative feedback mechanism. With very high doses of androgen the cell number attained before negative feedback is activated is higher than normal.[30] In the continued presence of androgens, the size of the prostate is maintained. However, removal of circulating androgens activates the autophagic mechanisms which cause cell death and organ involution.

As a corollary to this model, Bruchovsky et al.[31] have postulated that the ability of a hormone-sensitive tissue to involute is a property acquired by these cells as a consequence of growth and maturation in the presence of appropriate hormones. In the case of the prostate gland, this capacity to involute is gained during pubertal development.[32] Although the autophagic mechanism is apparently induced by androgen, it is only activated by withdrawal of androgen. As is illustrated in Figure 2, this biphasic control of cellular autolysis connotes that androgens act both as agonists to induce the autophagic mechanism and antagonists to prevent its activation.

2. Relaxation of Constraint Mechanisms

Bruchovsky and Van Doorn[33] have formulated a series of theoretical growth curves (reproduced as Figure 3) for the anticipated responses of target-cell neoplasms to endocrine therapy in the context of deletions in one or more of the three homeostatic constraint mechanisms. In tumors where only negative feedback control has been deleted, DNA synthesis and cell proliferation are stimulated owing to the fact that initiation control remains responsive to the circulating androgens (Figure 3A). Withdrawal of hormones via castration or other means causes tumor regression since the auto-

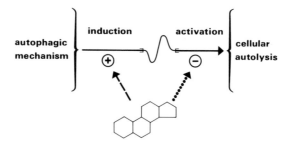

FIGURE 2.   Biphasic control of cellular autolysis. (From Bruchovsky, N. Rennie, P. S., Van Doorn, E., and Noble, R. L., *J. Toxicol. Environ. Health,* 4, 391, 1978. With permission.)

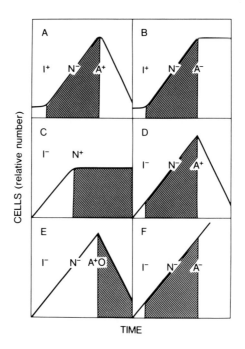

FIGURE 3.   Theoretical basic responses of neoplasms. Deletion of negative feedback (N) with or without further deletion of initiation (I) and autophagia (A) would have predictable consequences on growth patterns of cells as shown. Plus and minus symbols denote the presence and absence, respectively, of a given response; A'O indicates that the normally restricted pathway to cellular autolysis is unimpeded. (From Bruchovsky, N. and Van Doorn, E., *Recent Results in Cancer Research,* Springer-Verlag, Berlin, 1976. With permission.)

phagic control, which also remains intact, is activated. This pattern of androgen sensitivity has been observed in variants of the Shionogi mouse mammary carcinoma,[34,35] the prostatic adenocarcinoma of the Nb rat,[12,36] and in many prostatic tumors of humans.[1-3]

When both negative feedback and autophagic control are deleted, removal of androgens leads to a cessation of growth since the initiation control no longer receives the required hormonal stimulation (Figure 3B). While this type of response has been noted in some animal tumor models,[10,29,37] the fact that the tumor mass remains constant indicates that the successful response of a tumor to endocrine therapy is not limited to regression.[38] However, by clinical definition the slowing of growth would not be considered an objective response.

The growth patterns depicted in panels C, D, and E of Figure 3 predict the hypothetical growth responses of prostatic tumors to additive hormonal therapy, where androgens are given rather than removed. In the event that negative-feedback control remains intact (Figure 3C), it may be possible to achieve a stationary growth pattern, as observed in Noble's experiments,[9,10] by the administration of hormone. The acquisition of the autophagic mechanism through the conditioning effects of added hormone (Figure 3D) may account for the "rebound regression" which is occasionally observed after cessation of additive therapy in the treatment of metastatic breast cancer in postmenopausal women.[39,40] In cases where the administration of hormone directly results in tumor regression[39-41] (Figure 3E), the model would predict that the activation control of the biphasic autophagic mechanism, as outlined in Figure 2, has been deleted; thus the hormones act as agonists to induce the autophagic mechanism but not as antagonists to hinder its expression.

When all three homeostatic constraint mechanisms are lost, the growth of the tumor is completely refractory to androgens (Figure 3F). Since the emergence of androgen-resistant cells makes endocrine therapy ineffective and hence reduces the survival time of the host, a means of preserving or inducing dormant homeostatic constraint mechanisms would be of significant therapeutic value. The likelihood of achieving this goal is largely dependent on the nature and stability of the specific molecular changes that confer androgen resistance.

III. A MOLECULAR BASIS FOR ANDROGEN RESISTANCE

At present, it is not possible to clearly distinguish between those molecular changes which arise as a consequence of androgen resistance, from those which are related to the primary biochemical deletion or modification which directly causes androgen resistance. However, since the loss of androgen sensitivity is presumably related to a functional loss in a necessary component of the mechanism of action of androgens, most investigations in this area have attempted to dissect out the critical step in the biochemical events between the cellular uptake of hormone and the hormone-elicited response. A simplified scheme of the major steps in the mechanism of action of androgens is presented in Figure 4. In the blood, testosterone, the principal male sex hormone secreted by the testes, exists in equilibrium in an unbound form and a form bound to sex-hormone binding globulin (SHBG). Although most of the testosterone circulates as a steroid-protein complex, it is the unbound form that diffuses into cells. Upon entry into a target cell, testosterone is converted to dihydrotestosterone by the enzyme, 5α-reductase. Dihydrotestosterone binds with high affinity and specificity to a receptor protein in the cytoplasm to form an androgen-receptor complex which is then translocated into the target cell nucleus. During or after this process, the androgen-receptor complex is structurally modified. The binding of androgen-receptor complexes to specific chromatin loci, termed acceptor sites, is believed to be the definitive event which in some unknown manner, triggers the synthesis of specific mRNA molecules responsible for the appropriate cellular response. For a more comprehensive and detailed discussion of this mechanism, several excellent reviews are available.[28,42,43]

Within the framework of the mechanism of action of androgens four major categories of biochemical defects which may cause androgen resistance can be identified and are listed in Table 1. In each of these categories findings relevant to the development of androgen resistance are discussed below.

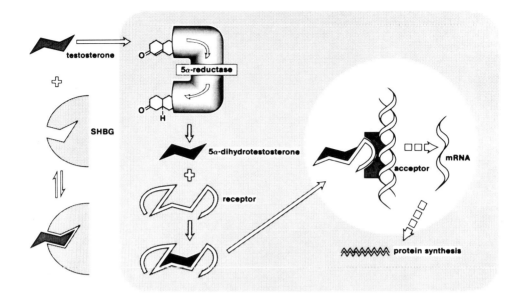

FIGURE 4.   Mechanism of action of androgens. (From Rennie, P. S. and Bruchovsky, N., *Male Accessory Sex Glands*, Vol. 4, Spring-Mills, E. and Hafez, E. S. E., Eds., Elsevier/North Holland Biomedical Press, Amsterdam, 1980. With permission.)

TABLE 1
BIOCHEMICAL CHANGES WHICH MAY CAUSE ANDROGEN RESISTANCE

A. Decreased Intracellular Concentration of Androgens
    Reductions in the transport of androgens
    Decreased enzyme activation of androgens
B. Failure to Interact with Active Site
    Reductions in the concentration of androgen receptors
    Dysfunctional androgen receptors
    Reduced nuclear uptake of androgen receptors
C. Reduced Direct Effect on Active Site
    Alterations in acceptor sites
    Increased concentration of acceptor sites
D. Development of Alternative Pathways
    Estrogen receptors
    Progesterone receptors

A. Decreased Intracellular Concentration of Androgens
1. Reduced Transport of Androgens
a. Transport in the Blood

In the plasma of sexually mature human males, the mean concentration of testosterone is approximately 500 ng/100 mℓ,[44] of which over 90% is bound to the serum protein, SHBG.[45,46] Since only the unbound form of steroid hormones is able to enter cells, the amount of testosterone and other androgens available to the target cells is, in part, regulated by the serum concentration of SHBG.[47] However, while the serum concentration of SHBG can be raised acutely by thyroid hormones[48] and reduced by androgens,[49] it is generally constant throughout adult life[49] and is probably not directly associated with the development of androgen resistance.

b. Permeability of the Plasma Membrane

The plasma membrane is the first site at which the target cell may regulate the passage of androgens into the cytoplasm. Owing to the lipophilic, nonionic character of steroids, it is assumed that steroids enter both target and nontarget cells indiscriminantly by passive diffusion. However, a differential uptake of androgens, estrogens, and steroidal antiandrogens has been observed in perfusion experiments with human and dog prostates in vitro.[50,51] While these results suggest the presence of a carrier-mediated process for the transport of steroids into the prostate, saturability of this carrier system could not be demonstrated; hence the existence of a facilitated diffusion or an active transport mechanism for steroid movement across the plasma membrane is doubtful.

After a study of the binding of estrogen to plasma membranes of rat uterine cells, Muller et al.[52] concluded that the membranes do not contain specific estrogen carrier proteins; rather the small number of estrogen-binding sites associated with uterine membranes is due entirely to contamination by cytosolic estrogen receptors. Furthermore, Giorgi and Stein[53] performed a detailed evaluation of the kinetics of steroid transport into cells and found that the passage of all steroids by passive diffusion alone occurs at such a fast rate and high capacity that it is unlikely that a supplementary transport mechanism would be a limiting factor in selectivity controlling the transport of any one hormone or determining its intracellular concentration.

Finally, if a carrier-mediated mechanism on the plasma membrane was of physiological importance for controlling the entry of steroids into target cells, then the occurrence of dysfunctional carriers as a result of mutations would yield cells with a restricted capacity to accumulated steroids in the cytoplasm. However, such mutations and their concomitant transport deficiencies have not been observed in either androgen- or other hormone-responsive tumor lines.[35,54] Thus the permeability of the plasma membrane is unlikely to be a critical factor in the development of androgen resistance.

2. Decreased Activation of Androgens

a. Activation by 5α-Reductase

After entry into the cytoplasm of a target cell, androgens are acted upon by cytoplasmic enzymes which metabolize these steroids through one or more steps to dihydrotestosterone.[55,56] The major metabolic pathways in this regard are shown in Figure 5. Since testosterone is normally the most plentiful androgen available, 5α-reductase (3-oxo-5α-steroid Δ4-dehydrogenase), the enzyme which irreversibly converts testosterone directly to dihydrotestosterone, assumes a key position for regulating the intracellular concentration of dihydrotestosterone. In general, the relative growth promoting potency of each androgen is correlated to the amount of intracellular dihydrotestosterone formed and subsequently incorporated into the target cell nucleus[28,29] Hence, any alterations in 5α-reductase activity will predictably affect the tissue accumulation of this androgen and ultimately cellular growth.

Benign prostatic hyperplasia (BPH), a disorder characterized by nonmalignant, hyperplastic growth of prostatic epithelial cells of men over 40 years of age, exemplifies a condition in which excessive tissue levels of dihydrotestosterone are linked to an elevated activity of 5α-reductase.[57-59] An example of results which support this relationship is presented in Figure 6. Paradoxically, the almost threefold elevation of 5α-reductase activity in BPH specimens relative to normal is wholly attributable to an increase in a stromal, rather than an epithelial form of this enzyme.[60-63] In normal, BPH, and carcinomatous prostates over 70% of the whole tissue level of 5α-reductase is in the stromal fraction, whereas other steroid metabolizing enzymes are more evenly divided between stroma and epithelium.[62] Since the Km of the epithelial enzyme in

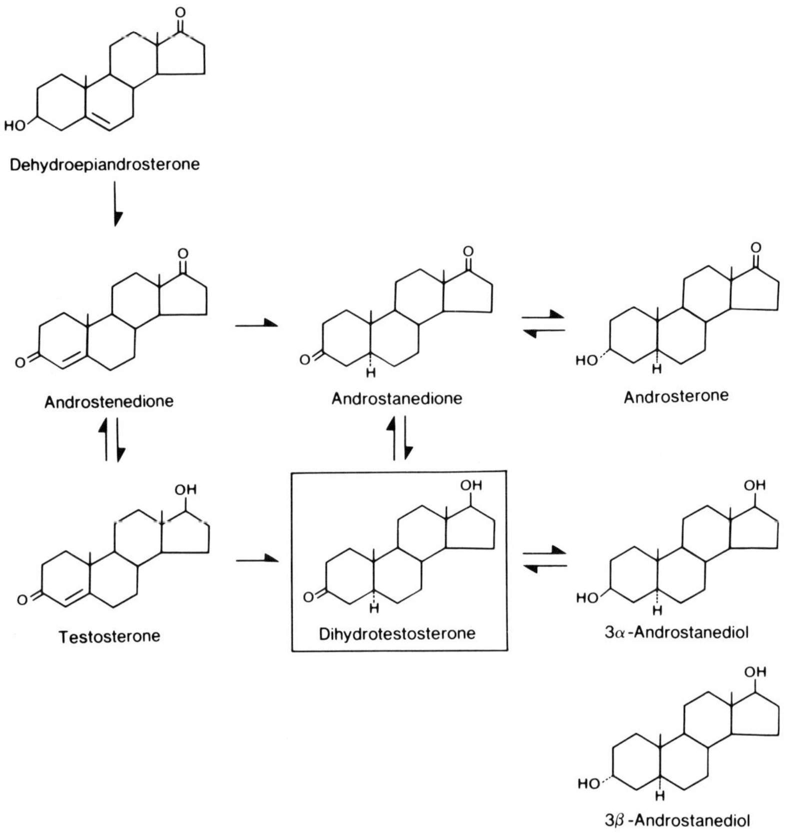

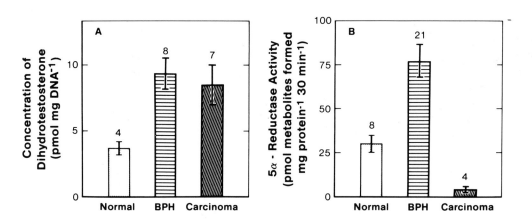

FIGURE 5.   Formation of dihydrotestosterone from natural androgens.

FIGURE 6.   Concentration of dihydrotestesterone and 5α-reductase activity in human prostate. Whole-tissue homogenates of prostatic tissue were analysed for (A) the concentration of dihydrotestesterone as determined by radioimmunoassay and (B) the activity of 5α-reductase. (From Bruchovsky, N., Rennie, P. S., and Wilkin, R. P., *Steroid Receptors, Metabolism and Prostatic Cancer,* Schroder, F. H. and DeVoogt, H. J., Eds., Excepta Medica, Amsterdam, 1980. With permission.)

BPH is close to the physiological concentration of testosterone in the blood, the functional significance of high stromal concentrations of 5α-reductase is not clear.[64] However, the latter finding supports McNeal's hypothesis[65] that prostatic stroma is involved in the initiation of the hyperplastic process.

The intracellular concentration of dihydrotestosterone is higher in prostatic carcinoma than in normal prostate (Figure 6), although the concentration of 5α-reductase activity is lower.[62,66,67] A reduced tissue level of 5α-reductase activity is also a common characteristic of many tumors in androgen target cells of animals.[68,69] Assays based on the measurement of 5α-reductase activity may permit discrimination between hyperplastic and neoplastic growth of the prostate, although their usefulness in the assessment of androgen resistance in tumors is less certain.[68,70,71] Since human prostatic tumors are able to retain higher than normal tissue concentrations of dihydrotestosterone despite reduced 5 α-reductase activity (Figure 6),[59,67] the cellular factors that regulate the retention of dihydrotestosterone are probably more involved with the intracellular concentration of active androgen than its rate of formation.

A decrease in 5α-reductase activity in target tissues has been implicated as the primary defect in the androgen resistance associated with one form of male pseudohermaphroditism.[72] 5α-Reductase can be readily detected in cultures of genital fibroblasts derived from normal males, but similar skin samples grown from individuals with the pseudohermaphrodite type 2 syndrome lack this enzyme.[73] Hence, while a direct connection between a deficiency in 5α-reductase activity and the androgen-resistant phenotype has not been observed in tumor cells, there is a biological precedent for this type of causal relationship.

b. Deactivation by 3α(β)-Hydroxysteroid Dehydrogenase

Owing to the irreversible nature of the 5α-reductase catalyzed reaction, the first step in the intracellular metabolic deactivation of dihydrotestosterone to less potent androgenic forms is conversion of dihydrotestosterone to either androstanedione or 3α-androstanediol (and to much lesser extent, 3β-androstanediol) by the enzmes 17β-hydroxysteroid dehydrogenase and 3α(β)-hydroxysteroid dehydrogenase respectively (Figure 5). In the prostate, the activity of the latter enzyme is higher than that of the former.[56] Since the reaction catalyzed by 3α(β)-hydroxysteroid dehydrogenase is reversible, the predominance of either the oxidative or reductive pathway will be determined by the availability of appropriate cofactors and steroid substrates.

In studies with normal, benign hyperplastic, and neoplastic prostates, 3α(β)-hydroxysteroid dehydrogenase activity was found to be evenly distributed between stroma and epithelium.[62,67] Moreover, unlike the fluctuations observed in 5α-reductase activity, the relative amounts of 3α(β)- hydroxysteroid dehydrogenase activity are approximately equivalent in each of these prostatic tissues.[67,74] At present there is no evidence that deactivation of dihydrotestosterone by steroid metabolizing enzymes is associated with androgen resistance.

B. Failure to Interact with the Active Site
1. Reduced Concentration of Androgen Receptors

Since the specific, high affinity binding of dihydrotestosterone to androgen receptors in the cytpolasm of target cells is fundamental to the mechanism of androgen action, a reduction or loss of androgen receptors should be indicative of androgen resistance. The finding that over 90% of human breast tumors which have low or undetectable levels of estrogen receptors are estrogen resistant, supports that hypothesis[75,76] However, since only 55-60% of breast tumors with a positive estrogen receptor test respond to endocrine therapy,[75,76] it cannot be assumed that the presence of steroid receptors is an absolute assurance of hormonal dependence.

Analyses of androgen receptors in cytoplasmic extracts from androgen-dependent and androgen-resistant tumor lines of both the Shionogi mammary carcinoma[35,68] and the Dunning prostatic carcinoma of Copenhagen rats[77] have substantiated the association of androgen resistance with decreased cytoplasmic concentrations of androgen receptors. However, while all the androgen-dependent variants of the Shionogi tumor lines have cytoplasmic androgen receptors, approximately 30% of the androgen-resistant tumors also have these proteins.[35]

The successful application of receptor assays for the detection of hormone resistance in human breast carcinomas and animal tumor models has provided a rationale for the measurement of androgen receptors in the cytoplasm of human prostates. Estimates of the concentration of androgen receptors in cytosolic extracts from hyperplastic, carcinomatous, and normal human prostates, which have been compiled from several different laboratories,[66,78-92] are presented in Table 2. From this tabulation it is evident that interpretation of this data is difficult because of differences in the manner in which the results are expressed, the lack of control studies dealing with normal prostate, and the wide interlaboratory variations in the values reported. While a precise estimate of the number of androgen receptors cannot be assigned to each type of tissue, the general trend implies that carcinomatous prostates have slightly lower concentrations of these molecules than do nonmalignant prostates. Since in most instances the carcinoma specimens were not subgrouped on the basis of androgen sensitivity, it is probable that many of the means listed in Table 2 are composites of both androgen-dependent and androgen-resistant tumors.

A direct relationship between androgen resistance and reductions in the cytoplasmic concentration of androgen receptors has not been unequivocally demonstrated with human prostate carcinomas.[93] One reason for this has been the technical problem of measuring androgen receptors in cytosol preparations which are invariably contaminated with serum SHBG, a protein which has an affinity for androgens similar to that of androgen receptors.[91] Since serum from rodents does not contain SHBG,[94] receptor measurements in tissues from these animals are somewhat less complicated. Fortunately, this problem has been largely solved by the introduction of the synthetic androgen, methyltrienolone (R1881), which binds with high affinity to androgen receptors but has a low affinity for SHBG.[78,95]

Another reason is that there are few reports in which the androgen-receptor status of individual tumors has been compared to the clinical response of the malignancy to endocrine therapy. Furthermore, with the data that is available there is no apparent consensus on the merits of androgen-receptor measurements as an index of androgen resistance in human prostatic tumors. Mobbs and associates[81] found that in cancer patients with low serum levels of androgens, a response to endocrine treatments was only observed when the concentration of androgen receptors in the prostatic cytoplasm was between 0.6 - 1.0 fmol/mg tissue; higher or lower values were indicative of androgen resistance. Similarly, Ekman et al.,[92] reported an 80% response rate to hormonal manipulations in patients with receptor positive prostatic carcinomas, whereas in patients with receptor negative tumors, only 20% responded. However, two other studies failed to demonstrate any consistent relationship between the quantity of androgen receptors in cytoplasmic extracts of human prostatic tumors and the response rate to endocrine therapy.[96,97] Clearly more data is required before a judgment can be made on the efficacy of androgen receptor measurements in the assessment of androgen resistance in human prostate carcinomas.

In contrast to ambiguities encountered with human prostatic tumors, a direct connection between an androgen-receptor deficiency and androgen resistance has been established in studies of testicular feminization (tfm); a form of male pseudoherma-

Table 2
CYTOSOLIC AND NUCLEAR CONCENTRATIONS
OF ANDROGEN RECEPTORS IN HUMAN
PROSTATE

A. CYTOSOL RECEPTOR

Prostate tissue	fmol/g tissue	fmol/mg Protein	fmol/mg DNA
BPH	120[a]	8 (0-20)[b]	566 (67-1270)[c]
	141 (7-250)[d]	12 (0-38)[e]	
	168 (0-320)[f]	27[g]	
	210 (0-640)[h]	35 (4-90)[c]	
	649[i]	46[j]	
	1380 (408-3460)[c]	48 (12-87)[i]	
		52[k]	
		80 (30-162)[l]	
Carcinoma	210 (0-480)[h]	20 (14-26)[b]	143 (51-318)[m]
	830 (287-2000)[m]	27 (8-74)[m]	
		31 (5-95)[c]	
Normal			609 (236-1120)[c]

B. NUCLEAR RECEPTOR

	fmol/g tissue	fmol/mg Protein	fmol/mg DNA
BPH	404 (138-555)[d]	39 (7-125)[n]	98[o]
	1638[j]	104 (40-151)[j]	127 (32-212)[p]
			290[k]
			765 (475-1324)[d]
Carcinoma	797[i]	80 (14-236)[n]	110 (75-138)[p]
		83[j]	269[j]
Normal		8 (6-10)[n]	112 (49-150)[p]

[a]　Bonne, C. and Raynaud, J. P., *Steroids,* 27, 497, 1976.
[b]　Snochowski, M., Pousette, A., Ekman, P., Bression, D., Andersson, L., Hogberg, B., and Gustafsson, J. A., *J. Clin. Endocrinol. Metab.,* 45, 920, 1977.
[c]　Ekman, P., Snochowski, M., Dahlberg, E., Bression, D., Hogberg, B., and Gustafsson, J. A., *J. Clin. Endocrinol. Metab.,* 49, 205, 1979.
[d]　Sirett, D. A. N. and Grant, J. K., *J. Endocrinol.,* 77, 101, 1978.
[e]　Krieg, M., Grobe, I., Voigt, K. D., Altenahr, E., and Klosterhalfen, H., *Acta Endocrinol.,* 88, 397, 1978.
[f]　Mobbs, B. G., Johnson, I. E., Connolly, J. G., and Clark, A. F., *J. Steroid Biochem.,* 8, 943, 1977.
[g]　Wagner, R. K., Schulze, K. H., and Jungblut, P. W., *Acta Endocrinol.,* Suppl., 193, 52, 1975.
[h]　Mobbs, B. G., Johnson, I. E., Connolly, J. G., and Clark, A. F., *J. Steroid Biochem.,* 9, 289, 1978.
[i]　Hicks, L. L. and Walsh, P. C. *Steroids,* 33, 389, 1979.
[j]　Menon, N., Tananis, C. E., Hicks, L. L., Hawkins, E. F., McLoughlin, M. G., and Walsh, P. C., *J. Clin. Invest.,* 61, 150, 1978.
[k]　Shain, S. A., Boesel, R. W., Lamm, D. L., and Radwin, H. M., *Steroids,* 31, 541, 1978.

Table 2 (continued)
CYTOSOLIC AND NUCLEAR CONCENTRATIONS OF ANDROGEN RECEPTORS IN HUMAN PROSTATE

l   Ghanadian, R., Auf, G., Chaloner, P. J., and Chisholm, G. D., *J. Steroid Biochem.*, 9, 325, 1978.

m   Ekman, P., Snochowski, M., Zetterberg, A., Hogberg, B., and Gustafsson, J. A., *Cancer (Philadelphia)*, 44, 1173, 1979.

n   Lehoux, J. G., Bernard, B., and Elhilali, M., *Arch. Androl.*, 5, 237, 1980.

o   Symes , E. K., Milroy, E. J. G., and Mainwaring, W. I. P., *J. Urol.*, 120, 180, 1978.

p   Rennie, P. S. and Bruchovsky, N., Male Accessory Sex Glands, *Human Reproductive Medicine*, 4, 265, 1980.

phroditism in which affected individuals have a male karyotype but a female phenotype. This condition may occur in several species including man and in most cases it has been shown that the androgen resistance is not due to a gonadal insufficiency but rather to an absence or a reduced concentration of androgen receptors in cytoplasm of the target cells.[98-100] In tfm mice, there is evidence that this disorder involves a mutation in an X-linked gene which regulates the production of androgen receptors.[101-103]

2. Dysfunctional Androgen Receptors

In addition to reductions in the cytoplasmic concentration of androgen receptors, androgen resistance may also be due to the production of abnormal forms of androgen receptors which fail to convey the necessary androgenic signal to the genome. In the Shionogi mouse mammary tumor system, altered molecular forms of androgen receptors have occasionally been observed in androgen-resistant lines.[35] However, molecular heterogeneity of androgen receptors as a primary cause or result of androgen resistance in neoplasms is probably unique to a few examples. In rat prostate multiple forms of androgen receptors have been observed, [104-106] although their recovery and molecular characteristics are strongly influenced by endogenous proteases[107,108] which complicate interpretation of these results. By most physiochemical and kinetic criteria, including estimates of equilibrium constants, androgen receptors isolated from the cytoplasm of human prostatic carcinomas and BPH samples are relatively homogeneous.[83-85,92]

Pinsky et al.[109] compared the physical and kinetic properties of androgen receptors isolated from genital skin fibroblasts cultured from patients with testicular feminization. In two patient samples with a normal complement of androgen receptors, a detailed examination of their receptors revealed subtle deviations from normal with respect to their rate constants for dissociation of dihydrotestosterone. In the absence of other detectable abnormalities, they concluded that such qualitative modifications of the androgen receptors are in some instances responsible for the androgen resistant phenotype.

3. Reduced Nuclear Uptake of Androgen Receptors

Since the nucleus is the cellular compartment in which androgen-receptor complexes initiate a response, the intranuclear presence of androgen receptors implies an intact and functional cellular apparatus for the processing of these molecules in the cytoplasm and for their translocation into the nucleus. Hence biochemical assays for androgen resistance which include the quantitation of both nuclear and cytoplasmic concentrations of androgen receptors are more informative than those involving measurement of cytoplasmic androgen receptors only.

Estimates of the nuclear concentration of androgen receptors in samples of human prostate tissue are shown in Table 2. As with measurements of cytoplasmic androgen receptors, there is a considerable range in the mean values of androgen receptors in nuclei from each of three types of prostate tissue. In the two examples where androgen receptors were measured in both the cytoplasm and nucleus, the nuclear concentration of these molecules is higher.[79,82] Carcinomatous nuclei generally have similar, or possibly lower, levels of androgen receptors than nuclei from BPH specimens.

Although there are no reports comparing the development of androgen resistance with the nuclear concentration of androgen receptors in human prostatic tumors, such comparisons have been made with the Shionogi carcinoma. Eleven variant lines of androgen-dependent and androgen-resistant Shionogi tumors were grouped into four classes on the basis of androgen requirements for growth, concentration of cytoplasmic receptor, uptake of androgens into the nucleus, and displaceable nuclear binding of androgens (Table 3).[35] All the androgen-dependent lines (Class 1) were positive for each of these biological markers. Class 2 tumors were androgen resistant and retained a normal complement of androgen receptors in the cytoplasm and a normal uptake of androgens into the nucleus but did not possess nuclear binding sites. Another androgen-resistant class (Class 3) lacked androgen receptors, nuclear uptake, and nuclear binding. A further androgen-resistant phenotype (Class 4) was deficient in cytoplasmic receptors and nuclear uptake of androgens, yet positive with respect to nuclear androgen-binding sites. Hence, when screening of these tumors included a test for both cytoplasmic androgen receptors and nuclear binding, androgen resistance could be predicted with 100% accuracy.

A study of androgen binding in nuclei from androgen-responsive and androgen-resistant prostatic tumors of Nb rats demonstrated a positive correlation between the concentration of receptors and androgen resistance.[110] Scatchard analysis of nuclear androgen-binding sites revealed that nuclei from the dorsal prostate have both high and low affinity sites, whereas nuclei from androgen responsive tumors derived from this organ, lack the high affinity sites and have reduced amounts of the low affinity sites. Nuclei from those tumors characterized by androgen-resistant growth had no high affinity sites and only trace amounts of the low affinity sites. These observations and those obtained with the Shionogi carcinoma suggest that reduced nuclear concentrations of androgen receptors are indicative of androgen resistance.

Radioimmunoassay measurements of androgens in nuclei from human and rat prostates have demonstrated that the nuclear concentration of dihydrotestosterone is several fold greater than the comparable nuclear concentration of androgen receptors,[67,111] With the latter tissue it was found that the nuclear concentration of androgen receptors is logarithmically related (correlation coefficient, 0.92) to the concentration of nuclear dihydrotestosterone.[111] Hence, while binding of androgens to receptors and the entry of dihydrotestosterone into target cell nuclei are probably closely linked events, it is less certain that the nuclear concentration of androgen is achieved solely through receptor-mediated processes. In view of the recent discovery of hormone-specific binding sites on the nuclear membrane[112,113] and nuclear matrix[114] of target cells, it is tempting to speculate that membrane or matrix sites are involved in the nuclear uptake of androgens. Since the retention of androgen receptors by chromatin is sensitive to fluctuations in the intranuclear concentration of dihydrotestosterone,[111,115] it is likely that the nuclear components responsible for ensuring high concentrations of this androgen will indirectly regulate receptor recycling.[116] Thus hypothetically, a type of androgen resistance may occur in cells which have an altered mechanism for the nuclear uptake of dihydrotestosterone.

Table 3
CLASSIFICATION OF ANDROGEN DEPENDENT AND RESISTANT
SHIONOGI TUMORS

Class	Growth	Cytoplasmic binding in vivo (molecules/cell)	Nuclear uptake in vivo (molecules/30 min/nucleus)	Displaceable nuclear binding in vitro (molecules/nucleus)	
				Control	After castration
1	Dependent	1400 ± 190 (25)	6500 ± 460 (43)	370 ± 70 (9)	10 ± 10 (3)
2	Resistant	1000 ± 370 (6)	7300 ± 660 (16)	80 ± 20 (3)	
3	Resistant	170 ± 30 (4)	400 ± 70 (5)	40 ± 20 (5)	
4	Resistant	180 ± 40 (8)	330 ± 70 (10)	380 ± 70 (8)	820 ± 220 (4)

Note: Values shown are mean ± SEM for the number of experiments in parentheses.

From Bruchovsky, N. and Rennie, P. S., *Cell,* 13, 273, 1978. With permission.

C. Reduced Direct Effect on Active Site
1. Altered Acceptor Sites

The two types of androgen-cell interactions which are considered basic to the mechanism of hormone action are: first, the binding of specific androgens to a cytoplasmic receptor; and second the binding of androgen receptor complexes to chromatin acceptor sites. It follows that a prostate tumor cell may have measurable androgen receptors but is androgen resistant due to nonfunctional or defective chromatin acceptor sites.

Relatively little is known concerning either the biochemical nature of acceptor sites or the molecular mechanism whereby these sites initiate specific cellular responses. Both DNA and chromosomal proteins have been implicated in the structure of the acceptor sites,[115,117-119] although specific DNA and protein components have not been isolated. Also it is uncertain whether there are discrete, heterogenous acceptor sites, each governing a particular response; or whether there is one class of relatively homogenous acceptor sites, whose degree of occupancy determines the type of cellular response.

In support for at least limited heterogeneity, Mainwaring et al.[118] found that nuclear extracts from rat prostate contain two distinct classes of acceptor sites — a small number of high affinity sites and a larger number of low affinity sites. Recently Davies et al.[119] reported that while there are almost 3 times as many acceptor sites in the transcriptionally inactive regions of the prostate genome than in the transcriptionally active fractions, the former sites had a lower affinity for androgen receptors than the latter. After reviewing the literature dealing with acceptor occupancy in hormone target cells and the initiation of mRNA synthesis, Leake[120] concluded that only about 2,000 of the occupied acceptor sites may actually be required for regulation of physiological responses; the remaining 8,000 to 18,000 may simply ensure sufficient availability of steroid hormone receptors in the nucleus.

In the regenerating rat prostate, the recruitment of cells into the growth fraction and the induction of 5α-reductase activity are both directly correlated to the average number of androgen receptors bound to the chromatin of each cell.[111] However, the induction of secretory acid phosphatase, a putative marker of differentiation,[121] is not directly synchronized with acceptor site occupancy. Rather, maximal activity of this enzyme is observed in the regenerating prostate when about 2,000 androgen receptors are bound to chromatin; as additional acceptor sites are filled the induction of secretory acid phosphatase is postponed and cell proliferation becomes the dominant response. When replication has ceased, due to activation of the negative feedback mechanism, secretory acid phosphatase,[31,111,121] is restored to its maximal activity. On the basis of these observations, it may be theoretically possible to induce desirable growth responses in prostatic neoplasms through differential titration of their acceptor sites.

At present there is insufficient data to prove whether there is a direct connection between aberrant acceptor sites and the development of hormone resistance. In the Shionogi carcinoma,[34,35] the prostatic adenocarcinoma of the Nb rat,[110] and many specimens of human prostatic tissue,[67,122] nuclear androgen receptors are recovered predominantly in a high molecular weight form. On the basis of measurements of association constant for androgens[35,110,122] and sensitivity to nucleases,[67,115] the large molecular form probably represents androgen receptors that are tightly bound to chromatin. Referring again to the results in Table 3, it is evident that the androgen resistance of classes 2 and 3 phenotypes is associated with reduced nuclear concentrations of androgen receptors due to either defective uptake and retention of receptors, or the absence of androgen receptors in the cytoplasm. On the other hand, Class 4 tumors have nuclear androgen binding sites that are similar in concentration to those measured in the androgen-dependent lines but different with respect to their sensitivity to androgen withdrawal. Unlike androgen-dependent tumors and normal rodent prostate,[116,123] the androgen receptors of the class 4 tumors are not recycled into the cytoplasm after castration.

Radioimmunoassays for dihydrotestosterone in nuclei from the class 4 variants of the Shionogi carcinoma indicate that these nuclei have the same endogenous concentration of dihydrotestosterone as do those from androgen dependent lines.[124] Although not evident in pulse experiments with radioactive androgens,[35,68] under steady state conditions dihydrotestosterone is able to enter the nucleus of the class 4 tumors but as a consequence of either reduced nuclear permeability or irreversible binding to acceptor sites, the androgen receptors are unable to exit. The nuclear trapping of androgen receptors presumably results in a constitutive form of constant androgenic stimulation which is unaffected by androgen withdrawal and is therefore, for practical purposes, androgen resistant.

2. Increased Concentration of Acceptor Sites

Since DNA is a major component of acceptor sites, any changes in the amount of DNA per cell will alter the functional domains which are under the control of these sites. Based on spectrophotometric analyses of DNA in prostatic carcinomas, a relationship between the cellular DNA content and the grade of malignancy has been inferred.[125] In a recent study using the technique of fluorometric flowcytometry with fine-needle aspirates of untreated prostatic tumors, it was found that the incidence of aneuploid DNA values increased with the degree of anaplasia.[126]

The results shown in Table 4 indicate that the average per nuclear concentration of DNA in specimens of well-differentiated, prostatic carcinoma is approximately twice that found in nuclei from normal human prostate. Owing to the higher amount of DNA in the carcinomatous nuclei, there is no apparent difference in the nuclear concentrations of dihydrotestosterone and androgen receptors in normal and neoplastic tissues when the estimates are normalized on a per mg of DNA basis. However, when this data is expressed as molecules per nucleus, the number of dihydrotestosterone and androgen receptor molecules in carcinomatous nuclei is almost double that measured in nuclei from normal prostate. These results imply that DNA exerts a positive influence on the nuclear retention of dihydrotestosterone and its receptor.

Whether the biological potency of the additional androgen receptors in nuclei of prostatic tumors is diluted or augmented by additional acceptor sites is not clear. Faithful duplication of the entire genome (polyploidy) presumably yields a ratio of recep-

Table 4

NUCLEAR CONCENTRATION OF ANDROGEN RECEPTORS AND
DIHYDROTESTOSTERONE

Tissue	DNA (pg/ nucleus)	Androgen receptors		Dihydrotestosterone	
		molecules/ nucleus	fmol/mg DNA	molecules/nucleus	fmol/mg DNA
Normal	15 ± 2 (4)	1000 ± 200 (5)	112	15,000 (2)	1670
Hyperplastic	18 ± 2 (12)	1400 ± 300 (11)	127	39,000 ± 3100 (8)	3540
Well-differentiated carcinoma	28 ± 3 (6)	1900 ± 200 (5)	110	25,000 ± 8000 (3)	1460

Note: Values shown are the mean ± SEM for the number of experiments in parentheses.

(From Rennie, P. S., and Bruchovsky, N., Male Accessory Sex Glands, Elsevier/North-Holland Biomedical Press, Amsterdam, 1980. With permission.)

tors: acceptors similar to that of the nonmalignant cell, whereas excess multiplication of only part of the genome (aneuploidy) will cause an imbalance in this ratio. As a consequence of this imbalance, regions of the genome will no longer be regulated by androgen receptors. Thus, the cells will escape androgenic control and become androgen resistant.

D. Development of Alternative Pathways

A further process through which androgen-dependent cells may lose their requirement for androgens is the development of alternative molecular pathways for growth regulation which are superimposed upon existing androgen responsive mechanisms. Since relatively little is known of the hormone-receptor specificity of acceptor sites and since receptors for nonandrogenic steroids have been detected in the prostate,[93] it is conceivable that under conditions of androgen deprivation other steroid receptor complexes may supplant or substitute for androgen receptors in stimulating the growth of the prostate. In this context, androgens would be redundant, and although the cells would still require steroid hormones for their maintenance and growth, phenotypically they would appear to be androgen resistant.

1. Estrogen Receptors

Although the prostate is not normally considered a target organ for estrogens, the occurrence of estrogen receptors in the cytoplasm of human and rat prostate has been reported.[83,85,127] Estrogen receptors have also been detected in primary carcinoma of the prostate,[85,96,97,128] but not in metastatic lesions.[129] The presence of estrogen receptors in BPH extracts has been demonstrated by some investigators,[63,85,96,130] but not by others,[83,131] and in one study,[63] a predominantly stromal localization of estrogen receptors was observed in this tissue.

There is some indication that the concentration of estrogen receptors in prostatic carcinomas is of clinical significance. De Voogt and Dingjan[96] reported that 3 out of 4 patients with prostate cancer who benefited from estrogen administration as a means of reducing circulating androgens, had tumors with a relatively high concentration of estrogen receptors prior to treatment. In a larger study, Sidh et al.[97] observed subjective and objective regression after endocrine treatment (estrogen administration, castration, or both) in 9 of 15 patients with prostatic tumors that had an estrogen binding capacity which exceeded that of the number of androgen binding sites. By contrast, the majority of those tumors that had an androgen binding capacity greater than the concentration of estrogen binding sites either remained stable (6 of 7 patients) or progressed (17 of 18 patients). One may speculate that high concentrations of estrogen receptors are not only a favorable prognostic marker but also an indication of a functioning estrogen receptor mechanism at the target cell level.

Whether estrogen receptors are biologically active in normal prostate is uncertain. Korenchevsky and Dennison[132,133] inferred that estrogens can partially inhibit involution of the prostate and that in this gland, they have a direct influence on stromal growth. A recent study by Corrales et al.[134] demonstrated that treatment of four-month-old Copenhagen rats with estradiol caused a twofold increase in the weight of the ventral prostates; however, this effect was not observed in older rats or in other strains of rats.

In some instances, the specific steroid requirements of a tumor can be changed from estrogens to androgens by manipulating the hormonal environment in which it matures. Noble reported[10,11] that after repeated androgen administration to Nb rats bearing estrogen-dependent prostatic tumors, which had regressed after removal of estrogen pellets, of the tumors that regrew, one line, Nb - 2Pr-A, was found to have switched its hormonal requirements from estrogen-dependent to androgen-responsive. Noble originally referred to this process as directed progression. A further example of this phenomenon is the production of an androgen-responsive tumor from an estrogen-dependent rat mammary carcinoma as described by Cutts.[135]

Although there are no reports of estrogen-dependent tumors arising from estrogen treated androgen-dependent tumors, the possibility that in some cases, androgen resistance is actually due to a switch to estrogen dependence as a consequence of prolonged estrogen therapy, cannot be discounted. Glick et al.[136] reported that 5 of 29 patients whose carcinomas of the prostate were refractory to prior hormonal manipulations with estrogens and castration, achieved an objective response to treatment with the antiestrogen, tamoxifen. However, since tamoxifen is, in vitro, an inhibitor of 5α-reductase activity,[137] and since the androgen responsive prostatic tumors of Nb rats also respond to tamoxifen,[11] the clinical observation may be due to the drug having anti-androgenic as well as antiestrogenic activity.

2. Progestin Receptors

Evidence documenting the occurrence of progesterone receptors in normal,[81,83] hyperplastic,[83,138,139] and carcinomatous prostates[129,140] has been without contradiction. As with the estrogen receptors in the prostate, the in vivo function of the progesterone receptors is not understood. In BPH specimens the concentration of progesterone receptors is apparently higher in stroma than in the epithelium[139] and also is correlated to the weight of the prostatic tissue.[141] However, there are no reports linking progesterone receptors to the outcome of endocrine therapy or to the development of androgen resistance.

IV. CONCLUSIONS

In neoplasms, the emergence of androgen resistant cells from a population of androgen dependent cells can be described in terms of both cellular and molecular events. At the cellular level, androgen resistance occurs as a result of tumor progression,[6,7] a process often associated with gradually decreasing cellular differentiation and increasing malignant and autonomous growth. Tumor progression is thought to be a consequence of either successive selection of individual clones or a sequence of adaptive or epigenetic accomodations of a single clone to its cellular environment. While it is uncertain which theory correctly accounts for the development of the androgen resistant phenotype, the observation that the onset of hormone resistance can be delayed or prevented by the fractional replacement of steroid hormones is contrary to the clonal selection theory of resistance.[9-12] Furthermore, the finding that the hormone require-ments of some animal tumors can be switched from estrogens to androgens[9,10,23,24] suggests that certain properties of neoplasms can be selectively manipulated by hor-monal treatments. Although this latter point does not prove that tumor progression occurs through an adaptive mechanism, it does imply that progression can be directed and that the malignant phenotype is not necessarily immutable.

Androgens and other steroid hormones are believed to regulate the growth of their target cells through the expression of three homeostatic constraint mechanisms (Figure 1),[28-30] which have been termed initiation of DNA synthesis, negative feedback, and autophagia. Using this model, patterns of abnormal cellular growth can be predicted on the basis of deletions in one or more of these intrinsic control mechanisms (Figure 3).[32] Since in most cases, tumors of androgen target tissues develop in hosts with nor-mal levels of circulating androgens, the original neoplastic transformation must in-volve the loss of negative feedback control which then permits unhindered stimulation of the initiation mechanism for DNA synthesis and cell proliferation. In the extreme case where all three constraint mechanisms are deleted, the cells are completely resist-ant to androgens. As most epithelial cells in nontarget tissues do not normally require androgens for viability, the loss of androgen sensitivity can be viewed as a reversion to a less specialized phenotype. Whether the constraint mechanisms are permanently lost or simply dormant in androgen resistant cells is not clear.

In terms of eradicating malignant cells and of gauging a clinical response to endo-crine therapy, a functioning autophagic mechanism is of major importance. In normal target tissues the capacity to undergo an autophagic response is acquired at puberty due to exposure to increased levels of circulating androgens.[32] Since activation of the autophagic mechanism is lethal, control of its expression must therefore be induced prior to the full maturation of this biphasic mechanism (Figure 2).[31] In the prostates of postpubertal animals inhibition of the autophagic mechanism is strongly correlated to the presence of androgen receptors in the nucleus whereas activation of autophagia occurs after androgen receptors move out of the nucleus and into the cytoplasm.[116,123] Since the *de novo* biosynthesis of androgen receptors is also stimulated by androgens, [116] it is likely then that the cellular production of these molecules precedes or is closely linked to the androgenic induction of the autophagic mechanism. Accordingly, only those cells that have demonstrable androgen receptors will retain the autophagic mech-anism.

In agreement with this prediction most tumors that are deficient in androgen recep-tors have also lost the capacity for autophagia.[35,68,77] However, the converse does not necessarily hold; many androgen resistant cells also have androgen receptors.[35] Thus diagnostically, the absence of androgen receptors in tumors, indicative of androgen resistance, conveys more information than their presence.

Since the acquisition of the autophagic mechanism in normal target tissues only occurs after maturation in the presence of hormone,[33] one might expect that neoplastic cells which grow in an androgen depleted environment may fail to develop this con-straint mechanism. The fact that hormone withdrawal therapy tends to accelerate tu-mor progression is in keeping with this hypothesis. Within the cell, any lesion in the pathway whereby androgens are normally processed and brought into direct contact with acceptor sites will also effectively reduce the androgenic stimulation of the cell and compromise the induction phase of the autophagic mechanism.

In the context of defined steps of androgen action in target cells, several biochemical events can be identified which may potentially limit the intracellular concentration and distribution of androgens. The most prominent agents in this regard are the androgen receptors. As mentioned, these molecules are presumed to play a key role in the regulation of autophagia as well as other intact constraint mechanisms.[116,123] In addition to a reduction in the cellular concentration of androgen receptors, the occurrence of dysfunctional forms of these proteins may also result in a diminished hormone stimulation of the genome.[109] Reductions in 5α-reductase activity will directly decrease the amount of dihydrotestosterone available to the receptors.[28,29] While deficiencies in this enzyme have been associated with congenital forms of androgen resistance,[72,73] it is less certain that 5α-reductase activity is a limiting factor in the development of this condition in neoplasms. Similarly, androgen resistance cannot, at present, be ascribed to changes in serum SHBG, the permeability of the plasma membrane, or increased metabolic reduction of dihydrotestosterone by the enzyme, 3α(β)-hydroxysteroid dehydrogenase — all of which could potentially alter the intracellular concentration of active androgen.

In tumors with an adequate concentration of androgen receptors, androgen resistance may be due to the failure of the receptors to interact successfully with the acceptor sites governing growth constraint mechanisms. On the basis of relative binding affinities three types of faulty receptor-acceptor interactions can be envisioned. First, the androgen receptors have a reduced affinity for the acceptor sites; consequently, they are unable to stimulate the genome and are also not retained within the nucleus. Second, the androgen receptors have an increased affinity for the acceptor sites; in this situation they provide a constant stimulation of DNA synthesis, as well as an inhibition of autophagia, and are unable to exit from the nucleus. Third, the androgen receptors have a normal affinity for the acceptor sites but the latter are not functionally integrated into the regions of the genome controlling the constraint mechanisms.

Examples illustrating each of the three types of aberrant interactions cannot be given with any degree of assurance since relatively little is known about the structural and functional characteristics of acceptor sites. However, pending a more complete knowledge of these sites, certain androgen resistant phenotypes have been observed that have properties consistent with defective acceptor sites. The class 2 tumors in Table 3 have androgen receptors which are not retained by nuclei possibly because of a reduced affinity for acceptor sites (type one interaction). The class 4 tumors in Table 3 have androgen receptors which are tightly bound to chromatin and which are unable to enter the cytoplasm (type two interaction). Since the synthesis of androgen receptors is induced by androgens, presumably through a mechanism involving specific acceptor sites, the general uncoupling of acceptor sites could also prevent induction and normal replenishment of these proteins. Thus the absence of androgen receptors in the class 3 tumors in Table 3 may be due to nonfunctional acceptor sites (type three interaction).

A modified version of the third type of interaction may occur in polypoid or aneuploid cells. In these cells the acceptor sites might continue to exercise control over the expression of large regions of the genome but not over the additional genetic material. In this hypothetical form of androgen resistance the number of androgen receptors per nucleus would probably equal that in nuclei of androgen dependent tumors whereas the concentration of androgen receptors on a per unit DNA basis would be lower. While evidence for this mechanism of hormone resistance has not been reported, prostatic tumors frequently have an elevated DNA content[125,126] and in well-differentiated carcinomas of the prostate, there is an apparent adjustment in the number of nuclear androgen receptors to compensate for increases in the concentration of DNA (Table 4).

While most forms of androgen resistance probably arise as a result of molecular changes associated with the mechanism of action of androgens, a further process may involve the development of an alternative pathway in which the hormone dependence of a tumor has changed from androgens to estrogens. In studies with animal tumor models the converse situation, the switching from estrogen to androgen responsiveness, has been observed after lengthy intervals of treatment with androgens.[10,11,135] Since many human prostate carcinomas contain high levels of estrogen receptors,[85,96,97,128] it is theoretically possible that these molecules may biologically substitute for androgen receptors during endocrine therapy with high doses of estrogens. However, even if such a transition can be induced, it is unlikely to be a common occurrence in human prostatic tumors since there are no clinical reports of tumor regressions following cessation of estrogen treatments, a result that would be expected in cases where the tumors had become estrogen dependent.

It is apparent that the cellular and molecular events directly responsible for the development of androgen resistance in neoplasms are not fully understood. Nevertheless, the information that is available suggests: first, that the androgen resistant state has many phenotypic variations; and second, that most, if not all androgen-resistant cells have defects involving aspects of androgen receptors and/or acceptor sites. Presumably assays based on both of the latter parameters would be of diagnostic value in accurately assessing the degree of androgen sensitivity retained by prostatic tumors and the likelihood of achieving tumor regression with endocrine therapy. Thus tests for androgen resistances would spare some patients from needless medical or surgical endocrine procedures and their associated morbidities.

If endocrine therapy is to have a major impact on the long-term survival of patients with prostatic cancer, it must be designed to reverse or to prevent the emergence of androgen-resistant cells. Whether precise knowledge of how androgen receptor-acceptor interactions regulate homeostatic constraint mechanisms will provide a means of fulfilling this goal is uncertain. However, there is some evidence that the malignant phenotype is not irreversible[25-27] and that the androgen-resistant phenotype in particular, can be blocked or delayed by careful conditioning with hormones alone or in combination with antihormones.[9-12] Conceivably, the hormonal titration of specific acceptor sites may provide a means for successfully preserving or activating dormant growth constraint mechanisms in tumors.

ACKNOWLEDGMENTS

I wish to thank Linda Wood for typing this manuscript. Financial assistance from the National Cancer Institute of Canada is gratefully acknowledged.

REFERENCES

1. Stoll, B. A. Endocrine therapy in cancer, *The Practitioner*, 222, 211, 1979.
2. Chisholm, G. D. and O'Donoghue, E. P. N., The nonsurgical treatment of prostatic carcinoma, *Vitam. Horm.*, 33, 377, 1975.
3. Brendler, H., Therapy with orchiectomy or estrogens or both, *JAMA*, 210, 1074, 1969.
4. Walsh, P. C., Physiologic basis for hormonal therapy in carcinoma of the prostate, *Urol. Clin. N. Amer.*, 2, 125, 1975.
5. Furth, J., Conditioned and autonomous neoplasms: a review, *Cancer Res.*, 13, 477, 1953.
6. Foulds, L., Mammary tumors in hybrid mice: Growth and progression of spontaneous tumors, *Br. J. Cancer*, 3, 345, 1949.
7. Foulds, L., The experimental study of tumor progression: a review, *Cancer Res.*, 14, 327, 1954.
8. Uriel, J., Cancer retrodifferentiation, and the myth of Faust, *Cancer Res.*, 36, 4269, 1976.

9. Noble, R. L., Hormonal control of growth and progression in tumors of Nb rats and a theory of action, *Cancer Res.,* 37, 82, 1977.
10. Noble, R. L., Sex steroids as a cause of adenocarcinoma of the dorsal prostate in Nb rats, and their influence on the growth of transplants, *Oncology,* 34, 138, 1977.
11. Noble, R. L., Development of androgen-stimulated transplants of Nb rat carcinoma of the dorsal prostate and their response to sex hormones and tamoxifen, *Cancer Res.,* 40, 3551, 1980.
12. Noble, R. L., Production of Nb rat carcinoma of the dorsal prostate and response of estrogen-dependent transplants to sex hormones and tamoxifen, *Cancer Res.,* 40, 3547, 1980.
13. Nowell, P. C., The clonal evolution of tumor cell populations, *Science,* 194, 23, 1976.
14. Schnabel, F. M., Concepts for systemic treatment of micrometastases, *Cancer (Philadelphia),* 35, 15, 1975.
15. Fidler, I. J., Tumor heterogeneity and the biology of cancer invasion and metabolism, *Cancer Res.,* 38, 2651, 1978.
16. Hakannson, L. and Troupe, C., On the presence within tumors of clones that differ in sensitivity to cytostatic drugs, *Acta Pathol. Microbiol. Scand. A,* 82, 32, 1974.
17. Sluyser, M. and Van Nie, R., Estrogen receptor content and hormone-responsive growth of mouse mammary tumors, *Cancer Res.,* 34, 3253, 1974.
18. Prehn, R. T., Analysis of antigenic heterogeneity within individual 3-methylcholanthrene-induced mouse sarcomas, *J. Natl. Cancer Inst.,* 45, 1039, 1970.
19. Killion, J. J. and Kollmorgen, G. M., Isolation of immunogenic tumor cells by affinity chromatography, *Nature (London),* 259, 674, 1976.
20. Kerbel, R. S., Implications of immunological heterogeneity of tumors, *Nature (London),* 280, 358, 1979.
21. Smolev, J., Heston, W., Scott, W. and Coffey, D., Characterization of the Dunning R-3327-H prostatic adenocarcinoma: An appropriate animal model for prostatic cancer, *Cancer Treat. Rept.,* 61, 273, 1977.
22. Smolev, J., Coffey, D., and Scott, W., Experimental models for the study of prostatic adenocarcinoma, *J. Urol.,* 118, 216, 1977.
23. Mineshita, T. and Yamaguchi, K., An androgen-dependent mouse mammary tumor, *Cancer Res.,* 25, 1168, 1965.
24. Kim, U. and Depowski, M. J., Progression from hormone dependence to autonomy in mammary tumors as an *in vivo* manifestation of sequential clonal selection, *Cancer Res.,* 35, 2068, 1975.
25. Stansly, P. G., Is there another approach to cancer therapy?-Workshop on the suppression of the malignant phenotype, *Cancer Res.,* 35, 1599, 1975.
26. Ponder, B. A. J., Genetics and Cancer, *Biochem. Biophys. Acta,* 605, 369, 1980.
27. Sachs, L., Control of normal cell differentiation and the phenotypic reversion of malignancy in myeloid leukaemia, *Nature (London),* 274, 535, 1978.
28. Bruchovsky, N., Lesser, B., Van Doorn, E., and Craven, S., Hormonal effects on cell proliferation in rat prostate, *Vitam. Horm.,* 33, 61, 1975.
29. Bruchovsky, N. and Lesser, B., Control of proliferative growth in androgen responsive organs and neoplasms, *Adv. Sex Horm. Res.,* 2, 1, 1976.
30. Isaacs, J. T. and Coffey, D. S., Androgenic control of prostatic growth: regulation of steroid levels, *UICC Technical Report Series,* 48, 112, 1979.
31. Bruchovsky, N., Rennie, P. S., Van Doorn, E., and Noble, R. L., Pathological growth of androgen sensitive tissues resulting from latent actions of steroid hormones, *J. Toxicol. Environ. Health,* 4, 391, 1978.
32. Brandes, D., The fine structure and histochemistry of prostatic glands in relation to sex hormones, *Int. Rev. Cytol.,* 20, 207, 1966.
33. Bruchovsky N. and Van Doorn, E., Steroid receptor proteins and regulation of growth in mammary tumors, in, *Recent Results in Cancer Research,* Vol. 57, St. Arneault, G., Band, P., and Israell, L., Eds., Springer-Verlag, Berlin, 1976, 121.
34. Bruchovsky, N., Sutherland, D. J. A., Meakin, J. W., and Minesita, T., Androgen receptors: relationship to growth response and to intracellular androgen transport in nine variant lines of the Shionogi mouse mammary carcinoma, *Biochem. Biophys. Acta,* 381, 61, 1975.
35. Bruchovsky, N. and Rennie, P. S., Classification of dependent and autonomous variants of Shionogi mammary carcinoma based on heterogenous patterns of androgen binding, *Cell,* 13, 273, 1978.
36. Noble, R. L., The development of prostatic adenocarcinoma in Nb rats following prolonged sex hormone administration, *Cancer Res.,* 37, 1929, 1977.
37. Noble, R. L. and Hoover, T., A classification of transplantable tumors in Nb rats controlled by estrogen from dormancy to autonomy, *Cancer Res.,* 35, 2935, 1975.
38. Bruchovsky, N. and Rennie, P. S., New considerations in the hormonal induction and regulation of animal tumors, *UICC Technical Report Series,* 48, 134, 1979.

39. Heuson, J. C., Hormones by administration, in *The Treatment of Breast Cancer*, Atkins H., Ed., University Park Press, Baltimore, 1974, 113.
40. Lee, Y. T. and Spratt, J. S., Rate of growth of soft tissue metastases of breast cancer, *Cancer (Philadelphia)*, 29, 344, 1972.
41. Stoll, B. A., *Hormonal Management in Breast Cancer*, Lippincott, Philadelphia, 1970, 13.
42. Liao, S., Cellular receptors and mechanisms of action of steroid hormones, *Int. Rev. Cytol.*, 41, 87, 1975.
43. Mainwaring, W. I. P., *The Mechanism of Action of Androgens, Monographs on Endocrinology, Vol. 10*, Springer-Verlag, New York, 1977, 1.
44. King, R. J. B. and Mainwaring, W. I. P., *Steroid-Cell Interactions*, Universty Park Press, Baltimore, 1974, 42.
45. Vermeulen, A. and Verdonck, L., Studies on the binding of testosterone to human plasma, *Steroids*, 11, 609, 1968.
46. Westphal, U., *Steroid-Protein Interactions, Monographs on Endocrinology, Vol. 4*, Springer-Verlag, New York, 1971, 1.
47. Lasnitzki, I. and Franklin, H. R., The influence of serum on the uptake, conversion and action of dihydrotestosterone in rat prostate glands in organ culture, *J. Endocrinol.*, 64, 289, 1975.
48. Dray, F., Mowszowicz, D., Ledru, M. J., Crepy, O., Delzant, G., and Sebaoun, J., Anomalies de l'affinite de liaison de testosterone dans le serum des sujects thyrotoxicosiques et dans le virilisme pilaire idiopathique, *Ann. Endocrinol. (Paris)*, Suppl., 30, 223, 1969.
49. DeMoor, P., Steeno, O., Heyns, W., and Van Baelen, H., The steroid binding beta-globulin in plasma: pathophysiological data, *Ann. Endocrinol. (Paris)*, Suppl., 30, 233, 1969.
50. Giorgi, E. P., Stewart, J. C., Grant, J. K., and Shirley, I. M., Androgen dynamics *in vitro* in the human prostate gland. Effect of oestradiol — 17β, *Biochem. J.*, 126, 107, 1972.
51. Giorgi, E. P., Studies on androgen transport into canine prostate *in vitro*, *J. Endocrinol.*, 68, 109, 1976.
52. Muller, R. E., Johnston, T. C., and Wotiz, H. H., Binding of estradiol to purified uterine plasma membranes, *J. Biol. Chem.*, 254, 7895, 1979.
53. Giorgi, E. P. and Stein, W. D., The transport of steroids into animal cells in culture, *Endocrinology*, 108, 688, 1981.
54. Higgins, S. J. and Gehring, U., Molecular mechanisms of steroid hormone action, *Adv. Cancer Res.*, 28, 313, 1978.
55. Bruchovsky, N. and Wilson, J. D., The conversion of testosterone to 5α-androstan-17β-ol-3-one by rat prostate *in vivo* and *in vitro*, *J. Biol. Chem.*, 243, 2012, 1968.
56. Bruchovsky, N., Comparison of the metabolites formed in rat prostate following the *in vivo* administration of seven natural androgens, *Endocrinology*, 89, 1212, 1971.
57. Siiteri, P. K. and Wilson, J. D., Dihydrotestosterone in prostatic hypertrophy. 1. The formation and content of dihydrotestosterone in the hypertrophic prostate of man, *J. Clin. Invest.*, 49, 1737, 1970.
58. Krieg, M., Bartsch, W., Herzer, S., Becker, H., and Voigt, K. D., Quantitation of androgen binding, androgen tissue levels, and sex hormone-binding globulin in prostate muscle and plasma of patients with benign prostatic hypertrophy, *Acta Endocrinol.*, 86, 200, 1977.
59. Geller, J., Albert, J., De la Vega, D., Loza, D., and Stoeltzing, W., Dihydrotestosterone concentration in prostate cancer tissue as a predictor of tumor differentiation and hormonal dependency, *Cancer Res.*, 38, 4349, 1978
60. Cowan, R. A., Cowan, S. K., Grant, J. K., and Elder, H. Y., Biochemical investigations of separated epithelial and stroma from benign hyperplastic prostatic tissue, *J. Endocrinol.*, 74, 111, 1977.
61. Sirett, D. A. N., Cowan, S. K., Janeczko, A. E., Grant, J. K., and Glen, E. S., Prostatic tissue distribution of 17β-hydroxy-5α-androstan-3-one and of androgen receptors in benign hyperplasia, *J. Steroid Biochem.*, 13, 723, 1980.
62. Wilkin, R. P., Bruchovsky, N., Shnitka, T. K., Rennie, P. S., and Comeau, T. L., Stromal 5α-reductase activity is elevated in benign prostatic hyperplasia, *Acta Endocrinol.*, 94, 284, 1980.
63. Krieg, M., Klotzl, G., Kaufmann, J., and Voigt, K. D., Stroma of human benign prostatic hyperplasia: preferential tissue for androgen metabolism and oestrogen binding, *Acta Endocrinol.*, 96, 422, 1981.
64. Bruchovsky, N., McLoughlin, M. G., Rennie, P. S., and To, M. P., Partial characterization of stromal and epithelial forms of 5α-reductase in human prostate, in press.
65. McNeal, J. E., Origin and evolution of benign prostatic enlargement, *Invest. Urol.*, 15, 340, 1978.
66. Krieg, M., Grobe, I., Voigt, K. D., Altenahr, E., and Klosterhalfen, H., Human prostatic carcinoma: significant differences in its androgen binding and metabolism compared to the human benign prostatic hypertrophy, *Acta Endocrinol.*, 88, 397, 1978.

67. Bruchovsky, N., Rennie, P. S., and Wilkin, R. P., New aspects of androgen action in prostatic cells: stromal localization of 5α-reductase, nuclear abundance of androstanolone and binding of receptor to linker deoxyribonucleic acid, in *Steroid Receptors, Metabolism and Prostatic Cancer*, Schroder, F. H., and De Voogt, H. J., Eds., Excepta Medica, Amsterdam, 1980, 57.

68. Bruchovsky, N. and Meakin, J. W., The metabolism and binding of testosterone in androgen-dependent and autonomous transplantable mouse mammory tumors, *Cancer Res.*, 33, 1689, 1973.

69. Shain, S. A., McCullough, B., Nitchuk, M., and Boesel, R. W., Prostate carcinogenesis in the AXC rat, *Oncology*, 34, 114, 1977.

70. Bruchovsky, N., Callaway, T., Lieskovsky, G., and Rennie, P. S., Markers of androgen action in human prostate: Potential use in the clinical assessment of prostatic carcinoma, in *Steroid Receptors and Hormone Dependent Neoplasia*, Wittliff, J. L. and Depunt, O., Eds., Masson Publishing, New York, 1980, 121.

71. Krieg, M., Bartsch, W., Janssen, W., and Voigt, K. D., A comparative study of binding, metabolism and endogenous levels of androgens in normal, hyperplastic and carcinomatous human prostate, *J. Steroid Biochem.*, 11, 615, 1979.

72. Walsh, P. C., Madden, J. D., Harrod, M. J., Goldstein, J. L., McDonald, P. C., and Wilson, J D., Familial incomplete male pseudohermaphroditism, type 2. Decreased dihydrotestosterone for mation in pseudovaginal perineoscrotal hypospadias, *N. Engl. J. Med.*, 291, 944, 1974.

73. Moore, R. J., Griffin, J. E., and Wilson, J. D., Diminished 5α-reductase activity in extracts of fibroblasts cultured from patients with familial incomplete male pseudohermaphroditism, type 2, *J. Biol. Chem.*, 250, 7168, 1975.

74. Bruchovsky, N. and Lieskovsky, G., Increased ratio of 5α-reductase: 3α(β)-hydroxysteroid dihydrogenase activities in the hyperplastic human prostate, *J. Endocrinol.*, 80, 289, 1979.

75. McGuire, W. L., Current status of estrogen receptors in human breast cancer, *Cancer*, 36, 638, 1975.

76. Bruchovsky, N., Rennie, P., and Van Doorn, E., Estrogen receptors — can they predict tumor response to hormone therapy?, *Mod. Med.*, 46, 64, 1978.

77. Isaacs, J. T. and Coffey, D. S., Spontaneous animal models for prostatic cancer, *UICC Technical Report Series*, 48, 195, 1979.

78. Bonne C. and Raynaud, J. P., Assay of androgen binding sites by exchange with methyltreienolone (R1881), *Steroids*, 27, 497, 1976.

79. Sirett, D. A. N. and Grant, J. K., Androgen binding in cytosols and nuclei of human benign hyperplastic prostatic tissue, *J. Endocrinol.*, 77, 101, 1978.

80. Mobbs, B. G., Johnson, I. E., Connolly, J. G., and Clark, A. F., Evaluation of the use of cyperoterone acetate competition to distinguish between high-affinity binding of [³H] dihydrotestosterone to human prostate cytosol receptors and to sex hormone-binding globulin, *J. Steroid Biochem.*, 8, 943, 1977.

81. Mobbs, B. G., Johnson, I. E., Connolly, J. G., and Clark, A. F., Androgen receptor assay in human benign and malignant prostatic tumor cytosol using protamine sulphate precipitation, *J. Steroid Biochem.*, 9, 289, 1978.

82. Hicks, L. L. and Walsh, P. C., A microassay for the measurement of androgen receptors in human prostatic tissue, *Steroids*, 33, 389, 1979.

83. Ekman, P., Snochowski, M., Dahlberg, E., Bression, D., Hogberg, B., and Gustafsson, J. A., Steroid receptor content in cytosol from normal and hyperplastic human prostates, *J. Clin. Endocrinol. Metab.*, 49, 205, 1979.

84. Snochowski, M., Pousette, A., Ekman, P., Bression, D., Andersson, L., Hogberg, B., and Gustafsson, J. A., Characterization and measurement of the androgen receptor in human benign prostatic hyperplasia and prostatic carcinoma, *J. Clin. Endocrinol. Metab.*, 45, 920, 1977.

85. Wagner, R. K., Schulze, K. H., and Jungblut, P. W., Estrogen and androgen receptor in human prostate and prostatic tumor tissue, *Acta Endocrinol.*, Suppl., 193, 52, 1975.

86. Menon, N., Tananis, C. E., Hicks, L. L., Hawkins, E. F., McLoughlin, M. G., and Walsh, P. C., Characterization of the binding of a potent synthetic androgen, melhyltrienolone (R1881) to human tissues, *J. Clin. Invest.*, 61, 150, 1978.

87. Shain, S. A., Boesel, R. W., Lamm, D. L., and Radwin, H. M., Characterization of unoccupied (R) and occupied (RA) androgen binding components of the hyperplastic human prostate, *Steroids*, 31, 541, 1978.

88. Ghanadian, R., Auf, G., Chaloner, P. J., and Chisholm, G. D., The use of methytrienolone in the measurement of the free and bound cytoplasmic receptors for dihydrotestosterone in benign hypertrophied human prostate, *J. Steroid Biochem.*, 9, 325, 1978.

89. Lehoux J. G., Bénard, B., and Elhilali, M., Dihydrotestosterone receptors in human prostate. I. Nuclear concentration in normal, benign, and malignant tissues, *Arch. Androl.*, 5, 237, 1980.

90. Symes, E. K., Milroy, E. J. G., and Mainwaring, W. I. P., The nuclear uptake of androgen by human benign prostate *in vitro:* action of antiandrogens, *J. Urol.*, 120, 180, 1978.

91. Rennie, P. S. and Bruchovsky, N., Measurement of androgen receptors, in *Male Accessory Sex Glands, Human Reproductive Medicine,* Vol. 4, Spring-Mills, E. and Hafez, E. S. E., Eds., Elsevier/North-Holland Biomedical Press, Amsterdam, 1980, 265.

92. Ekman, P., Snochowski, M., Zetterberg, A., Hogberg, B., and Gustafsson, J. A., Steroid receptor content in human prostatic carcinoma and response to endocrine therapy, *Cancer (Philadelphia),* 44, 1173, 1979.

93. Rennie, P. S. and Bruchovsky N., Hormone receptors in prostatic tissue, in, *Research on Steroids,* Vol. 9, Proceedings of the Ninth Meeting of the International Study Group for Steroid Hormones, Adercreutz, H., Bulbrook, R. D., Van der Molen, M. J. Vermeulen, A., and Sicarra, F., Eds., Excerpta Medica, Amsterdam, 1980, 120.

94. Murphy, B. E. P., Binding of testosterone and estradiol in plasma, *Canad. J. Biochem.,* 46, 299, 1968.

95. Ojasoo, T. and Raynaud, J-P., Unique steroid congeners for receptor studies, *Cancer Res.,* 38, 4186, 1978.

96. De Voogt, J. H. and Dingjan, P., Steroid receptors in human prostatic cancer. A preliminary evaluation, *Urol. Res.,* 6, 151, 1978.

97. Sidh, S. M., Young, J. D., Karmi, S. A., Powder, J. R., and Bashirelahi, N., Adenocarcinoma of prostate: Role of 17β-estradiol and 5α-dihydrotestosterone binding proteins, *Urology,* 13, 597, 1979.

98. Bullock, L. P., Bardin, C. W., and Ohno, S., The androgen insensitive mouse: absence of intranuclear androgen retention in the kidney, *Biochem. Biophys. Res. Commun.,* 44, 1537, 1971.

99. Stanley, A. J., Gumbreck, L. G., Allison, J. E., and Easley, R. B., Male pseudohermaphroditism in the laboratory rat, *Recent Prog. Horm. Res.,* 29, 43, 1973.

100. Attardi, B. and Ohno, S., Cytosol androgen receptor from kidney of normal and testicular feminized (Tfm) mice, *Cell,* 2, 205, 1974.

101. Lyon, M. F. and Hawkes, S. G., X-linked gene for testicular feminisation in the mouse, *Nature (London),* 227, 1217, 1970.

102. Ohno, S., Simplicity of mammalian regulatory systems inferred by single gene determination of sex phenotypes, *Nature (London),* 234, 134, 1971.

103. Ohno, S., Major regulatory genes for mammalian sexual development, *Cell,* 7, 315, 1976.

104. Rennie, P. and Bruchovsky, N., *In vitro* and *in vivo* studies on the functional significance of androgen receptors in rat prostate, *J. Biol. Chem.,* 247, 1546, 1972.

105. Katsumata, M. and Goldman, A. S., Separation of multiple dihydrotestosterone receptors in rat ventral prostate by a novel micro-method of electrofocusing. Blocking action of cyproterone acetate and uptake by nuclear chromatin, *Biochem. Biophys. Acta,* 359, 112, 1974.

106. Lea, O. A., Wilson, E. M., and French, F. S., Characterization of different forms of androgen receptor, *Endocrinology,* 105, 1350, 1979.

107. Bruchovsky, N. and Craven, S., Prostatic involution: effect on androgen receptors and intracellular androgen transport, *Biochem. Biophys. Res. Commun.,* 62, 837, 1975.

108. Wilson, E. M. and French, F. S., Effects of proteases and protease inibitors on the 4.5S and 8S androgen receptor, *J. Biol. Chem.,* 254, 6310, 1979.

109. Pinsky, L., Kaufman, M., and Summitt, R. L., Congenital androgen insensitivity due to a qualitatively abnormal androgen receptor, In Press.

110. Rennie, P. S., Bruchovsky, N., Noble, R. L., and Mo, S., Nuclear binding of androgens and acid phosphatase activity in prostatic tumors of Nb rats, *Biochem. Biophys. Acta,* 632, 428, 1980.

111. De Larminat, M-A., Rennie, P. S., and Bruchovsky, N., Radioimmunoassay measurements of nuclear dihydrotestosterone in rat prostate: relationship to androgen receptors and androgen-regulated responses, *Biochem. J.,* 200, 465, 1981.

112. Lefebvre, Y. A. and Novosad, Z., Binding of androgens to a nuclear-envelope fraction from the rat ventral prostate, *Biochem. J.,* 186, 641, 1980.

113. Smith, P. and Von Holt, C., Interaction of the activated cytoplasmic glucocorticord hormone receptor complex with the nuclear envelope, *Biochemistry,* 20, 2900, 1981.

114. Barrack, E. R. and Coffey, D. S., The specific binding of estrogens and androgens to the nuclear matrix of sex hormone responsive tissues, *J. Biol. Chem.,* 255, 7265, 1980.

115. Rennie, P. S., Binding of androgen receptor to prostatic chromatin requires intact linker DNA, *J. Biol. Chem.,* 254, 3947, 1979.

116. Van Doorn, E. and Bruchovsky, N., Mechanisms of replenishment of nuclear androgen receptor in rat ventral prostate, *Biochem. J.,* 174, 9, 1978.

117. Mainwaring, W. I. P. and Mangan, F. R., The specific binding of steroid-receptor complexes to DNA: evidence from androgen receptors in rat prostate, *Adv. Biosci.,* 7, 165, 1971.

118. Mainwaring, W. I. P., Symes, E. K., and Higgins, S. J., Nuclear components responsible for the retention of steroid-receptor complexes especially from the standpoint of the specificity of hormonal responses, *Biochem. J.,* 156, 129, 1976.

119. Davies, P., Thomas, P., Borthwick, N. M., and Giles, M. G., Distribution of acceptor sites for androgen-receptor complexes between transcriptionally active and inactive fractions of rat ventral prostate chromatin, *J. Endocrinol.*, 87, 225, 1980.
120. Leake, R. E., Problems associated with dose response in steroid-hormone activation of structural genes, *Molec. Cells Endocrinol.*, 21, 1, 1981.
121. Rennie, P. S., Bruchovsky, N., and Hook, S. L., Androgenic regulation of a tissue specific isoenzyme of acid phosphatase in rat ventral prostate, *J. Steroid Biochem.*, 9, 585, 1978.
122. Lieskovsky, G. and Bruchovsky, N., Assay of nuclear androgen receptor in human prostate, *J. Urol.*, 121, 54, 1979.
123. Van Doorn, E., Craven, S., and Bruchovsky, N., The relationship between androgen receptors and the hormonally controlled responses of rat ventral prostate, *Biochem. J.*, 160, 11, 1976.
124. Bruchovsky, N., personal communication, 1981.
125. Tavares, A. S., Costa, J., and Costa Maia, J., Correlation between ploidy and prognosis in prostatic carcinoma, *J. Urol.*, 109, 676, 1973.
126. Rönström, L., Tribukait, B., and Esposti, P-L., DNA pattern and cytological findings in fine-needle aspirates of untreated prostatic tumors. A flowcytofluorometric study, *The Prostate*, 2, 79, 1981.
127. Dubois, R., Dubé, J. Y., and Tremblay, R. R., Presence of three different estradiol binding proteins in rat prostate cytosol, *J. Steroid Biochem.*, 13, 1467, 1980.
128. Bashirelahi, N. and Young, J. D., Specific binding protein for 17β-estradiol in prostate with adeno-carcinoma, *Urology*, 8, 553, 1976.
129. Ekman, P., Snochowski, M., Dahlberg, E., and Gustafsson, J-A., Steroid receptors in metastatic carcinoma of the human prostate, *Europ. J. Cancer*, 15, 257, 1979.
130. Hawkins, E. F., Nijs, M., and Brassinne, C., Steroid receptors in human prostate. 2. Some properties of the estrophilic molecule of benign prostatic hypertrophy, *Biochem. Biophys. Res. Commun.*, 70, 854, 1976.
131. Murphy, J. B., Emmott, R. C., Hicks, L. L., and Walsh, P. C., Estrogen receptors in the human prostate, seminal vesicle, epididymis, testis, and genital skin: a marker for estrogen-responsive tissues, *J. Clin. Endocrinol. Metab.*, 50, 938, 1980.
132. Korenchevsky, V. and Dennison, M., The effect on oestrone on normal and castrated male rats, *Biochem. J.*, 28, 1474, 1934.
133. Korenchevsky, V. and Dennison, M., Histological changes in organs of rats injected with oestrone alone or simultaneously with oestrone and testicular hormone, *J. Pathol. Bacteriol.*, 41, 323, 1935.
134. Corrales, J. J., Hoisaeter, P. A., Kadohama, N., Murphy, G. P., and Sandberg, A. A., A model for studies on the response of the ventral prostate to oestrogens, *Acta Endocrinol.*, 97, 125, 1981.
135. Cutts, J. H., Unusual response to androgen of estrogen dependent mammary tumors, *J. Natl. Cancer Inst.*, 42, 485, 1969.
136. Glick, J. H., Wein, A., Padavic, K., Negendank, W., Harris, D. and Brodovsky, H., Tamoxifen in refractory metastatic carcinoma of the prostate, *Cancer Treat. Rep.*, 64, 813, 1980.
137. Habib, F. K., Rafati, G., Robinson, M. R. G., and Stitch, S. R., Effects of tamoxifen on the binding and metabolism of testosterone in human prostatic tissue and plasma *in vitro*, *J. Endocrinol.*, 83, 369, 1979.
138. Asselin, J., Labrie, F., Gourdeau, Y., Bonne, C., and Raynaud, J-P., Binding of [³H] methyltrien-olone (R1881) in rat prostate and human benign prostatic hypertrophy (BPH), *Steroids*, 28, 449, 1976.
139. Cowan, R. A., Cowan, S. K., and Grant, J. K., Binding of methyltrienolone (R1881) to a progester-one receptor-like component of human prostatic cytosol, *J. Endocrinol.*, 74, 281, 1977.
140. Gustafsson, J-A., Ekman, P., Pousette, A., Snochowski, M., and Högberg, B., Demonstration of a progestin receptor in human benign prostatic hyperplasia and prostatic carcinoma, *Invest. Urol.*, 15, 361, 1978.
141. Tilley, W. D., Keightley, D. D., and Marshall, V. R., Oestrogen and progesterone receptors in benign prostatic hyperplasia in humans, *J. Steroid Biochem.*, 13, 395, 1980.

Chapter 6

BIOCHEMICAL ASPECTS OF ESTROGEN RESISTANCE IN MAMMARY TUMORS

Pierre Paul Baskevitch and Henri Rochefort

TABLE OF CONTENTS

I. INTRODUCTION

It is now well-established that estrogens are promoters for the induction of mammary tumors and that in vivo the growth of some human breast cancers is stimulated by ovarian hormones.[1] Hormone dependence in mammary tumors has been studied in experimental animal tumors induced by chemical carcinogens such as: 7,12-dimethylbenz(a) anthracene (DMBA); 3-methylcholanthrene (MCA); nitrosomethylurea (NMU); or by oncogenic viruses such as MMTV (mouse mammary tumor virus) (Table 1). Taking advantage of the recent progress in the understanding of the mechanism of action of estrogens,[2,3] we will review the work that has been performed on experimentally induced tumors with the aim of explaining why some breast cancers have lost their sensitivity to estrogens. In this chapter, estrogen resistance is loosely defined as the inability of malignant cells to be stimulated by estrogens. We recognize that this is a minimal criterion since hormone dependence may also encompass growth retardation and regression as described later in this chapter and also in Chapters 5 and 8.

II. TUMOR PROGRESSION FROM ESTROGEN DEPENDENCE TO ESTROGEN RESISTANCE

It is generally agreed that estrogens are required for the induction of breast cancer, and that most epithelial mammary cells are estrogen-responsive at that time. The mechanism of estrogen resistance of mammary tumors might, therefore, be found during the evolution of an already developed tumor.[4] It is important to understand the mechanism of the transition from a hormone-responsive tumor into a hormone-unresponsive tumor, in order to be able to avoid and eventually to reverse progression. Tumor progression is generally considered as the transition of a tumor "from bad to worse"[4] since the prognosis of estrogen-independent cancer is worse than that of estrogen-dependent cancer. Hormone resistance is a property of the tumor and not of the organism, which may bear both hormone-dependent and independent tumors, as has been shown in the rat DMBA model.[5] Progression is considered as evolutive and the resistant state as irreversible.

Several hypotheses have been raised in an attempt to explain the cellular process by which a hormone-dependent mammary tumor becomes independent. The tumor may start with several clones of hormone-dependent and independent cells. More likely, the tumor is first monoclonal, well-differentiated and hormone-responsive. It then becomes heterogeneous by the continuous emergence of new clones, some of which may be hormone-independent. These clones, which generally grow more rapidly[6] and without a requirement for hormone, are progressively selected for and overgrow the responsive clones.[9,5] Finally, the tumor becomes a homogeneous, hormone-independent tumor. In mammary glands, the preneoplastic state is assumed to be hormone-dependent. For instance hyperplastic alveolar nodules in mice[4] and with some hyperplastic nodules of fibrocystic disease in humans[7] contain high concentrations of estrogen receptor. When the tumor has reached a clinical stage, it is generally cytologically heterogeneous and it becomes progressively autonomous *via* a gradual selection of hormone-resistant clones. Thus, a major hurdle in interpreting the biochemical studies carried out on whole tumor tissue is that it may be heterogeneous and made up of a mixture of cell populations with differing proportions of estrogen receptor positive and negative cells. However, it is known that some models are mainly estrogen-dependent, such as the DMBA-induced tumors in rats, while others (such as the tumors induced by MMTV in mice) are mainly hormone-independent. These tumors and the increasing number of available cloned cell lines will facilitate future studies.

Table 1
EXPERIMENTAL MAMMARY TUMORS IN RODENTS

Species	Strain	Cytosol Concentration of estrogen receptor (fmol/mg protein)	Effect of ovariectomy on growth	Progesterone receptor induced by 17β-estradiol	Tumor induction
Mouse	C3H	20[a]	no	no	MMTV[b]
	GR ind.	5-10[c]	no	no	MMTV[d]
	GR dep.	30[c,d]	yes		MMTV[d]
	C53B1/DBA2	[e]	no[e]		Urethan[e]
	(MXT)	200			
Rat	R3230 AC	20[f]	yes		DMBA[g,h]
	DMBA ind.	100[i,f]	no	yes	DMBA[g,h]
	DMBA resp.	100[i,f]	yes	yes	DMBA[g,h]
	DMBA dep.	150[j,f]	yes	yes	DMBA[g,h]
	MTW9	40[k]	yes		MCA[l]
	MTW9/MTTW10	50[l]	no	yes	MCA[l]
	NMU	70[m]	yes		NMU[m]

[a]   Richards, J. E., Shyamala, G., and Nandi, S., *Cancer Res.,* 34, 2764, 1974.
[b]   Muhlbock, O., *Acta Endocrinol.,* 3, 105, 1949.
[c]   Sluyser, M. Evers, S. G., and De Goeij, C. C. J., *Nature (London),* 263, 386, 1976.
[d]   Sluyser, M. and Van Nier, *Cancer Res.,* 34, 3253, 1974.
[e]   Watson, C., Medina, D., and Clark, J. H., *Cancer Res.,* 37, 3344, 1977.
[f]   McGuire, W. L. and Julian, J. A., *Cancer Res.,* 31, 1440, 1971.
[g]   Huggins, C. L., Grand, C., and Brillantes, F. P., *Nature (London),* 189, 204, 1961.
[h]   Haslam, S. R. and Bern, H. A., *Proc. Nat. Acad. Sci.,* 74, 4020, 1977.
[i]   Vignon, F. and Rochefort, H., *Endocrinology,* 98, 722, 1976.
[j]   Jensen, E. V. and De Sombre, E. R., *Ann. Rev. Biochem.,* 41, 203, 1972.
[k]   Hollander, V. P. and Diamond, E. J., *Endocrine Control in Neoplasia,* Raven Press, New York, 1978, 93.
[l]   Kim, V. and Furth, J., *Proc. Soc. Exp. Biol.,* 103, 640, 1960.
[m]   Turcot-Lemay, L. and Kelly, P., *J. Nat. Cancer Inst.,* 66, 97, 1981.

One of the major goals in cancer therapy is to prevent or to reverse tumor progression. Since hormone-independent tumors are generally less differentiated than the hormone-dependent ones, the use of agents which induce differentiation has been proposed.[8] Reversion of the malignant phenotype may go as far as the normalization of cancer cells, an effect already demonstrated in tissue culture.[9,10]

Attempts have been made to stabilize hormone-dependent tumors by maintaining a hormone level sufficiently low to prevent a stimulation of dependent cells, but high enough to suppress further selection of resistant cells. This interesting work by Noble is described in Chapter 8.

Insight into the control of progression can therefore be anticipated from studies which attempt to define the biological factors (proteins or others) responsible for maintaining and inducing a fully differentiated state of cells.

III. BIOCHEMICAL ACTION OF ESTROGEN IN HORMONE-RESPONSIVE MAMMARY TUMORS

Estrogens can trigger responses in mammary tumors *via* separate mechanisms:

1.   They can stimulate tumor growth: this effect is the most important clinically even though its mechanism is unknown.
2.   They can induce specific proteins by a mechanism which is better understood, but this effect is not always related to tumor growth.

In terms of growth response, estrogen-dependent tumors are ones which remain dormant or regress in the absence of estrogens. By contrast, estrogen-responsive tumors regress following initiation of estrogen-replacement therapy; but this type of response is not observed in animal tumor models. Estrogen-stimulated tumors grow in the absence of hormone, but the rate of growth is more rapid in its presence. Estrogen-independent tumors grow at the same rate with or without estrogens (Figure 1); they are therefore autonomous for growth, and the mechanism controlling tumor growth is altered at a maximal (constitutive) level. A distinction should be made between tumors which totally regress after ovariectomy and those which only stop growing. The mechanism of regression is likely to be more complex than a simple lack of growth stimulation. Tumor autophagy or tumor cell lysis is observed in hormone-dependent malignancy following ovariectomy and thus hormone resistance could also be due to the absence of the autophagic mechanism.[11]

Tumors may also be estrogen-sensitive or resistant in terms of induced proteins. When estrogens regulate tumor growth, they also induce specific proteins; this is the case of the ovarian-dependent DMBA tumor in the rat (Table 1). By contrast, a tumor protein can still be induced by estrogens while tumor growth is autonomous: for example, some DMBA tumors which are resistant for growth, are in fact estrogen-sensitive for the induction of progesterone receptor.[12-14] This is also found in the MTW9-B system in which the tumor does not regress upon ovariectomy although the hormone withdrawal treatment makes the progesterone receptor disappear;[15] conversely, 17β-estradiol is able to restore the progesterone receptor but does not modify tumor growth.

In human breast cancer, even though 77% of patients whose tumors are positive for both estrogen and progesterone receptors respond to endocrine treatment, 23% remain unresponsive;[16] thus, it is important to look for other estrogen markers, more amenable to routine assay and closely related to tumor growth.[17-19]

The mechanism of regulation of mammary tumor growth by estrogens may be direct on the malignant cells themselves,[20] or indirect, *via* the liberation at a distance, of hormone or growth factors.[21] In addition, the mechanism may vary according to species. In rodents, it is generally agreed that estrogens and prolactin are the major hormones stimulating tumor growth.[22-23] Prolactin can promote the growth of a mammary tumor in an ovariectomized-adrenalectomized rat for a short period of time[23,24] but estrogen alone cannot sustain the growth of a rat mammary tumor after hypophysectomy[25,26] or after antiprolactin treatment.[27] However, the long-term growth of the tumors appears to require estrogen.[28] The synergism between the two hormones can be explained through the regulation of receptor concentrations: 17β-estradiol increases the concentration of estrogen receptor,[13,29,30] progesterone receptor,[12,13] and prolactin receptor[13] and prolactin increases the concentration of estrogen receptor.[29,31]

In human beings, the situation is quite different since 17β-estradiol appears to be the predominant hormone sustaining the growth of mammary tumors in vivo,[23] while there is no evidence that prolactin stimulates breast cancer growth. However, other growth factors or proteins are candidates to mediate the effect of estrogens.

In rodents, the effect of 17β-estradiol on tumor growth may be mediated by factors (estromedins) extracted from uterus, kidney, and mammary tumors, which are estrogen target organs. These growth factors appear to be induced in vivo by 17β-estradiol[21] and they are able to promote the growth of the estrogen-dependent MTW9-PL mammary tumor cell line. Conversely, α-fetoprotein has been found to decrease the growth of estrogen-dependent pituitary tumors in culture.[32] 17β-Estradiol in vitro does not reverse this inhibitory effect of α-fetoprotein[32] but it may be involved in vivo to alleviate the suppressive action of α-fetoprotein.[33] However, this explanation pertains only

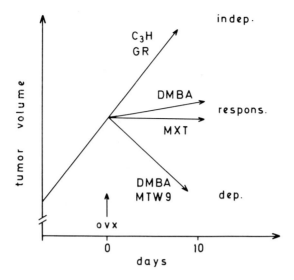

FIGURE 1. Effect of Ovariectomy on mammary tumor growth. When female mice (GR; C3H; MXT) or rats (DMBA; MTW9) carrying mammary tumors are castrated (OVX), three kinds of tumor can be schematicallly discriminated according to the evolution of their size. The independent tumor which grows at the same rate as initially, the responsive tumor which grows slower and the hormone dependent tumor which totally regresses.

when α-fetoprotein is secreted, i.e., in the newborn and in cancers secreting α-fetoprotein, and is therefore unlikely in human breast cancer.

IV. BIOCHEMICAL ALTERATIONS IN ESTROGEN-RESISTANT MAMMARY TUMORS

Since the mechanism by which estrogens stimulate the cell proliferation in the breast is unknown, the growth of breast tumors may escape from estrogen control through any mechanism involving:

1. A defect in estrogen action
2. An alteration in the pathway of any other growth factor
3. A defect of cell differentiation leading to the constitutive release of mitogenic agents

In fact, an estrogen-independent tumor may grow as rapidly as, or even faster than, a dependent tumor which is being stimulated by estrogen. The loss of the requirement for estrogen is often accompanied by a decrease in cell differentiation. Both changes could be due to the presence at a constitutive level of growth factors, proteins or hormones which themselves are capable of stimulating cell growth. These mitogenic agents might be first regulated by estrogen and thereafter synthesized at constitutive levels in the hormone-resistant tumor. Virtually nothing is known about such potential mechanisms of resistance.

By contrast, since the effect of 17β-estradiol on the induction of certain well-characterized proteins appears to be receptor dependent,[17,34] probably direct on cancer cells and located at the gene level, it is likely that the pathway leading to the hormone resistance of specific gene regulation will be defined in the near future. Unfortunately, in many studies, no distinction has been made between the inability of 17β-estradiol to stimulate cell growth and to regulate gene expression. To avoid ambiguity in our review, we will mention whether estrogen resistance was assessed through tumor growth or induced proteins; however, we will focus on the inability of estrogen to regulate the biosynthesis of specific proteins in resistant tumors. Since induced proteins are synthesized at very low levels in hormone-resistant tumors, most workers have looked at the estrogen receptor mechanism of the tumor cell to see whether one of the steps leading to the action of 17β estradiol could be altered or lacking in an already developed hormone-independent tumor, as compared to a hormone-dependent tumor.

A. Alterations at the Level of the Estrogen Receptor

The central dogma of the mechanism of action of estrogen is that estrogens act only through their specific receptor. This mechanism involves several steps,[2,3] as shown in Figure 2 and the blockage of any of these should be sufficient to make the tumor estrogen resistant. Briefly, the action of 17β-estradiol in target cells involves its entry into the cell and its binding to a cytosol receptor; this binding triggers the activation of the estrogen-receptor complex and its subsequent transfer into the cell nucleus. The complex combines with a DNA and protein-containing acceptor site (acc$^+$); this interaction alone is thought to be inadequate to initiate transcription which may require a coupling of the receptor-acceptor complex with an effector site (eff$^+$). Although the final steps in the mechanism of regulation of gene expression remain obscure, it is clear that the estrogen receptor is capable of inducing the synthesis of several specific proteins in addition to increasing protein synthesis more generally. Estrogen resistance may *a priori* be due to a block located at any step between the entry of the hormone into the cell and the final expression of the induced proteins.

1. Decrease in the Concentration of Estrogen Receptor

It is well-established that, without estrogen receptors, 17β-estradiol is inactive. Several mammary tumor cell lines, notably RBA[35] and NMU[35] in rats and BT20[36] and Evsa T[36] in humans, contain no detectable estrogen receptor (r- phenotypes) and do not respond to estrogens either for growth or for induced proteins. In attempting to predict the estrogen resistance of human breast cancer, Jensen's group[37] measured the cytoplasmic form of estrogen receptor in breast cancer biopsies, and clearly demonstrated[16] that about 90% of the receptor-negative patients failed to respond to therapy and their tumors were assumed to be estrogen-resistant. However, among the receptor-positive patients only 50% responded to therapy; this observation indicated that estrogen receptor is necessary, but not sufficient for a full estrogenic response.[16]

In human breast cancer, the prediction of hormone-dependence appeared to be directly correlated with the concentrations of estrogen receptor.[16,38] This may be due to two factors:

1. Breast tumors are heterogeneous and contain different kinds of cells with varying concentrations of estrogen receptors; indeed, it has been proposed that tumor tissue is a mosaic of receptor-positive responding cells and receptor-negative resistant cells.[39,40]
2. There may be a threshold estrogen receptor level for estrogen activity.

In human beings, this level has been arbitrarily defined as 10 fmol/mg cytosol protein, i.e., about 300 to 400 sites per cell. However, the limit may vary according to the assay method, the type of response which is being evaluated and the hormonal status of the patient. The correlation between receptor content and responsiveness sug-

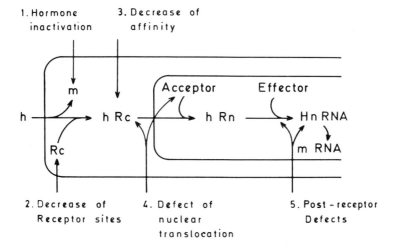

FIGURE 2.   Schematic representation of the mechanism of action of estrogens in one target cell and possible steps involved in the estrogen resistance of mammary tumors for protein induction. h = estrogen; m = metabolite; Rc = cytosol estrogen receptor (ER) and Rn = nuclear estrogen receptor. Acceptor and effector sites of the chromatin are defined in the text; HnRNA: first transcript of heterogeneous nuclear RNA. To our knowledge the only demonstrated defect in the receptor mechanism is the absence of cytosol estrogen receptor (r⁻ variants). The mechanism of the r⁺ resistant variants may involve defective activation and nuclear translocation or post receptor defects.

gests that, if the receptor concentration could be increased, it might be possible to increase the responsiveness of the tumor. In fact several hormones, especially 17β-estradiol and prolactin can increase the concentration of estrogen receptor in the hormone-dependent DMBA tumor.[13,29] However, the regulation of receptor sites may be altered in the hormone-resistant state since, in the ovarian-independent mammary tumors of the rat[29] and the C3H mouse,[41] ovariectomy did not decrease the concentration of sites although it did so in the ovarian-dependent tumors.[12] These results suggest that the normal regulation of estrogen binding sites has been lost during tumor progression. Conversely, in the estrogen-unresponsive C3H mammary tumor, pituitary grafts can increase the estrogen receptor content of the tumor three-fold without reversing its estrogen resistance.[41]

In summary, the absence of estrogen receptor usually denotes an estrogen-resistant condition of a tumor; the corollary is not true, however, since the presence of estrogen receptor only identifies a hormone-dependent phenotype in about 50% of cases. The functional status of the receptor in the other 50% is assumed to be abnormal.

2. Decrease in the Affinity Between Estrogen Receptor and its Ligand

All studies on mammary tumors to date have failed to reveal an alteration in the affinity of estrogen receptor for 17β-estradiol, which is invariably characterized by a K_D of approximately 0.2 nM. Recently, however, an apparent defect of this type was observed in an estrogen independent Leydig cell tumor:[42] this tumor did not grow or regress after ovariectomy. In vitro studies showed the presence, in the cytosol, of a low affinity estrogen binder; when small molecules with a molecular weight of less than 500 were removed from the cytosol, a molecule appeared which resembled the estrogen receptor. It was characterized by a Stokes radius only slightly different from normal and was able to bind to DNA.[42] Thus, estrogen resistance was associated with small components which decreased the in vitro binding of 17β-estradiol to a receptor-like molecule.

Generally speaking, whenever the binding of 17β-estradiol has been measured in either human or rodent neoplastic mammary tissue, Scatchard plots invariably have displayed a low number of binding sites with unchanged affinity. In addition, competitive experiments have shown no modification of the binding specificity for different ligands. There is therefore no strong evidence that an alteration in receptor-ligand affinity can explain the resistance of mammary cancers.

3. Defect of Estrogen Receptor Activation and Nuclear Translocation

Receptor activation is a modification of the receptor protein induced by the binding of the steroid, which facilitates the retention of receptor in the nucleus in vivo and enhances the binding to DNA or nuclei in vitro. The phenotype of a normal target cell is nt+ (presence of nuclear transfer). In the glucocorticoid-sensitive lymphoma, modifications of this phenotype such as nt⁻ (absence of nuclear transfer), ⁻ntⁱ (increased binding of the receptor to the nucleus) have been noted.[45] The observations are reviewed in detail in Chapter 4. It has been suggested that estrogen receptor activation and nuclear transfer are multistep processes[44,45] implying the potential existance of at least two defects of receptor activation, namely, absence (act⁻) or lability (actⁱ).[46]

In contrast to the glucocorticoid receptor systems, no similar defects in the estrogen receptor activation and nuclear transfer of receptors have been found consistently in mammary tumors. An absence of receptor translocation has been described in vitro in the GRS/A mouse mammary tumor;[47] however, in the C3H mouse tumor, translocation took place when studied in vivo.[48] Activation was also found to be normal in the DMBA-induced mammary tumor,[12] as was translocation.[48,49] There are many in vitro studies of the interaction of estrogen receptor with DNA and chromatin, but very few workers have studied its translocation in vivo by measuring the cytosol and nuclear estrogen receptor, before and after the injection of 17β-estradiol into the animal. Results of in vitro binding studies vary according to the authors and the systems used: it has been a common practice to use a DNA-cellulose binding assay[50] to test the binding of the cytosol form of estrogen receptor in mammary tumors. In the W/Fu rat, the MTW9 tumor is estrogen-dependent for growth and its receptor is able to bind to DNA-cellulose. When the prolactin-secreting pituitary tumor MtTW10 is grafted onto the MTW9 tumor-bearing animal, the mammary tumor becomes estrogen-independent for growth[51] and simultaneously the DNA-binding ability of estrogen receptor seems to decline since the amount capable of binding to DNA-cellulose is reduced threefold[52] while the overall receptor concentration is not modified. Removal of the MtTW10 graft reverts the MTW9 tumor to its previous estrogen-dependent phenotype.

Several authors have described variants of human breast cancer which are characterized by an impaired nuclear transfer of estrogen receptor in vivo.[53-55] Such tumors, which represented 20 to 40% of all receptor-positive tumors, were found to contain cytosol estrogen receptor but no nuclear estrogen receptor and did not respond to endocrine therapy. Whether receptor proteolysis takes place in the nucleus or whether the processing of receptor is blocked in such tumors is unknown. Resistance to the antiestrogen Tamoxifen has been described by Nawata et al.[56] in a variant clone derived from MCF-7 human breast cancer cells. The variant retains substantial estrogen responsiveness while having lost inhibitory responses to antiestrogen. Studies on the time course of translocation of estrogen receptor suggest that some event distal to the initial binding of Tamoxifen to receptor may be defective in the resistant cells. This was shown by the substantial decrease in processing of antiestrogen receptor complexes as compared to that in wild-type cells. Also, the reduced binding of estrogen receptor complex from the resistant cells to DNA-cellulose was compatible with a defect in a single receptor or its activating system. Since these phenotypic alterations parallel those which occur in glucocorticoid resistant lymphoma cells, a malfunctioning receptor mechanism is likely to be a common and major cause of hormone resistance in tumor cells. However, in such systems, it is known that the DNA binding site of a receptor can be destroyed by a partial proteolysis,[57] and consequently, it is difficult to ascertain whether the decrease of DNA binding ability, which is observed in some variants, is a biological property or an artifact observed in vitro.

4. Different Molecular Forms of Estrogen Receptor

Using sedimentation rate analysis in low salt gradients,[58] it is possible to identify several forms of uterine estrogen receptor: the "native" 8S form which is able to bind to DNA, the molybdate-stabilized 9-10S form which has lost this ability, the "activated" form which aggregates in low salt sucrose gradients, and several partially proteolyzed forms characterized by a sedimentation coefficient of 3 to 5 S in low salt. All these forms have saturable high affinity 17β-estradiol binding sites and can thus be considered authentic. Proteolysis can prevent the binding of estrogen receptor to DNA without altering its affinity for estrogens. Endogenous proteases are known to be present in mammary tumors and thus, may give rise to artifactual results in cell-free experiments. On the other hand, the possibility that proteolysis might constitute a biologically significant phenomenon deserves serious consideration.

In mouse[59] and rat[49,60] mammary tumors it is possible to separate, in low salt gradients, two different saturable estrogen binding proteins characterized by sedimentation rates of 4S and 8S. In human breast cancers also, the 4S form alone has been found in estrogen-independent tumors and a mixture of 4S and 8S forms in dependent tumors.[61,62] The significance of the 4S form has not been established and doubts remain about its relationship to plasma protein, proteolysed estrogen receptor and nonspecific protein binders.

In addition to the classical form of estrogen receptor, which has a high affinity for 17β-estradiol and can be translocated into the nucleus, Clark and co-workers[63,64] have identified another 17β-estradiol binding site in the nucleus. The affinity of the second site for 17β-estradiol was clearly lower than that of the native estrogen receptor. Of interest was the observation that the growth response of uterine tissue seemed to correlate more strongly with the low affinity binding site rather than with the estrogen receptor.[63]

In summary, r^-, nt^-, nt^i and act^- phenotypes have been suggested in hormone resistant tumors. Among them, only r^- variants have been clearly proven at present, thus suggesting that the defect accounting for the resistance of the r^+ tumor must be located distal to the translocation step.

B. Nonreceptor Mechanisms
1. Beyond the Receptor Translocation Step

Since virtually nothing is known about the coupling of the receptor-hormone complex with chromatin and the consequences of this interaction, it is *a priori* difficult to explain why the complex might become inactive in estrogen unresponsive cells. However, there are examples of lack of response to estrogens with an apparently normal nuclear estrogen receptor and several explanations have been proposed. First, the estrogen receptor complex may have a defect that is undetectable by our methods. Second, the interaction of estrogen receptor with specific or nonspecific sites in chromatin may be altered. For example, if the specific effector sites are present in very small numbers, they may be masked by the more abundant but less specific acceptor sites.[65] Third, the cell-free interaction between estrogen receptor and chromatin acceptor sites may, in fact, be entirely nonspecific[66] since test results are independent of whether nuclei from target or nontarget cells are used. More affirmative observations have been made with the chick oviduct system; Spelsberg[67] has shown that the progesterone receptor is able to bind an acidic chromatin protein present in target cell nuclei and has suggested that this protein might be the effector site. One approach to screen for the absence of effector sites in tissue (eff⁻) is to look for cells or tumor variants which are estrogen-insensitive for the induction of specific proteins, while having no detectable defect in estrogen receptor content and nuclear transfer ability. This appears to be the situation in the C3H mouse mammary tumor and in the cloned estrogen resistant variant of MCF-7 human breast cancer cells.[56] Hence, the latter tissues may prove ideal for unmasking anomalous receptor-chromatin interactions.

2. Before the Cytosol Receptor

Defects in the permeability of the cell membrane for entry of estrogens, or an increase in the metabolism and inactivation of estrogens in the cells can also be proposed to explain the estrogen-resistance of r⁺ cells. Moreover, an alteration in the vascularization of the tumor may decrease the accessibility of 17β-estradiol to the cell and thus to its receptor. In such cases, estrogen receptor would be functional as soon as it could bind to it in vivo.

Any of these proposed mechanisms, receptor-mediated or not, can potentially explain why tumors might be estrogen-resistant for stimulating or inducing specific gene products such as the progesterone receptor. However, they do not account for the ultimate failure of hormones to influence the growth rate of hormone-resistant tumors.

V. OTHER MODELS TO APPROACH ESTROGEN RESISTANCE MECHANISMS

A. Pharmacology and Antiestrogens

Through the use of different agonists and drugs, estrogen responsive tissues can be manipulated in vivo and in vitro to become unresponsive. The mechanism of this provoked resistance can sometimes be traced to the cytosol estrogen receptor. This is the case with the classical antiestrogens such as Tamoxifen and Nafoxidine, which act as competitive inhibitors most likely through their high affinity metabolites[68] and by stimulating an activation of estrogen receptor which is different from that produced by 17β-estradiol.[69] We will not review the action of antiestrogens here. Complete information is available from other sources.[70,71] Suffice it to say that the spontaneous estrogen resistance of mammary tumors is unlikely to be due to the in vivo occupation of estrogen receptor by inactive ligands. On the other hand, the receptor-altering inhibitor pyridoxal phosphate[72] which prevents translocation, or the intercalating drug ethidium bromide,[73] which changes the structure of nuclear acceptor sites, and their analogues, should evolve into useful agents for elucidating the nt⁻ phenotype of mammary tumors.

Since the majority of the resistant tumors studied, at least in rodents, appear to be r⁺ and nt⁺, any agent which prevents the action of 17β-estradiol without altering the receptor activation and nuclear translocation steps would expedite studies of hormone resistance. Recently, we have been able to grow MCF-7 human breast cancer cells in the presence of BUdR, thereby substituting the thymidine in DNA by this analogue.[74,75] The BUdR substituted cells became estrogen unresponsive[76] since they were unable to synthesize and secrete an estrogen-specific protein.[77] Since the estrogen receptor displayed a greater affinity for the BUdR-substituted DNA and nuclei,[74,75,78] the receptor-chromatin interaction was apparently altered by the modification yielding an nt^i phenotype. In this case, the acceptor sites and not the estrogen receptor were clearly changed.

B. Physiological Transition from Resistance to Responsivenesss
During the normal differentiation processes, a specific target tissue may progressively acquire hormone sensitivity or lose this sensitivity indefinitely or temporarily.

1. Ontogeny of Estrogen Sensitivity
The ontogeny of each step of the mechanism of action of estrogens is sometimes dissociated. In the fetal guinea pig uterus, estrogen receptor is undetectable until the 34th day of gestation, whereupon it increases until birth to reach a concentration of 500 fmol/mg of protein;[79,80] a steady decrease follows until the adult stage development. The receptor is able to translocate into the nucleus as soon as it appears in tissue, but it induces the appearance of the progesterone receptor only after the 50th day of gestation.[81] Between the 34th and 50th days of gestation,[81] the uterus is therefore not fully responsive to estrogen.
The development of the rat uterus for the most part differs only in the time course: the estrogen receptor is present at birth and translocation occurs as early as the 7th postnatal day[82], followed by the stimulation of 17β-estradiol induced protein at 7 to 10 days.[82,83] However, long-term responses, such as growth are delayed until days 15 to 20 of the postnatal period.[83] The partial and transitory resistance observed between the short- and long-term response might be due to either a receptor or an effector site that has not matured into a fully active state, or to a suboptimal amount of estrogen receptor complex which would only be able to induce short-term responses. In the latter case, a low concentration of either 17β-estradiol or estrogen receptor would be responsible for the apparent resistance of the tissue.
In the chick, the liver contains estrogen receptor about 10 days before hatching; the receptor is able to translocate into the nucleus, but vitellogenin inducibility appears much later at 13 to 15 days after hatching.[85] In Xenopus liver, the acquisition of estrogen-responsiveness, followed by the inducibility of vitellogenin, is also progressive. [86] First, estradiol is able to increase the synthesis and secretion of all proteins exclusive of vitellogenin. Subsequently, the expression of the vitellogenin gene becomes manifest by its inducibility with 17β-estradiol. At metamorphosis, the effect of 17β-estradiol on vitellogenin induction is maximal.[86,87] Thus the guinea pig uterus at 34 to 50 days of gestation, the 10 to 15 day postnatal rat uterus, the fetal chick liver, and possibly the developing Xenopus liver may all represent estrogen-resistant tissues in which there is a postreceptor blockade of function.

2. Hormone Resistant Genes According to Tissue Localization and Differentiation
In the chick, conalbumin and transferrin have identical sequences and may therefore be transcribed by similar, if not identical genes. The former is synthesized in the oviduct under estrogen control; the latter, synthesized and secreted in the liver, is also induced by 17β-estradiol but the effect is not as great in the liver as in the oviduct. Thus, there may be differences between the effect of 17β-estradiol on similar or identical genes in different tissues which both have measurable and fully active estrogen receptors. Furthermore, the chick liver is estrogen-responsive for apolipoprotein B[88] and vitellogenin[89] (and thus eff⁺), but more resistant for transferrin regulation (eff⁻). Similar results have been obtained with the chick oviduct for the ovalbumin-like genes X and Y.[90]

3. Transitory Estrogen Resistance During Pregnancy and Lactation
In virgin mammary glands the estrogen receptor is able to induce the appearance of the progesterone receptor . During pregnancy this responsiveness decreases[91] while the estrogen receptor content and the gland size increase. Estrogen receptor becomes inefficient in the lactating gland for progesterone receptor induction.[92,93] Therefore, a tis-

sue which proceeds through a cyclic differentiation can successively be estrogen responsive and unresponsive, the estrogen resistant state being reversible. The molecular mechanism of this physiological estrogen resistance is unknown.

VI. CONCLUSIONS

The study of hormone resistance in breast cancer can be approached by looking for defects in the estrogen-inducibility of specific proteins related to or responsible for tumor growth . The progesterone receptor is the only protein currently being assayed on a routine basis and, unfortunately, is not totally correlated with tumor growth or response to treatment.[12-14] The discovery of induced proteins better related to clinical response parameters would therefore be a major landmark in breast cancer treatment.[17]

A mammary cancer is usually heterogeneous and different clones can be selected for during tumor progression. The fact that the progression of a mammary tumor leads to its estrogen resistance argues for the early detection of breast cancer at a stage where the tumor will most likely be responsive to hormonal treatment.

REFERENCES

1. Beatson, G. T., On the treatment of inoperable cases of carcinoma of the mamma: suggestions for a new method of treatment, with illustrative cases, *Lancer,* 2, 104, 1896.
2. Jensen, E. V. and de Sombre, E. R., Mechanism of action of the female sex hormones, *Ann. Rev. Biochem.,* 41, 203, 1972.
3. Katzenellenbogen, B. S., Dynamics of steroid hormone receptor action, *Ann. Rev. Physiol.,* 42, 17, 1980,.
4. Medina, D., Tumor progression, in *Cancer,* Vol. 3, Becker, F. F., Ed., Plenum Press, New York, 1975, 99.
5. Huggins, C. L., Grand, C., and Brillantes, F. P., Mammary cancer induced by a single feeding of polynuclear hydrocarbons and its suppression, *Nature (London),* 189, 204, 1961.
6. Briand, P., Thorpe, S. M., and Daehnfeldt, J. L., Difference in growth of hormone dependent and hormone independent mammary tumors of GR mice *in vivo* and *in vitro, Acta Pathol. Microbiol. Scand.,* A87, 427, 1979.
7. Haagensen, C. D., Cystic disease of the breast, in *Diseases of the Breast,* 2nd ed., W. B. Saunders, Philadelphia, 1971, 155.
8. Sachs, L., Constitutive uncoupling of pathways of gene expression that control growth and differentiation in myeloid leukemia: a model for the origin and progression of malignancy, *Proc. Nat. Acad. Sci., USA,* 77, 6152, 1980.
9. Honna, Y. Kasukabe, T., Okabe, J., and Hozumi, M., Prolongation of survival time of mice inoculated with myeloid leukemia cells by inducers of normal differentiation, *Cancer Res.,* 39, 3167, 1979.
10. Sachs, L., Control of normal cell differentiation and the phenotypic reversion of malignancy in myeloid leukemia, *Nature (London),* 274, 535, 1978.
11 . Bruchovsky, N., Rennie, P. S., Van Doorn, E., and Noble, R. L., Pathological growth of androgen-sensitive tissues resulting from latent actions of steroid hormones, *J. Toxicol. Environ. Health,* 4, 391, 1978.
12. Vignon, F., Ph. D., Thesis, Etapes Initiales du Mecanisme D'action des Oestrogenes Dans les Tumeurs Mammaires, 1979.
13. Arafah, B. M., Manni, A., and Pearson, O. H., Effect of hypophysectomy and hormone replacement on hormone receptor levels and the growth of DMBA-induced mammary tumors in the rat, *Endocrinology,* 107, 1364, 1980.
14. Koenders, A. J. M., Geurts-Moesport, A., Zolingers, J., and Benraad,T. J., Progesterone and estradiol receptors in DMBA-induced mammary tumors before and after ovariectomy and after subsequent estradiol administration, in *Progesterone Receptors in Normal and Neoplastic Tissues,* McGuire, W. L., Raynaud, J. P., Baulieu, E. E., Eds., Raven Press, New York, 1977, 71.

15. Ip, M., Milholland, R. J., Rosen, F., and Kim, U., Mammary cancer: selective action of the estrogen receptor complex, *Science,* 203, 361, 1979.
16. McGuire, W. L., Steroid hormones receptors in breast cancer treatment strategy, in *Recent Progress in* Hormone Research, Vol. 36, Greep, R. O., Ed., Academic Press, New York, 1980, 135.
17. Rochefort, H., Garcia, M., Vignon, F., and Westley, B., Proteins induced by the estrogen receptor in uterus and breast cancer cells, in *Steroid Induced Uterine Proteins,* Beato, M., Ed., Elsevier, Amsterdam, 1980, 171.
18. Edwards, D. P., Adams, D. J., Savage, N., and McGuire, W. L., Estrogen induced synthesis of specific proteins in human breast cancer cells, *Biochem. Biophys. Res. Commun.,* 93, 804, 1980.
19. Lyttle, C. R. and de Sombre, E. R., Generality of estrogen stimulation of peroxidase activity in growth responsive tissues, *Nature (London),* 268, 337, 1977.
20. Lippman, M. E., Monaco, M. E., and Bolan, G., Effects of estrone, estradiol and estriol on hormone responsive human breast cancer in long-term tissue culture, *Cancer Res.,* 37, 1901, 1977.
21. Sirbasku, D. A., Estrogen induction of growth factors specific for hormone-responsive mammary, pituitary, kidney tumor cells, *Proc. Nat. Acad. Sci. USA,* 75, 3786, 1978.
22. McGuire, W. L., Physiological principles underlying endocrine therapy of breast cancer, in *Breast Cancer: Advances in Research and Treatment,* McGuire, W. L., Ed., Plenum Press, New York, 1977, 217.
23. Pearson, O. H., Llerena, O., Molina, A., and Butler, T., Prolactin-dependent rat mammary cancer: a model for man, *Trans. Assoc. Am. Phys.,* 82, 225, 1969.
24. Clemens, J. A., Welsch, C. W., and Meites, J., Effect of hypothalamic lesions on the induction and growth of mammary tumors in carcinogen-treated rats, *Proc. Soc. Exp. Biol. Med.,* 127, 969, 1968.
25. Sterental, A., Dominguez, J. M., Weissman, C., and Pearson, O. H., Pituitary role in the estrogen dependency of experimental mammary cancer, *Cancer Res.,* 23, 481, 1963.
26. Welsch, C. W. and Rivera, E. M., Differential effects of estrogen and prolactin on DNA synthesis in organ cultures of DMBA-induced rat mammary carcinoma, *Proc. Soc. Exp. Biol. Med.,* 139, 623, 1972.
27. Rose, D. P. and Pruitt, B., Modification of the effect of a gonadoliberin analog on DMBA-induced rat mammary tumors by hormone replacement, *Cancer Res.,* 39, 3968, 1979.
28. Dao, T. L. and Sinha, D., Estrogen and prolactin in mammary carcinogenesis: *in vivo* and *in vitro* studies, in *Prolactin and carcinogenesis,* Boyns, A. R. and Griffiths, K., Eds., Alpha Omega Alpha, Cardiff, 1972, 189.
29. Vignon, F. and Rochefort, H., Regulation of the estrogen receptor in ovarian-dependent mammary tumors; effect of ovariectomy and prolactin, *Endocrinology,* 98, 722, 1976.
30. Pavlik, E. J. and Coulson, P. B., Modulation of estrogen receptors in four different target tissues: differential effects of estradiol *versus* progesterone, *J. Steroid Biochem.,* 7, 369, 1976.
31. Leung, B. S. and Sasaki, S., On the mechanism of prolactin and estrogen action in DMBA-induced mammary carcinoma in the rat: II, *in vivo* tumor responses and estrogen receptor, *Endocrinology,* 97, 564, 1975.
32. Soto, A. M. and Sonnenschein, C., Control of growth of estrogen-sensitive cells: role of α-fetoprotein, *Proc. Nat. Acad. Sci., U.S.A.,* 77, 2084, 1980.
33. Sonnenschein, C. and Soto, A. M., The mechanism of estrogen action, the old and a new paradigm, in *Estrogens in the Environment,* McLachlan, J. A., Ed., Elsevier, New York, 1980, 169.
34. Garcia, M. and Rochefort, H., Androgen effects mediated by the estrogen receptor in DMBA-induced rat mammary tumors, *Cancer Res.,* 38, 3922, 1978.
35. Vignon, F., Chan, P. C., and Rochefort, H., Hormonal regulation in two rat mammary cancer cell lines: glucocorticoid and androgen receptors, *Molec. Cell. Endocrinol.,* 13, 191, 1979.
36. Engel, L. W. and Young, N. A., Human breast carcinoma in continuous culture: a review, *Cancer Res.,* 38, 4327, 1978.
37. Jensen, E. V., Block, G. E., Smith, S., Kyser, K., and de Sombre, E. R., Estrogen receptors and hormone dependency, in *Estrogen Target Tissues and Neoplasia,* Dao, T. L., Ed., University of Chicago Press, 1972, 23.
38. Paridaens, R., Sylvester, R., Heuson, J. C., and Leclercq, G., Concentration des recepteurs oestrogenes et hormonodependance, in *Recepteurs Hormonaux et Pathologie Mammaire,* Martin, P. M., Ed., Medsi, Paris, 1980, 167.
39. Sluyser, M., Hormone-responsive mammary tumors in GR mice, *Reviews on Endocrine-Related Cancer,* Suppl. April, 285, 1978.
40. Kim, U. and Depowski, M. J., Progression from hormone dependence to autonomy in mammary tumors as an *in vivo* manifestation of clonal selection, *Cancer Res.,* 35, 2068, 1975.
41. Coezy, E. and Rochefort, H., Effect of pituitary isografts on the concentration of estrogen and glucocorticoid receptors in C3H mice mammary tumors, *Eur. J. Cancer,* 15, 1185, 1979.

42. Sato, B., Maeda, Y., Noma, K., Matsumoto, K., and Yamamura, Y., Estrogen binding component of mouse Leydig cell tumor: an *in vitro* conversion from non-receptor to receptor like molecule, *Endocrinology,* 108, 612, 1981.

43. Gehring, U., Cell genetics of glucocorticoid responsiveness, in *Biochemical Action of Hormones,* Vol. 7, Litwack, G., Ed., Academic Press, New York, 1980, 205.

44. Bailly, A., Le Fevre, B., Savouret, J. F., and Milgrom, E., Activation and changes in sedimentation properties of steroid receptors, *J. Biol. Chem.,* 255, 2729, 1980.

45. Rochefort, H., Andre, J., Baskevitch, P. P., Garcia, M., Raynaud, A., and Westley, B., Interaction of steroid receptors with chromatin, in *Endocrinology,* Cumming, I., Ed., Elsevier/North-Holland, Amsterdam, 1980, 66.

46. Schmidt, T. J., Harmon, J. M., and Thompson, E. B., "Activation labile" glucocorticoid-receptor complexes of a steroid-resistant variant of CEM-C7 human lymphoid cells , *Nature (London),* 286, 507, 1980.

47. Shyamala, G., Estradiol receptors in mouse mammary tumors: absence of the transfer of bound estradiol from the cytoplasm to the nucleus, *Biochem. Biophys. Res. Commun.,* 46 , 1623, 1972.

48. Vignon, F. and Rochefort, H., Nuclear translocation of estradiol receptor in the autonomous C3H mammary tumors, *Cancer Res.,* 38, 1808, 1978.

49. McGuire, W. L. and Julian, J. A., Comparison of macromolecular binding of estradiol in hormone-dependent and hormone-independent rat mammary carcinoma, *Cancer Res.,* 31, 1440, 1971.

50. Yamamoto, K. R., Stampfer , M. R., and Tomkins, G. M., Receptors from glucocorticoid-sensitive lymphoma cells, and two classes of insensitive clones: physical and DNA-binding properties, *Proc. Nat. Acad. Sci. USA,* 71, 3901, 1974.

51. Hollander, V. P. and Diamond, E. J., Hormonal control in animal breast cancer, in *Endocrine Control in Neoplasia,* Sharma, R. K. and Criss, W. E., Eds., Raven Press, New York, 1978, 93.

52. Sukur, K., Feldman, M., and Hollander, V. P., The biological significance of estrogen receptor binding to DNA, *Cancer Res.,* 40, 1050, 1980.

53. Laing, L., Smith, M. G., Calman, K. C., Smith, D. C., and Leake, R. E., Nuclear estrogen receptors and treatment of breast cancer, *Lancet,* 2, 168, 1977.

54. Garola, R. E. and McGuire, W. L., An improved assay for nuclear estrogen receptor in experimental and human breast cancer, *Cancer Res.,* 37, 3333, 1977.

55. Romic-Stojkovic, R. and Gamulin, S., Relationship of cytoplasmic and nuclear estrogen receptors and progesterone receptors in human breast cancer, *Cancer Res.,* 40, 4821, 1980.

56. Nawata, H., Bronzert, D., and Lippman, M., Isolation and characterization of a tamoxifen-resistant cell line derived from MCF7 human breast cancer cells, *J. Biol. Chem.,* 256, 5016, 1981.

57. Andre J. and Rochefort, H., Estrogen receptor: loss of DNA binding ability following trypsin or Ca^{++} treatment, *FEBS Lett.,* 32, 330, 1973.

58. Toft, D. and Gorski, J., A receptor molecule for estrogens: isolation from the rat uterus and preliminary characterization, *Proc. Nat. Acad. Sci. USA,* 55, 1574, 1966.

59. Shyamala, G. and Yeh, Y. F., Estradiol receptor of mammary glands: a molecular analysis of the cytoplasmic estrogen binding proteins, in *Multiple Molecular Forms of Steroid Hormones Receptors,* Agarwal, M. K., Ed., Elsevier /North-Holland, Amsterdam, 1977, 129.

60. Chamness, E. R. and McGuire, W. L., Estrogen receptor in the rat uterus. Physiological forms and artifacts, *Biochemistry,* 11, 2466, 1972.

61. Wittliff, , J. L., Beaty, B. W., Savlov, E. D., Patterson, W. B., and Cooper, R. A., Estrogen receptors and hormone dependency in human breast cancer, in *Recent Results in Cancer Research,* Vol. 57, 1976, 59.

62. Muldoon, T. G., Mouse mammary tissue estrogen receptor ontogeny and molecular heterogeneity, in *Ontogeny of Receptors and Reproductive Hormone Action,* Hamilton, T., Clark, J. H., and Sadler, W. A., Eds., Raven-Press, New York, 1979, 225.

63. Clark, J. H., Markaverich, B., Upchurch, S., Eriksson, H., Hardin, J. W. and Peck, E. J., Heterogeneity of estrogen binding sites: relationship to estrogen receptors and estrogen response, in *Recent Progress in Hormone Research,* Vol. 36, Greep, R. O., Ed., Academic Press, New York, 1980, 135.

64. Watson, C. S. and Clark, J. H., Heterogeneity of estrogen binding sites in mouse mammary cancer, *J. Receptor Res.,* 1, 91, 1980.

65. Yamamoto, K. R. and Alberts, B., In vitro conversion of estradiol receptor protein to its nuclear form: dependence on hormone and DNA, *Proc. Nat. Acad. Sci. USA,* 69, 2105, 1972.

66. Chamness, G. C., Jennings, A. W., and McGuire, W. L., Oestrogen receptor binding is not restricted to target nuclei, *Nature (London),* 241, 458, 1973.

67. Spelsberg, T. C., Webster, R., and Pickler, G. M., Multiple binding sites for progesterone in the hen oviduct nucleus: evidence that acidic proteins represent the acceptors, in *Chromosomal Proteins and Their Role in the Regulation of Gene Expression,* Stein, G. S., Kleinsmith, L. J., Eds., Academic Press, New York, 1975, 153.

68. **Borgna, J. L. and Rochefort, H.,** Hydroxylated metabolites of tamoxifen are formed in vivo and bound to estrogen receptor in target tissues, *J. Biol. Chem.,* 256, 859, 1981.

69. **Rochefort, H. and Borgna, J. L.,** Differences of receptor activation by estrogens and antiestrogens, *Nature (London),* 292, 257, 1981.

70. **Agarwal, M. K., Ed.,** *Antihormones,* Elsevier, New York, 1979.
    ney; Academic Press, New York, 1980.

72. **Muller, R. E., Traish, A., and Wotiz, H. H.,** Effects of pyridoxal phosphate on uterine estrogen receptor. I: Inhibition of nuclear binding in cell free system and in rat uterus, *J. Biol. Chem.,* 255, 4062, 1980.

73. **Andre, J., Vic, P., Humeau, C., and Rochefort, H.,** Nuclear translocation of the estrogen receptor: partial inhibition by ethidium bromide, *Mol. Cell. Endocrinol.,* 8, 225, 1977.

74. **Baskevitch, P. P. and Kallos, J.,** *In vivo* nuclear retention to the estradiol-receptor complex to the 5- BUdR substituted DNA in a human breast cancer cell line, *Cancer Treat. Reports,* Abstr. no. 61, 63, 1157, 1979.

75. **Kallos, J., Hollander, V. P., Baskevitch, P. P., and Rochefort, H.,** Study of the photo attachment of the estrogen receptor to the nuclear acceptor sites in human breast cancer cells, *Ann. N. Y. Acad. Sci.,* 346, 415, 1980.

76. **Garcia, M., Westley, B., and Rochefort, H.,** 5-BUdR specifically inhibits the synthesis of estrogen-induced proteins in MCF-7 cells, *Eur. J. Biochem.,* 116, 297, 1981.

77. **Westley, B. and Rochefort, H.,** A secreted glycoprotein induced by estrogen in human breast cancer cell lines, *Cell,* 20, 353, 1980.

78. **Kallos, J., Hollander, V. P., Fasy, T. M., and Bick, M. D.,** Estrogen receptor binds more tightly to BUdR-substituted DNA, *Proc. Nat. Acad. Sci., USA,* 75, 4898, 1978.

79. **Sumida, C. and Pasqualini, J. R.,** Determination of cytosol and nuclear estradiol binding sites in fetal guinea pig uterus by tritiated estradiol exchange, *Endocrinology,* 105, 406, 1979.

80. **Pasqualini, J. R., Sumida, C., Gelly, C., and Nguyen, B. L.,** Specific tritiated estradiol binding to the fetal uterus and testis of guinea pig; quantitative evolution of tritiated estradiol receptors in the different fetal tissues during fetal development, *J. Steroid Biochem.,* 7, 1031, 1976.

81. **Pasqualini, J. R., Sumida, C., Nguyen, B. L., Tardy, J., and Gelly, C.,** Estrogen concentrations and effect of estradiol on progesterone receptors in the fetal and newborn guinea pig, *J. Steroid Biochem.,* 12, 65, 1980.

82. **Somjen, D., Somjen, G., King, R. J. B., Kaye A. M., and Lindner, H. R.,** Nuclear binding of estradiol and induction of protein synthesis in the rat uterus during post-natal development, *Biochem. J.,* 136, 25, 1973.

83. **Katzenellenbogen, B. S.,** Regulation of uterine responsiveness to estrogen: developmental and multihormonal factors, in *Ontogeny of Receptors and Reproductive Hormone Action,* Hamilton, T. H., Clark, J. H., and Sadler, W. A., Eds., Raven Press, New York, 1979, 79.

84. **Hunt, M. E. and Muldoon, T. G.,** Factors controlling estrogen receptor levels in normal mouse mammary tissue, *J. Steroid Biochem.,* 8, 181, 1977.

85. **Lazier, C. M.,** Ontogeny of the vitellogenic response to estradiol and of the soluble nuclear estrogen receptor in embryonic chick liver, *Biochem. J.,* 174, 143, 1978.

86. **Skipper, J. K. and Hamilton, T. H.,** Xenopus liver: ontogeny of estrogen responsiveness, *Science,* 206, 693, 1979.

87. **Knowland, J.,** Induction of vitollegenin synthesis in Xenopus laevis tadpoles, *Differentiation,* 12, 47, 1978.

88. **Capony, F. and Williams, J. L.,** Apolipoprotein B of avian VLDL: characteristics of its regulation in non-stimulated and estrogen-stimulated rooster, *Biochemistry,* 19, 2219, 1980.

89. **Burns, A. T. H., Deeley, R. G., Gordon, J. I., Udell, D. S., Mullinix, K. P., and Goldberger, R. F.,** Primary induction of vitellogenin mRNA in the rooster by 17β-estradiol, *Proc. Nat. Acad. Sci., USA,* 75, 1815, 1978.

90. **Lemeur, M., Glanville , N., Mandel, J. L., Gerlinger, P., Palmiter, R., and Chambon, P.,** The ovalbumin gene family: hormonal control of X and Y gene transcription and mRNA accumulation, Cell, 23, 561, 1981.

91. **Haslam, S. L. and Shyamala, G.,** Progesterone receptor in normal mammary gland: receptor modulations in relation to differentiation, *J. Cell Biol.,* 86, 730, 1980.

92. **Shyamala, G. and McBlain, W. A.,** Distinction between progesterone and glucocorticoid binding sites in mammary glands. Apparent lack of cytoplasmic progesterone receptors in lactating mammary glands, *Biochem. J.,* 178, 345, 1979.

93. **Richards, J. E., Shyamala, G., and Nandi, S.,** Estrogen receptors in normal and neoplastic mouse mammary tissues, *Cancer Res.,* 34, 2764, 1974.

94. **Muhlbock, O.,** The sensitivity of the mammary gland to oestrone in different strains of mice with and without mammary tumor agent, *Acta Endocrinol.,* 3, 105, 1949.

95. Sluyser, M., Evers, S. G., and De Goeij, C. C. J., Sex hormone receptors in mammary tumors of GR mice, *Nature (London)*, 263, 386, 1976.

96. Sluyser, M. and Van Nie, R., Estrogen receptor content and hormone responsive growth of mouse mammary tumors, *Cancer Res.*, 34, 3253, 1974.

97. Watson, C., Medina, D., and Clark, J. H., Estrogen receptor characterization in a transplantable mouse mammary tumor, *Cancer Res.*, 37, 3344, 1977.

98. Haslam, S. R. and Bern, H. A., Histopathogenesis of DMBA-induced rat mammary tumors, *Proc. Nat. Acad. Sci., USA*, 74, 4020, 1977.

99. Kim, U. and Furth, J., Relation of mammary tumors to mammotropes, *Proc. Soc. Exp. Biol.*, 103, 640, 1960.

100. Turcot-Lema, L. and Kelly, P., Response to ovariectomy of NMU-induced mammary tumors in the rat, *J. Nat. Cancer Inst.*, 66, 97, 1981.

Chapter 7

CELLULAR FACTORS IN THE DEVELOPMENT OF RESISTANCE TO HORMONAL THERAPY*

John T. Isaacs

TABLE OF CONTENTS

* Supported by Grant #CA 15416-07 from The National Cancer Institute

I. OVERVIEW OF THE DEVELOPMENT OF RESISTANCE TO HORMONAL THERAPY

One of the fundamental concepts concerning cancer is that malignant tumors characteristically lose their normal responsiveness to growth factors which regulate cellular proliferation. This does not mean, however, that tumors are completely unresponsive and therefore autonomous to all growth factors. On the contrary, it has been known since the pioneering work of Charles Huggins in the 1940s that many types of human tumors do respond to normal growth factors in relation to their proliferation. Indeed, this response is often very similar to that of the normal tissue of origin for the particular tumor type. For tumors of endocrine-dependent tissue, these growth factors are often specific trophic hormones. For example, like the normal prostate which requires a continuous supply of androgen to maintain both cell number and secretory activity, prostatic cancers often retain a similar androgen requirement for stimulation of its growth. This form of cancer is thus often highly responsive to androgen ablation therapy. While approximately 60 to 70% of all men with metastatic prostatic cancer treated by androgen ablation do respond, indicating that their cancers are initially androgen responsive, essentially all of these men eventually relapse to a state unresponsive to further antiandrogen therapy.[1] What is the mechanism for this relapse phenomenon wherein a cancer initially responsive to specific trophic hormonal stimulation for its growth progresses following hormonal therapy to a hormone-resistant state no longer requiring such hormonal stimulation? The answer to this basic question is critical since, depending on the exact mechanism, it may or may not be possible to prevent the development of such resistance. The significance of such a possibility is obvious since once the resistance to hormonal therapy has occurred, any possibility of curing the patient solely with hormonal therapy is lost.

In an attempt to understand how this resistance to hormonal therapy might develop, a series of tumor cell and host factors will be discussed. Initially a general overview of the process will be presented followed in the latter part of the chapter by some experimental animal studies which will be used to illustrate the validity of these general concepts. It is important, however, before undertaking such a discussion to clarify four essential starting points. First, the term *hormone-dependent vs. hormone-independent* tumor cell will be used throughout this paper. A hormone-dependent tumor cell is defined as a cell which requires the same specific trophic hormonal stimulation for its proliferative growth as the normal tissue of origin for the particular tumor (e.g., androgen-dependent prostatic cancer cells, estrogen-dependent breast cancer cells, etc.). Conversely, a hormone-independent tumor cell is defined as a cell which does not require the same specific trophic hormonal stimulation as the normal tissue of origin for its proliferative growth. Such an independent cell can be either completely insensitive to hormonal stimulation for its growth or it can be sensitive, growing faster in the presence of hormonal stimulation, but not absolutely requiring such hormonal stimulation. The need for such operational definitions is obvious when it is recalled that while tumor cells can be defined as dependent or independent on the basis of their response to the specific trophic hormones for the particular tissue of origin, this definition is rather arbitrary since these same cells may or may not respond to a large variety of other more general hormones (e.g., insulin, hydrocortisol, thyroxin, etc.). Therefore, as defined, hormone-dependent and -independent are thus not absolute but relative terms. Second, the term *hormonal therapy* will be used throughout this chapter. Hormone therapy is any therapy (surgical or chemical) which results in the prevention of the specific trophic hormonal stimulation of the growth of hormone-dependent tumor cells regardless of the mechanism for such prevention. This therapy may thus affect the hormone-dependent tumor cells directly or indirectly by lowering the endogenous level of trophic hormones. For the purpose of the present discussion, only the development of resistance to hormonal therapy due to change in the tumor itself will be discussed. Apparent resistance due to suboptimal hormonal therapy wherein trophic hormonal stimulation of growth is not maximally prevented will not be discussed. Third, any mechanism proposed to explain the development of resistance to hormonal therapy must account for the observation that once resistance to hormonal therapy has developed, discontinuation of hormonal therapy does not simply reverse the hormonal resistance of the tumor. The development of resistance to hormonal therapy may involve a permanent irreversible change in the tumor.[2] Fourth, the entire issue of the development of resistance to hormonal therapy is based upon the fact that at least a portion of cells present within a tumor before therapy is begun is indeed dependent on trophic hormonal stimulation for its proliferative growth. If a tumor does not have at least some cells which initially require hormonal stimulation for their growth, then no response to subsequent hormonal therapy would be clinically observable. Indeed, the only detectable clinical response to hormonal therapy which allows a tumor to be defined as hormone responsive is that following hormonal therapy the tumor either stops growing or partially or completely regresses. This response thus requires that there are at least some cells within the tumor which stop proliferating and actually die as a result of hormonal therapy. If a tumor was composed of cells which were not hormone-dependent for growth but were only hormone-sensitive (i.e., grew faster in the presence of trophic hormones but did not die when hormonal stimulation was inhibited), then treatment of such a tumor with hormone therapy would not affect a clinically detectable response since such therapy would not stop, only slow, the continuing growth of the tumor. Such a tumor would therefore be clinically defined as a hormone-unresponsive tumor even though it contained hormone-sensitive tumor cells. Therefore when discussing the development of clinical resistance to hormonal therapy *a priori* we are discussing, regardless of the mechanism, the process of the emergence of hormone-independent tumor cells in a tumor which before hormonal therapy had at least some hormone-dependent tumor cells present.

II. PATHWAYS FOR THE EMERGENCE OF HORMONE-INDEPENDENT TUMOR CELLS FOLLOWING HORMONAL THERAPY

Theoretically, there are two basic ways in which hormone-independent cells can emerge following hormonal therapy. This can occur either by the development during therapy of hormone-independent tumor cells from a pool of initially homogeneously hormone-dependent tumor cells or alternatively by the selective outgrowth (i.e., clonal selection) during therapy of preexisting hormone-independent tumor cells present within an initially heterogeneously hormone-sensitive tumor population. These two pathways for the emergence of hormone-independent tumor cells will be presented separately; however, as will be discussed later, it is highly likely that the fundamental processes involved in both pathways are very similar. The basic difference between the two pathways, however, does have profound therapeutic implications. If the initial tumor, before therapy is begun, is homogeneously hormone-dependent, then it might be possible by a variety of therapeutic means to prevent the subsequent development during therapy of these hormone-independent cells and thus hormonal therapy could be curative. On the other hand, if the initial tumor, before therapy is begun, is heterogeneously composed of preexisting clones of hormone-dependent and -independent tumor cells, then therapy based solely upon a hormonal approach would not be curative since it only affects a portion of the tumor population. This latter situation would thus require, early in the treatment, the use of additional modalities (i.e., radiation, nonhormonal chemotherapy, etc.) specifically targeted at the hormone-independent tumor cells.

III. DEVELOPMENT DURING HORMONAL THERAPY OF HORMONE-INDEPENDENT TUMOR CELLS WITHIN AN INITIALLY HOMOGENEOUS HORMONE-DEPENDENT TUMOR

The clonal origin of many tumors wherein a single transformed tumor cell with a particular abnormal phenotype gives rise to a genetically homogeneous tumor has been confirmed chromosomally in many studies.[3,4] If this initially transformed cell is hormone-dependent, the subsequent tumor which such a transformed cell produces by clonal growth would be also homogeneously hormone-dependent. During hormonal therapy of such a homogeneous hormone-dependent tumor, most of the dependent tumor cells would stop proliferating and die thus producing a clinically observable loss of tumor volume indicative of a positive response to hormonal therapy. If after some period of positive response, the tumor again begins to expand its volume this indicates that development of resistance to hormonal therapy has occurred and that some of the initially hormone-dependent cells during the responsive period have progressed to become hormone-independent. This means that at some time during this responsive period the tumor went from being homogeneously hormone-dependent to heterogeneously hormone sensitive. During this heterogeneously hormone sensitive state both hormone-dependent and -independent tumor cells coexisted within the same tumor. This heterogeneously sensitive state is only temporary, however, since the hormone-independent tumor cells, once they develop, have a complete growth advantage, due to hormonal therapy, over the nonproliferating hormone-dependent tumor cells. Eventually this growth advantage leads, via clonal selection, to the complete loss of hormone-dependent tumor cells and thus to the irreversible development of a homogeneous hormone-independent tumor. It is this irreversible development which is the basis for the resistance to hormonal therapy.

While it is thus possible to outline the general pathway involved in the development of resistance to hormonal therapy, the basic question still remains as to how tumor cells which are initially hormone-dependent become transformed into hormone-independent cells during therapy. The exact mechanism responsible for this basic alteration of tumor cell phenotype has not been completely resolved, but must involve changes in the structure and/or regulation of the tumor genome. Regardless of the detailed mechanism, it is known that such a change in phenotype is both irreversible and inheritable.[2] This requires that some type of basic genetic change occurs in these cells. Genetic change is defined here as a heritable alteration of phenotype whether resulting from gene mutations, chromosomal alterations, or alterations in gene regulation. The ability of initially homogeneous hormone-dependent tumor cells to undergo such genetic changes demonstrates that these tumor cells become genetically unstable (i.e., genetically changeable) at some time during hormonal therapy. The development of this tumor genetic instability can lead to the addition of a series of genetically changed clones of tumor cells, each with a distinct phenotype. Only such newly developed clones in which the new phenotype allows these cells to proliferate without the requirement for trophic hormonal stimulation (i.e., hormone-independent cells) are important in the development of resistance to hormonal therapy. Once these hormone-independent clones develop during therapy, they have a complete growth advantage over all the other newly developed tumor clones which still retain hormonal dependence in addition to any original hormone-dependent cells still present in the tumor. Eventually, such a growth advantage, induced by hormonal therapy, leads via clonal selection to the development of resistance to hormonal therapy as described previously.

The basic question thus becomes what causes the development of genetic instability of the initially hormone-dependent tumor cells during hormonal therapy. One possibility is that the changing host environmental conditions following hormonal therapy are critically involved in inducing the development of this genetic instability. Exactly how this could occur is not completely understood. It is known, however, that exposure of tissue culture cells to medium deficient in single essential amino acids results in a decrease in cellular proliferation with a specifiic inhibition of the cell cycle during the S-phase. This inhibition has also been shown to induce the development of genetic instability such that eventually, demonstrable chromosomal aberrations occur.[5] The net result of this environmentally induced genetic instability is that genetically novel progeny are produced from the original parent cell precursors. Since one of the characteristic responses of dependent cells to trophic hormonal deprivation is a substantial decrease in their cellular proliferation, such hormonal deprivation might induce genetic instability in the initially hormone-dependent tumor cells via a very similar mechanism.

In addition to the mechanism just described in which the changing host hormonal environment following hormonal therapy plays a direct inductive role in the development of genetic instability of the initially hormone-dependent tumor cells, an alternative but related mechanism is possible. In this alternative explanation, random changes in the tumor microenvironment, independent of the environmental changes induced by hormonal therapy, could occur during hormonal therapy. These microenvironmental changes could lead, via inhibition of the cell cycle, to the same process of genetic instability of the initially hormone-dependent tumor cells such that genetically distinct hormone-independent cells could be added to the tumor.

A third explanation is also possible in which changes in host environment, whether dependent or independent of hormonal therapy, do not play a direct inductive role in the development of genetic instability of the initially hormone-dependent tumor cells during hormonal therapy. Instead, it is possible that the development of genetic instability of the hormone-dependent tumor cell occurs as a stochastic event related to the basic nature of the tumor cells themselves. How such genetic instability could develop independent of environmental factors is not entirely known. One possibility is that one of the earliest events in malignant transformation might involve activation of a gene locus which increases the likelihood of subsequent mitotic errors.[6,7] Indeed, such genes have been demonstrated in *Drosophila*.[8] In addition, such genes have been suggested in certain human families with "chromosomal breakage syndromes" (e.g., Bloom's syndrome, Fanconi's anemia, ataxia telangiectasia, and xeroderma pigmentosum) in which chromosomal breaks and rearrangements are increased as a result of inherited defects.[9,10]

In summary, a common pathway for the development of resistance to hormonal therapy appears to exist for tumors homogeneously composed, before therapy, of hormone-dependent tumor cells, Figure 1. This common pathway involves a sequential process initiated during the period of positive response to hormonal therapy in which the initially hormone-dependent tumor cells develop genetic instability by a variety of means, as outlined previously. The acquired genetic instability of these dependent cells results in the eventual development of genetically novel clones of hormone-independent tumor cells. The addition of these hormone-independent cells to the previously present hormone-dependent cells produces a heterogeneously sensitive tumor. This heterogeneously sensitive state is only temporary, however, since, via the process of clonal selection, brought about by the highly selective growth advantages induced by hormonal therapy, the hormone-independent tumor cells eventually produce a homogeneous hormone-independent tumor. When this occurs, the tumor is completely resistant to any form of hormonal therapy.

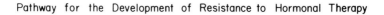

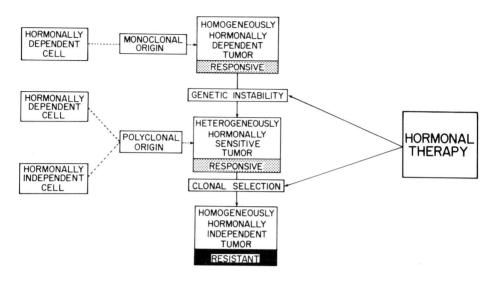

FIGURE 1.   Pathway for the development of resistance to hormonal therapy.

IV. THE EMERGENCE FOLLOWING HORMONAL THERAPY OF HORMONE INDEPENDENT TUMOR CELLS WITHIN AN INITIALLY HETEROGENEOUS HORMONE-SENSITIVE TUMOR

In the previous section, the common pathway for the development of resistance to hormonal therapy was discussed for a tumor which was initially homogeneous composed of hormone-dependent cells. Over the last few years it has become increasingly clear, however, that tumors are often not homogeneous but highly heterogeneous in their cellular composition. This tumor cell heterogeneity has been demonstrated with regard to the following: karyotype properties,[12,13,22] metastatic potential,[14] drug resistance,[15] antigenic properties,[12,16,17] growth rates,[12,18] hormone receptor content,[19] and pigment production.[20,21] In addition, as will be discussed in detail later, there is evidence that tumors can be heterogeneously composed of a mixture of preexisting clones of both hormone-dependent and -independent tumor cells even before hormonal therapy is begun.[22,23] Hormonal therapy, in such a heterogeneous context, would result in the death of the hormone-dependent cells, thus producing an observable initial response to therapy without, however, affecting the continuous growth of the other hormone-independent cells also present within the tumor. These independent cells would continue to proliferate following hormonal therapy such that even if these independent cells initially represented a small fraction of the prehormone-treated tumor, they would eventually not only replace any tumor loss due to the death of hormone-dependent cells, but progressively expand the tumor producing an observable relapse to hormonal therapy. Therefore the subsequent development of resistance to hormonal therapy of an initially heterogeneous hormone-sensitive tumor is explainable by the same process of clonal selection discussed in the previous section of the paper, Figure 1. The only difference is that in the heterogeneous tumor this heterogeneity developed before therapy was instituted.

How does a tumor become heterogeneously hormone-sensitive even before hormonal therapy is begun? One possibility is that instead of a monoclonal origin for the original tumor, the tumor initially arose as a polyclonal mixture of hormone-dependent and -independent tumor cells. Indeed, such a possibility has been proposed for human prostatic cancer. This suggestion is based upon the observation, obtained by careful pathological step-sectioning of primary human prostatic cancers, that many prostates have anatomically distinct multifocal areas of tumor involvement.[24] If some of these distinct tumor areas are hormone-dependent and others independent, then, a heterogeneous sensitive tumor would exist even before hormonal therapy began. Another possibility for the origins of heterogeneous sensitive tumors is that while the tumors may have been homogeneous hormone-dependent initially this tumor subsequently developed genetic instability before therapy leading to the development of hormone-independent tumor cells. In such a context, the development of genetic instability could be induced by changes in the tumor microenvironment or alternatively, it could develop simply as a stochastic event related to the basic instability of the initially hormone-dependent tumor cells as described previously. The only essential difference between this process and that previously described for the development of hormone-independent tumor cells during therapy is in the timing of the development of genetic instability in these two situations. Otherwise the overall process appears to follow the same common pathway outlined in Figure 1.

V. EXPERIMENTAL STUDIES DEMONSTRATING THE VALIDITY OF THE PROPOSED PATHWAY FOR THE DEVELOPMENT OF RESISTANCE TO HORMONAL THERAPY

In order to test if the common pathway outlined in Figure 1 is a valid model for the development of hormonal resistance, some type of experimental system is required. Fortunately there is available a series of animal models which experimentally demonstrate the development of resistance to hormonal therapy. Only one of these animal models, the Dunning R-3327 rat prostatic model, will be presented in detail.

In 1961, Dr. W. F. Dunning observed at necropsy a tumor of the dorsal lobe of the prostate of a 22-month-old Copenhagen male rat.[25] Pathological examination of this spontaneous primary tumor revealed a well-differentiated prostatic adenocarcinoma composed of distinct well-formed acini and glandular formations, including secretory material, corresponding to the dorsal-type lobe of the rat prostate. Fortunately Dr. Dunning was successful in serially passaging the original tumor subcutaneously into both pure Copenhagen and the Copenhagen male X Fisher female F_1 hybrid male rats. This serially transplantable tumor originally termed the R-3327, was further shown by Drs. Voigt and Dunning[26,27] to be a slow growing, androgen-sensitive, well-differentiated adenocarcinoma having both the high affinity androgen-specific receptor and the ability via 5α-reductase to metabolize testosterone to dihydrotestosterone.

This parent Dunning tumor received the suffix -H (R-3327-H) to denote its hormone sensitivity and has been shown to be an important model for human prostatic cancer since it mimics many of the properties of the human disease.[28] One of its important similarities is its response to androgen ablation.[23] When 1.5×10^6 viable H-cells are injected subcutaneously into intact adult F_1 male rats, H tumors become palpable approximately 40 to 50 days postinoculation. Once palpable, the growth of these tumors is continuous as revealed by the plot of the tumor volume vs. days post tumor inoculation, Figure 2. This linear growth curve can be replotted as the log of tumor volume vs. days post tumor inoculation to demonstrate that between 50 to 180 days the growth of the H tumor in intact male rats is exponential as shown by the fact that the tumor doubling time of 21 ± 6 days is constant during this period, Figure 2.

At 150 days postinoculation of 1.5×10^6 viable H-tumor cells into intact male hosts, the tumors, approximately 1-2 cc in volume, are growing exponentially and are histologically uniform, well-differentiated adenocarcinomas with essentially no area of ne-

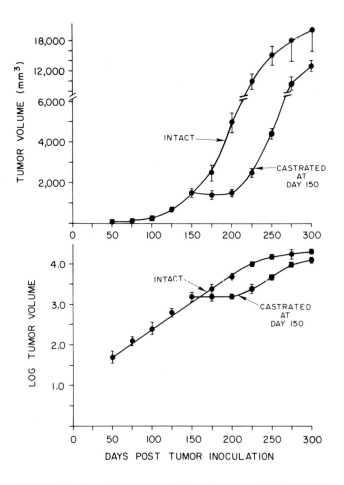

FIGURE 2.   Growth response of the androgen-sensitive R-3327-H
tumor to hormonal therapy. Initially 24 intact male rats were each
inoculated with 1.5×10^6 viable H tumor cells. A control group of 12
male rats was allowed to remain intact during the entire tumor growth
period while the remaining 12 test rats were castrated after 150 days
postinoculation. Upper panel - linear growth plots. Lower panel -
semilogarithmic plot of the tumor growth in the control and test animals.

crosis, Figure 3a. The tumors are composed of prominent well-developed acini, the
lumen of which are filled with periodic acid-Schiff's reagent (PAS) positive secretions
indicative of mucopolysaccharides. In addition, each tumor acini is surrounded by
well-developed stromal elements. If intact rats bearing such exponentially growing H-
tumors are castrated at day 150, the tumor abruptly stops its exponential growth and
for approximately 60 days does not increase its volume, Figure 2. This positive response to androgen ablation demonstrates that the H-tumor is highly androgen-sensitive. This sensitivity is revealed not only by the cessation of progressive tumor volume
growth but also by the histological appearance of the tumor during this androgen ablation responsive period. One month following castration, not only is there an increase
in the proportion of the tumor which is necrotic but even in areas that appear well
preserved grossly, there are now large relatively accellular areas in which very few
tumor acini are found, Figure 3b. These areas are essentially composed of only the
stromal element of the tumor (i.e., collagen and fibroblasts). These areas, depleted of

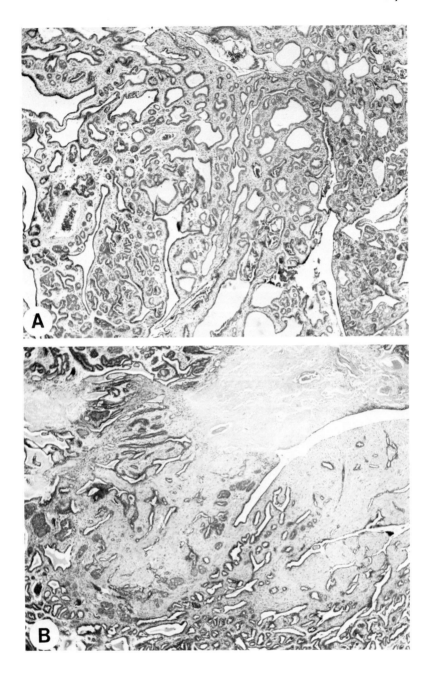

FIGURE 3A and B

tumor acini, are adjacent to large areas where tumor acini are perfectly maintained with no evidence of acinar involution or cellular death. The acini in these well maintained areas are fully secretory as revealed by the presence of PAS-positive secretions in their lumens. Approximately 2 months following castration, this initial response to androgen ablation is subsequently followed by a renewal of proliferative growth, indicating that the tumor has become resistant to hormonal therapy, Figure 2. The semilog plot of tumor volume vs. days postinoculation demonstrates that the growth of

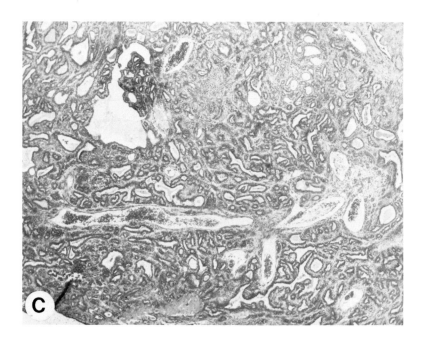

FIGURE 3.   Histologies of the R-3327-H tumor before, during and after response to androgen ablation. A. Tumor growing exponentially in intact male rats before castration: B. tumor not growing one month following castration; C. relapse tumor growing exponentially again two months following castration. All photomicrographs are at a 40× magnification.

this relapse tumor is exponential as illustrated by its constant tumor doubling time of 23 ± 8 days between day 200 to 275 postinoculation. The histological picture of the tumor when it has relapsed to androgen ablation, as judged by its renewed exponential growth, is now uniformly well-differentiated with very few areas depleted of tumor acini, Figure 3c.

To determine whether the development of resistancee to hormonal therapy of the H tumor is due to development during therapy of hormone-independent cells or due to the fact that the H tumor is heterogeneously hormone-sensitive before therapy was begun, fluctation analysis was performed on the H tumor. If the H tumor is initially heterogeneous, being composed of substantial areas of androgen-dependent and -independent tumor cells, then small trocar pieces of the H tumor of identical size (10 mg) taken at random throughout the tumor should vary widely in their individual ratios of androgen-dependent to -independent cells. Therefore, if such trocar pieces are used to individually inoculate rats, each animal will receive a constant number of total tumor cells composed, however of a highly variable number of androgen-independent cells. If allowed to grow in intact animals, all such trocar inoculums should grow to produce tumors of 1 cc volume with essentially identical times since the total number of starting cells in each case is identical and, under such conditions, both androgen-dependent and -independent cells grow equally well. In direct contrast to the consistency in the time required for trocar pieces to grow to 1 cc in intact rats, individual trocar pieces, when inoculated into castrate rats, should require widely fluctuating times to grow to 1 cc if the original H tumor is heterogeneous, since each trocar piece would have varying starting numbers of androgen-independent cells. If the H tumor is not heterogeneous but is instead composed of homogeneously androgen-dependent cells and castration actively induces the development of hormone-independent tumor cells, then individual trocar pieces of identical cell number should each have the same frequency of this induction and, therefore, the time required to grow to 1 cc should be very similar for all trocar pieces. Therefore, the fluctuation in the time required for individual trocar pieces to grow to 1 cc in castrate rats can be used to differentiate between these two different mechanisms for the development of hormonal resistance. As a control to judge the normal baseline fluctuations in growth response due to technical problems of tumor passage, the entire H tumor remaining after removal of the trocar pieces was enzymatically dissociated into tumor cells. These cells are then carefully mixed so that each cell suspension inoculation will have the same number of starting viable tumor cells as that of the trocar pieces. When these uniform cell suspensions are injected into intact vs. castrate rats, the time required for the tumors to grow to 1 cc should be much longer in the castrate hosts. However, the fluctuation in the time to grow 1 cc between individual castrate animals inoculated with these uniform cell suspensions should be small since each receives a constant number of viable cells of identical average composition. Therefore, the magnitude of the fluctuation in the time required for these uniform cell suspension inoculations to produce 1 cc tumors in castrate rats can be used to define the upper limit of the random fluctuation expected due simply to technical problems of tumor passage only. The data in Figure 4 demonstrates the actual fluctuation in the time required for tumors to grow to 1 cc in 10 intact and 10 castrate rats individually inoculated with either trocar tumor pieces or uniform tumor cell suspensions. For graphic purposes, each of the tumors was assigned an individual number on the basis of increasing time for the respective tumor to reach 1 cc postinoculation.

In this way, the variation in time between tumors number 1 and number 10 graphically illustrates the full range of fluctuation seen for each group. A horizontal line would indicate identical growth rates for all ten samples. In contrast, an increased slope reflects the degree of fluctuation in the samples. Examination of Figure 4 reveals that the fluctuation for the 10 intact animals inoculated with trocar pieces or uniform cell suspension is identical; the mean time to 1 cc for the trocar piece inoculations being 130 ± 18 days as compared to 135 ± 16 days for uniform cell suspension inoculations in intact rats. In direct contrast, Figure 4 reveals that the fluctuation for the 10 castrate rats inoculated with trocar pieces, as compared to castrate rats inoculated with cell suspensions, is not identical. Clearly, the fluctuation in the time required to produce 1 cc tumors in the 10 castrate animals inoculated with trocar pieces is much larger than that seen for the 10 castrate rats inoculated with comparable tumor cell suspensions. The mean time for the castrate group inoculated with trocar pieces to produce tumors of 1 cc is 250 ± 8 days (S.D.) which is, however, essentially identical to the mean value of 240 ± 25 days found for the castrate group inoculated with cell suspensions. The more than threefold increase in the standard deviation of the mean seen in the castrate group inoculated with trocar pieces (± 80) as compared to that of the castrate rats inoculated with cell suspensions (± 25), again demonstrates that this large fluctuation is not simply due to technical problems of tumor passage but to the basic nature of the H tumor. These results are not compatible with the idea that the H tumor before castration is homogeneous androgen-dependent and that androgen ablation induces the new development postcastration of androgen-independent tumor cells. If this had occurred, the fluctuation in the time required to produce 1 cc tumors should have been very similar between the castrate animals inoculated with trocar pieces as compared to those inoculated with uniform cell suspensions. These results, therefore, demonstrate that the H tumor is heterogeneous androgen-sensitive even before androgen ablation therapy is begun.

The development of resistance to hormonal therapy of the H tumor thus involves the process of clonal selection of a preexisting population of androgen-independent

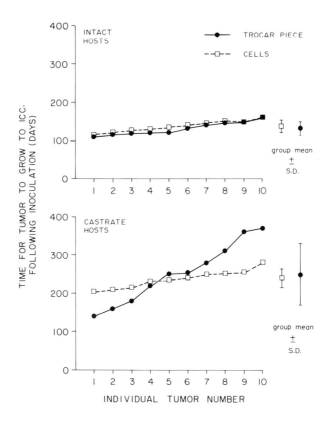

FIGURE 4.   Fluctuation in the time required for inoculations of solid trocar pieces (10 mg) —●— or cell suspensions (1.5 × 10⁶ viable cells) ---□--- of the R-3327H tumor to grow to a size of 1 cc in intact vs. castrate male rats. Initially, 10 intact and 10 castrate male rats were separately inoculated with tumor cell suspensions and then 10 different intact and 10 different castrate male rats were separately inoculated with solid trocar pieces of tumor. Each tumor was assigned an individual tumor number on the basis of increasing time required for the respective tumor to reach 1 cc postinoculation.

tumor cells present within the initially heterogeneous androgen-sensitive H tumor.[23] It is continuous growth of the androgen-independent clone of tumor cells, even during the period of positive response to hormonal therapy, which eventually kills the host animals. In hundreds of animals bearing the R-3327-H tumor, castration alone has never cured any animal. In this regard, the H tumor mimics very closely the clinical response seen in stage D human prostatic cancer, where too, initial response to androgen ablation therapy is almost universally followed by subsequent relapse to a hormone-resistant state.

While these experimental findings demonstrate the validity of the general concepts of tumor cell heterogeneity and clonal selection in the development of resistance to hormonal therapy, is there evidence to support the idea of acquired genetic instability as proposed in Figure 1? Again, the H tumor can be used to illustrate that a genetically stable tumor can develop genetic instability under certain conditions. The value of using the H tumor for such experimental studies is that this tumor has a normal karyotype composed of a diploid number of chromosomes (i.e., 42) with no marker.[29,30] Therefore, any change in this normal karyotype is definitive proof that genetic instability has occurred. The normal genetic stability of the H tumor is demonstrated by the fact that it has been possible to maintain the original characteristics of the H tumor

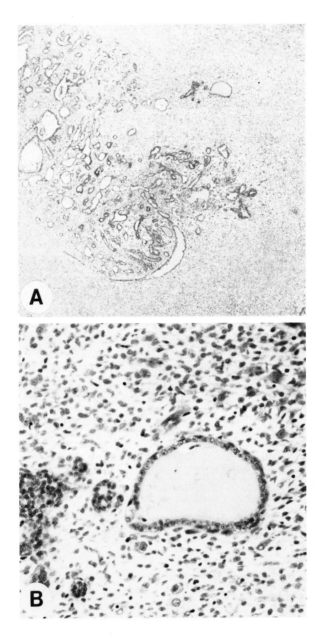

FIGURE 5.   Histology of the "unusually fast growing" H tumor.
A. Low magnification (40 ×); B. High magnification (200 ×).

(i.e., diploid chromosomal number, slow growth rate, androgen sensitivity, and well differentiated morphology) for over 20 years in serial passage. At several distinct sub-passages during the last 6 years, however, a few random H tumors developed definitive genetic instability. This genetic instability was initially demonstrated by the fact that these H tumors, growing in intact male rats, began growing at rates 8 to 10 times faster than normal. In these unusual animals, the tumor volume doubling times increased from approximately 20 to less than 3 days. Histological examination of these unusually fast growing tumors at a time when they are still less than 5 cc revealed heterogeneous tumors composed of distinct areas of well-differentiated glandular acini and areas of poorly differentiated anaplastic cells, Figure 5. When such heterogeneous tumors were passaged, the subsequent tumors uniformly became palpable after only 10 days postin-oculation instead of the usual 40 to 50 day period for normal H tumors. These unu-sually fast growing tumors often grew to the size of the host rat within 60 days. His-tological examination of these unusually fast growing tumors revealed uniformly anaplastic tumors with no indication of any areas of well-differentiated tumor cells. These fast growing anaplastic tumors were thus termed AT tumors.

The first of these anaplastic tumors to be maintained in serial passage was termed the AT-1 tumor. Once developed, the AT-1 was completely androgen-insensitive with relation to its growth; it grew equally well in intact or castrate male hosts with a tumor volume doubling time of 2.5 ± 0.2 days. This loss of androgen sensitivity occurred even though the AT-1 tumor originated in an intact male host demonstrating that changes in the host hormonal environment are not necessarily required for either the acquisition of genetic instability or the subsequent development of hormone-independ-ent tumor cells.

Once developed, the androgen-independent AT tumor cells, via the process of clonal selection brought about by their ninefold greater growth rate, quickly outgrow the slow growing, well-differentiated H tumor cells producing a homogeneously anaplastic tumor. Such a process of clonal selection also explains why these AT tumors are com-pletely resistant to hormonal therapy. In the earlier serial passages, the AT-1 tumor had a very low rate of distant metastases (< 5%). The average survival time of 51 ± 6 days following injection of 1.5×10^6 viable AT-1 tumor cells into intact male rats, however, is less than 1/7 of the total survival time found for male rats inoculated with H tumor cells at a comparable dose (mean H tumor survival time = 352 ± 58 days) demonstrating the increased malignancy of the AT-1 tumor. Biochemically, as well as histologically, the AT-1 tumor was also much less differentiated than the parent H tumor. The AT-1 tumor had no detectable levels of either high affinity androgen-spe-cific receptor or prostatic-specific acid phosphate and the levels of 5α-reductase were only about 10% of those seen for the H tumor.[31]

After 60 continuous serial passages in the Hopkins laboratories, the AT-1 tumor eventually became highly metastatic spreading to both the lymph nodes and lungs in nearly 100% of all inoculated animals.[32] This tumor was thus termed the MAT-LyLu tumor to denote its metastatic site specificity. Continuous serial passage of the AT-1 tumor in Dr. W. D. W. Heston's laboratory at Washington University, St. Louis, also eventually led to a highly metastatic tumor; however, this tumor metastasizes almost exclusively to the lung and was thus termed the MAT-Lu tumor.[33] Unfortunately, the original AT-1 before it became highly metastatic was not karyotyped. Direct analysis of the DNA content/cell, determined by biochemical assay, did reveal, however that the AT-1 tumor before become highly metastatic was not diploid but polyploid.[29] Chromosomal analysis performed on the MAT-LyLu and MAT-Lu tumors demon-strated that both of these anaplastic tumors are hypotetraploid.[30] For the MAT-LyLu tumor the modal chromosomal number is 66 with a range of 51-71; in addition, there were numerous chromosomal markers including loss and gain of chromosomes and structural abnormalities. The consistent abnormalities were loss of the X chromosomes and 5 kinds of structural abnormalities which include a translocation of a portion of one of the #4 to one of the #1 chromosomes [t(1;4)] and a translocation of a portion of an unidentified chromosome to one of the #4 chromosomes [t(3;4)].[30] For the MAT-Lu tumor the modal chromosomal number is 67 to 69 with a range of 61 to 72; again, there was both gain and loss of chromosomes and chromosomal structural abnormal-ities. The consistent abnormalities for the MAT-Lu tumor were the loss of a Y chro-mosome and 5 kinds of structural rearrangements including a t(4;7).[30] There is no common karyotypic abnormality characterizing the MA-LyLu and MAT-Lu tumors, however, other than the fact that both tumors are hypotetraploid and that both tumors are chromosomally distinct from the parent slow-growing H tumor.

During the last year, an additional anaplastic tumor spontaneously developed within one passage of the slow-growing H tumor. This anaplastic tumor too was completely androgen-insensitive even though it was always passaged in intact male rats. This anaplastic tumor, termed AT-2 to distinguish it from the previous AT-1 tumor, like the latter tumor was fast growing (doubling time of 2.2 ± 0.2 days) and in its early passage had a low metastatic potential ($< 5\%$). Flow cytometric analysis of the AT-2 tumor, in its 5th serial passage in intact male rats, demonstrated cells of both diploid and tetraploid amounts of DNA.[29] If the AT-2 tumor cells are cultured in vitro, however, only the tetraploid cells are obtained, indicating that the diploid component of the AT-2 tumors seen in vivo are nontumor supporting cells. This is further supported by the fact that the tetraploid AT-2 cells grown in culture, when inoculated back into rats, produce tumors with identical characteristics as the noncultured AT tumors (e.g., identical histology, growth rates, etc.). In addition, chromosomal analysis of the AT tumor at its fifth passage demonstrated the tumor to be tetraploid with a modal chromosomal number of 84 with a range from 77 to 85.[29] Karyotypes of cells from the fifth passage showed tetrasomy (4 chromosomes) in almost all chromosomal groups, though deviation from tetrasomy (gain or loss) was observed in a few chromosomes; in addition, there were two unidentified minute chromosomes.[30] Further chromosomal changes continued to develop with subsequent serial passage of the AT-2 tumor. By its 10th passage, aneuploidization from tetraploidy (i.e., loss of chromosomes) and the development of structural abnormalities was observed in the AT-2 tumor; the modal chromosomal number decreased to a value of 75 with a range of 67-80.[30]

These results demonstrate that the H → AT tumor progression, each time it has occurred, has consistently involved the development of genetic instability as evidenced by the subsequent development of new androgen-independent tumor cell progeny that are genetically different from their parental H-cell precursors. That definitive genetic differences do exist between parental and progeny Dunning tumor cells when such genetic instability develops, has been consistently demonstrated by the direct comparison of the respective karyotypes. The development of the genetic instability of the H tumor appears to be a dormant characteristic which is only expressed sporadically under unidentified conditions. This might explain why the H tumor expresses its genetic instability in what appears to be a discontinuous function of time. The discontinuous nature of this genetic instability is illustrated by the following two observations. First, there is no consistent relationship between the number of serial tumor passages (i.e., cell divisions) and the development of genetically novel tumor cell clones. For example, anaplastic tumors have developed on several occasions at a variety of H tumor passage numbers with no reproducible periodicity. Second, in specific tumor passages, in which genetic instability is demonstrated in some of the tumors, not all the tumors of that specific passage necessarily develop genetically novel clones of cells. Indeed, it has been through such selective genetic instability that it has been possible to not only generate new Dunning tumor sublines but also to maintain the properties of the original parent H tumor. In addition, it does not appear that the development of genetic instability necessarily requires a change in host hormonal environment since the development of the AT tumor occurred in intact host rats. This does not mean, however, that hormonal therapy might not also be able to induce the development of genetic instability, only that such an event has not been observed with the Dunning system of tumors.

In summary, these animal studies experimentally demonstrate the validity of the general concept that tumors can become genetically unstable during their continuous growth. Regardless of what specifically causes the discontinuous expression of this genetic instability, an important consequence of this instability is that new clones of hormone-independent tumor cells are capable of being added to the hormone-dependent tumor population at any time. These additions can occur either before or during hormonal therapy; however, regardless of the exact timing, the net result is the development of a heterogeneous hormone-sensitive tumor. It is this heterogeneously sensitive tumor state which forms the basis for the common pathway for the development of resistance to hormonal therapy as proposed in Figure 1.

VI. CONCLUSIONS AND FUTURE DIRECTION

Hormonal therapy has been an important modality for the treatment of disseminating cancer of endocrine-dependent tissues for over 40 years. Unfortunately, however, such therapy when given alone is rarely curative. The failure of hormonal therapy to cure such tumors, even though it can induce an initially positive response, is not due to a change in the systemic effectiveness of such a treatment. Instead the development of resistance to such therapy is related to changes in the tumor itself. Experiments by a large number of investigators have identified several of the important tumor cell and host factors involved in these tumor changes. Through the identification of these factors, a concept has evolved that there may be a common pathway for the development of resistance to hormonal therapy, as presented in Figure 1. While such a common pathway can be described in phenomenological terms, the detailed molecular biology of such a process is still unknown. It is clear, however, that the essential feature of the development of hormonal resistance is the emergence of hormone-independent tumor cells. The critical question for future studies, therefore, is exactly how do hormone-independent cells develop? If this question can be answered, it might be possible to design therapies which prevent the development of these independent tumor cells. Only under such conditions would hormonal therapy, used as a single modality, become potentially curative. However, even if therapeutic means can be developed to prevent the emergence of hormone-independent tumor cells, this type of blocking therapy would have to be performed before such development had already occurred to be effective. Therefore, before such therapy was begun, some type of clinical test to determine that the tumor did not already have some hormone-independent tumor cells present (i.e., the tumor was not already heterogeneous hormone-sensitive), would additionally be required. Since at present, neither a method for determining the homogeneous vs. heterogeneous nature of the hormonal requirements of a particular tumor nor a method for prevention of the development of hormone-independent tumor cells from dependent cells is available, these should be critical areas for extensive future study. Any advancement in either of these important areas would have profound consequences on the more effective use of hormonal therapy. Until these advancements are made, it would appear appropriate that hormonal therapy be utilized in combination with other modalities of treatment (e.g., radiation and/or other chemotherapy, etc.) which are specifically targeted at the hormone-independent cells either initially present or developing during hormonal therapy. In such combination approaches, it will be critical to evaluate the importance of both the timing (early vs. late) and the order (sequential or simultaneous) of hormonal therapy in relation to the other modalities utilized.

REFERENCES

1. **Menon, M. and Walsh, P. C.**, Hormonal therapy for prostatic cancer, in *Prostatic Cancer,* Murphy, G. P., Ed., PSP Publishing Co., Littleton, Mass., 1979, 175.
2. **Foulds, L.**, Tumor progression and neoplastic development, in *Cellular Control Mechanisms and Cancer,* Emmelot, P. and Muhlfork, O., Eds., Elsevier, Amsterdam, 1964, 242.
3. **Rowley, J. D.**, Chromosome abnormalities in cancer, *Cancer Genet. Cytogenet.,* 2, 175, 1980.
4. **Sandberg, A. A.**, Chromosomes and cancer, in *The Chromosomes in Human Cancer and Leukemia,* Elsevier, Amsterdam, 1980, 426.
5. **Freed, J. J. and Schatz, S. A.**, Chromosomal aberrations in cultured cells deprived of single essential amino acids, *Exp. Cell Res.,* 55, 393, 1969.
6. **Cairns, J.**, Mutation selection and the natural history of cancer, *Nature (London),* 255, 197, 1975.
7. **Nowell, P. C.**, The clonal evolution of tumor cell populations, *Science,* 194, 23, 1976.
8. **Green, M. M.**, Transposable elements in *Drosophila* and other diptera, *Ann. Rev. Genet.,* 14, 109, 1980.
9. **German J.**, Genes which increase chromosomal instability in somatic cells and predispose to cancer, *Prog. Med. Genet.,* 8, 61, 1972.
10. **Cairns, J.**, The origins of human cancers, *Nature (London),* 289, 353, 1981.
11. **Feinberg, A. P. and Coffey, D. S.**, An evaluation of the concept of DNA rearrangement in human carcinogenesis, submitted for publication, 1981.
12. **Dexter, D. L., Kowalski, H. M., Blazar, B. A., Fligiel, Z., Vogel, R., and Heppmer, G.**, Heterogeneity of tumor cells from a single mammary tumor, *Cancer Res.,* 38, 3174, 1978.
13. **Vindelov, L. L., Hansen, H. H., Christensen, I. J., Spang-Thomsen, M., Hirsch, F. R., Hansen, M., and Nissen, N. I.**, Clonal heterogeneity of small-cell anaplastic carcinoma of the lung demonstrated by flow-cytometric DNA analysis, *Cancer Res.,* 40, 4295, 1980.
14. **Fidler, I. J.**, Tumor heterogeneity and the biology of cancer invasion and metastasis, *Cancer Res.,* 38, 2651, 1978.
15. **Hakannson, L. and Troupe, C.**, On the presence within tumors of clones that differ in sensitivity to cytostatic drugs, *Acta Pathol. Microbiol. Scand. A.,* 82, 32, 1974.
16. **Prehn, R. T.**, Analysis of antigenic heterogeneity within individual 3-methylcholanthrene-induced mouse sarcomas, *J. Natl. Cancer Inst.,* 45, 1039, 1970.
17. **Killion, J. J. and Kollmorgen, G. M.**, Isolation of immunogenic tumor cells by affinity chromatography, *Nature (London),* 259, 674, 1976.
18. **Schnabel, F. M.**, Concepts for systemic treatment of micrometastases, *Cancer,* 35, 15, 1975.
19. **Sluyser, M. and VanNie, R.**, Estrogen receptor content and hormone-responsive growth of mouse mammary tumors, *Cancer Res.,* 34, 3253, 1974.
20. **Gray, M. J. and Pierce, G. B.**, Relationship between growth rate and differentiation of melanoma in vivo, *J. Natl. Cancer Inst.,* 32, 1201, 1964.
21. **Fidler, I. J. and Hart, J. R.**, Biological and experimental consequences of the zonal composition of solid tumors, *Cancer Res.,* 41, 3266, 1981.
22. **Kim, U. and Depowski, M. J.**, Progression from hormone dependent to autonomy in mammary tumors as an *in vivo* manifestation of sequential clonal selection, *Cancer Res.,* 35, 2068, 1975.
23. **Isaacs, J. T. and Coffey, D. S.**, Adaptation vs. selection as the mechanism responsible for the relapse of prostatic cancer to androgen therapy as studied in the Dunning R-3327-H adenocarcinoma, *Cancer Res.,* 41, 5070, 1981.
24. **Byar, P. and Mostofi, F.**, Carcinoma of the prostate: prognostic features in 208 radical prostatectomies; examination of the step-selection technique, *Cancer,* 30, 5, 1972.
25. **Dunning, W. F.**, Prostatic cancer in the rat, *Natl. Cancer Inst. Monogr.,* 12, 351, 1963.
26. **Voigt, W. and Dunning, W. F.**, *In vivo* metabolism of testosterone-³H in R-3327, an androgen-sensitive rat prostatic adenocarcinoma, *Cancer Res.,* 34, 1447, 1974.
27. **Voigt, W., Feldman, M., and Dunning, W. F.**, 5α-Dihydrotestosterone-binding proteins and androgen sensitivity in prostatic cancers of copenhagen rats, *Cancer Res.,* 35, 1840, 1975.
28. **Isaacs, J. T. and Coffey, D. S.**, Animal models in the study of prostatic cancer, *Cancer Detect. Prev.,* 2, 587, 1979.
29. **Isaacs, J. T., Wake, N., Coffey, D. S., and Sandberg, A. A.**, Genetic instability coupled to clonal selection as a mechanism for tumor progression in the dunning R-3327 rat prostatic adenocarcinoma system, *Cancer Res.,* 42, 2353, 1982.
30. **Wake, N., Isaacs, J., and Sandberg, A.**, Chromosomal changes associated with progression of the dunning R-3327 rat prostatic adenocarcinoma system, *Cancer Res.,* (in press), 1982.
31. **Isaacs, J. T., Isaacs, W. B., and Coffey, D. S.**, Models for development of nonreceptor methods for distinguishing androgen-sensitive and -insensitive prostatic tumors, *Cancer Res.,* 39, 2652, 1979.

32. **Isaacs, J. T., Yu, G. W., and Coffey, D. S.,** The characterization of a newly identified highly meta-static variety of the dunning R-3327 rat prostatic adenocarcinoma system: the MAT-LyLu tumor, *Invest. Urol.,* 19, 20, 1981.

33. **Lazan, D. W., Heston, W. D. W., Kadman, D., and Fair, W. R.,** Inhibition of metastases of the R-3327-MAT-Lu copenhagen rat prostatic tumor by diethylstilbestrol, *Cancer Res.,* (in press), 1982.

34. **Michalides, R., Wagenaar, E., Slayer, M.,** Mammary tumor virus DNA as a marker for genetic variance within hormone-responsive 6R mammary tumors, *Cancer Res.,* 42, 1154, 1982.

Chapter 8

TUMOR PROGRESSION - ENDOCRINE REGULATION AND CONTROL

Robert L. Noble

TABLE OF CONTENTS

I. PROLOGUE - ABOUT PROGRESSION

The term progression is widely used in general medicine to indicate a continuing change in a patient's health, specific disease, response to treatment, etc. It is used more specifically to refer to changes in the response of tumors to hormones, particularly tumors of the endocrine system. All kinds of cell responses, however, may exhibit a gradual change which might be referred to as a type of progression. The development of resistance to drugs used in chemotherapy and to hormones are both examples of progression directed at cell survival or mitogenesis. Foulds[1] originally defined neoplastic progression as "the development of a tumor by way of permanent qualitative changes in one or more of the characters of the cells." As malignant tumor cells progress, they tend to escape from their normal regulated and limited capacity for proliferation. They respond, therefore, to decreasing levels of a hormone until it is ineffective and growth becomes continuous but uncontrolled. Similarly, a tumor whose growth is inhibited initially by hormone treatment may gradually escape from the inhibiting effect. Progression takes place from a cellular change which is constant and predictable and seems to occur in all cells at the same time, and which ultimately results in a selfreplicating cell population behaving as of monoclonal origin. It is remarkable that progression is a constant, not random change, which is the same in tumors of all types, and in different organs, whether carcinomas or sarcomas. Progression is a continuous, gradual, irreversible process and not through a series of separate individual steps, although various levels of progression may be defined for descriptive purposes. There is little experimental evidence that progression is related to an abrupt random mutation. Progression in tumors has frequently been confused with changes in the growth rate. Although the latter may be used as an indication of some stages of progression, the two properties are independent. Foulds[1,2] in 1964 stated "there is little experimental evidence or none that sustained proliferation *per se* enhances progression and some evidence to the contrary." As will be emphasized in this review, it is becoming increasingly apparent that changes in the rate of malignant progression of a tumor result from alterations in the level of the stimulating or inhibiting hormone in its environment. Progression takes place most rapidly if tumor growth is slowed by removal of the stimulating hormone or treatment with an inhibiting hormone. It seems to be triggered by any interruption of cell mitogenesis, although gross tumor regression is not essential. Hormone-dependent tumor cells have an individual threshold of hormone for growth. If this is not attained by the host, the cells remain dormant and do not commence growth throughout a normal life span. Cells requiring less hormone for the activation of growth may remain dormant for prolonged periods but gradually progress to a stage where growth commences. Conversely, rapidly growing cells show little evidence of progression. The cellular mechanism involved in progression is not known. It has been assumed that it might logically be related to some type of continuing cumulative minor mutations.[3] It may be manifest by genetic transpositions, changes not believed to be the result of conventional mutagens.[4,5] Chromosome transpositions may be demonstrated in growing bacteria. They have been shown to be involved, however, in only a minor way in rapidly multiplying bacteria,[6] but are a major factor in stationary cultures.[7] As will be described, progression from controlled to autonomous growth does not occur in rapidly dividing hormone-dependent tumor cells in culture, or in vivo, but does so if the growth rate is reduced by withdrawal of the hormone.[8] The control of growth responses to hormones in normal cells is related to negative feedback mechanisms of the host. In contrast, progression is related to the direct effects of hormones on the tumor cell. The recent development of hormone-dependent tumor models in Nb rats which exhibit progressive growth changes in response to hormones, both in vitro and in vivo, has offered a new approach to the study of progression.[8] Progression in tumor cells is a defineable separate entity and should be considered so clinically. It is subject to different types of hormonal control which may favorably affect the prognosis of patients with some forms of malignancy.

II. HISTORICAL INTRODUCTION

Beatson[9] in 1896 and Lett[10] shortly afterwards, both encountered progression of the cancer process after they had demonstrated that bilateral ovariectomy in patients with inoperable breast cancer frequently led to a dramatic regression of the primary tumor or its metastases. The disease, however, was not cured but was followed by progression of surviving tumor cells and the return of an uncontrollable growth in spite of the absence of ovarian function. Lett showed that removal of the ovaries in 75 premenopausal patients led to improvement in 31 cases in contrast to postmenopausal patients who did not respond. Both Scottish surgeons observed progression of the disease with its inevitable return in an intractable form, although Lett listed 5 patients in whom tumors remained in a regressed state and did not recommence growth for at least 4 years. The circumstances leading to the first experimental demonstration of regression in estrogen-dependent breast carcinoma in Dr. J. B. Collip's laboratory at McGill University in 1941 have been described. The response of the tumor bearing rats mimicked the original observations on the effects of ovariectomy in humans, since complete regression of the tumor was followed by regrowth.[11] It could not be established, however, if the final tumors were autonomous as at that time transplants would not grow in the random-bred strain of hooded rats. This was readily shown later when inbred Nb animals became available in 1960.[12] Leslie Foulds[13] in 1954 summarized his observations on similar progressive types of reactions in the mammary glands of mice during successive pregnancies. In two books he described the progression of malignancy as a biological entity, emphasizing its importance in the experimental and clinical approach to the cancer problem. Like spontaneous tumors of the breast in rats those induced by carcinogenic hydrocarbons or nitroso methyl urea may show progression to autonomy. In such experiments estrogens are permissive for tumor production in the breast and the resulting growth may be influenced by hormones, particularly in the case of nitroso compounds.[15] Huggins[16] and collaborators who have championed models produced by hydrocarbons have described tumor extinction, and even cures, by hormone manipulation. Progression in tumor cells has a similarity to promotion of the cancer process in normal cells in which the change has been initiated by a carcinogen. The classic concepts of Berenblum and Shubik, however, are based on chemical carcinogenesis in a normal cell rather than progression in a malignant cell as affected by hormones. If progression towards malignancy occurs in a normal cell, however, then it might be affected by promoting agents. A historical, thumbnail-sketch of the pioneers of progression would picture Beatson,[9] who first encountered it, Lett[10] who made it statistically acceptable, their breast cancer patients who experienced it,[17] Foulds,[1] who defined it, Furth,[18] who expanded it, Huggins[19] who exploited it in prostatic cancer, aided by Dodds' discovery of the orally effective synthetic estrogens[20] and Jensen,[21] who made it receptive. This review will consider mainly experiments using Nb rats, which emphasize that progression is inevitably associated with endocrine and possibly other forms of malignancy. No attempt will be made to review the many papers referring to progression which have appeared since comprehensive reviews were made in 1957[22] and in 1964[23] although some more recent pertinent reviews will be cited. This chapter will summarize observations on a wide spectrum of unique tumors encountered over a period of some 20 years in Nb rats. (A closed colony of animals from which exposure to chemical, viral, or physical carcinogens have been excluded). Transplantable lines of many tumors have been established to serve as "models" for studies on progression which are continuing at the cellular and molecular levels in the Department of Cancer Endocrinology at the Cancer Control Agency of British Columbia. The conclusion that progression is inevitable and irreversible in tumors responsive to hormones suggests that the most practical treatment of such tumors should be directed at a control of the tumor's rate of progression to an unresponsive state, and not at attempts to kill all tumor cells by hormone manipulation. Foulds has stated that - "There is a disturbing possibility that therapy by suppressing or retarding growth may favor progression from the responsive to the unresponsive independent state. This important matter, closely relevant to the management of human patients by endocrine therapy or chemotherapy, deserves thorough investigation".[1] Foulds' apprehension concerning present day historically oriented endocrine therapy will be strongly reinforced by experiments to be described in Nb rats.

III. TUMOR GROWTH IN RESPONSE TO HORMONES

A. Methods

The methods used in most of our studies have been described in detail.[24] Certain items, however, seem particularly pertinent to the problem of progression and will be reiterated in greater detail. The original experimental objective was to follow the normal development of tumors in a closed colony of rats and to study the effects of hormones. Over the years, therefore, any exposure of the rats to chemical and other carcinogens has been carefully avoided. The colony has not been made pathogen free but the black-hooded rats have been bred randomly through litter mates since about 1960. Cutts originally started single pair breeding but subsequently the offspring were bred as brother/sister matings. The Nb rat therefore does not meet the full criteria for an inbred strain but the early lines accepted skin grafts over 20 years ago. The animals have never shown any evidence of tumor rejection or resistance following tumor removal and animals accept multiple grafts of different tumors. The Nb rat probably arose from Long Evans rats. In a number of experiments F_1 hybrids of Nb/Wistar and Nb/Fischer animals accepted transplants of tumors arising in Nb rats. Transplants of tumors in F_1 hosts showed the same responses in progression as found in Nb rats. Tumors which have appeared spontaneously were transplanted to normal and estrogenized hosts of the same sex to test for hormone dependent growth and were thereafter maintained in normal and hormone treated animals. Tumors which followed hormone treatment were processed in the same manner. Transplants were made from a small area of healthy-looking, growing-tumor tissue and cut into 1 mm³ pieces to allow injections with a trochar into the back of the neck under brief ether anesthesia. At the same time a hormone pellet was implanted subcutaneously into the flank. Cultured cells were injected subcutaneously - usually 3×10^6 cells in 0.5 cc of medium. Hormones were administered in the form of hard compressed 10 mg pellets (approx.) made with 10% cholesterol (as a binder) and 90% hormone. In some cases the hormone was reduced in specific amounts and the cholesterol increased accordingly. A 90% estrone pellet (EP) was best tolerated and used routinely, although pellets of estradiol, estriol or diethylstilbestrol gave similar results when allowance was made for varying solubility. Similarly, a 90% androgen pellet contained 90% testosterone propionate (TPP). Pellets of testosterone were more soluble. A single 10 mg EP lost approximately 1/2 its weight after a year in the rat. On the other hand, TPP dissolved more rapidly and were replaced every 2-3 months. In the case of hormone-dependent tumors the animal with the most rapidly growing tumor was used to maintain the tumor line. Pellets could be removed surgically at any time to completely remove the hormone. Postmortem and histological data is available from 1964-1979 on over 18,000 normal rats and 19,000 rats which received hormone treatment (at approximately the same sex ratio) and form the basis of the observations reviewed in this paper.

B. Tumor Incidence - Breast and Adrenal Cortex

The incidence of the three most common tumors in Nb rats in 3 different age groups is presented in Table 1. Estrogen treated rats are compared with normal animals over the 15 years of the study. It may be seen that spontaneous tumors or those following hormone treatment have been found to occur most frequently in the aged rat (1 year or more). The prolonged and continuous slow hormone absorption from pellets may be an important factor in the production of the unusually high incidence of tumors.[25] Rats bearing an EP absorb approximately 5 mg of estrone in a year. This represents a daily dose of 12-15 μg, greatly in excess of the physiological level which is probably in the order of 1 μg daily. Tumors which are related to the presence of an EP therefore would not occur naturally and might be considered as artifacts. However, the present evidence indicates that the behavior of these tumors is qualitatively identical to that found in those occurring spontaneously. As would be anticipated, however, the tumor incidence following exogenous hormones is higher and tumor appearance somewhat sooner than is found with spontaneous tumors. Exogenous levels of hormones (EP) are used as an experimental tool to obtain larger numbers of tumors and shorten the time needed for studies on their growth.

Table 1 includes the usual findings of tumors in the case of adrenal and breast carcinomas in Nb rats such as the increasing incidence with age in both spontaneous tumors and in estrogen treated rats. The effect was significantly greater in males. Such differences in tumor incidence are seen in all types of estrogen-dependent tumors arising in other organs. Fibroadenomas of the breast represent the most frequently encountered spontaneous tumor in the rat. They are unique, since the highest incidence of tumors occur in virgin females and the incidence falls progressively as estrogen levels are increased. Breast fibroadenomas in the rat are the only type of tumor where it can be conclusively demonstrated that tumor frequency *decreases* with estrogen treatment.

C. EP and Age

In some experiments (results not included in Table 1) particular methods of EP treatment were followed to produce the maximum incidence of tumors. The age of the rat at which EP treatment is started was critical for the development of breast carcinoma. An EP introduced into animals of up to 3 weeks of age resulted in carcinoma (usually multiple) in 100% of rats of either sex. If the start of treatment, however, was delayed to 7-8 weeks, the incidence of tumors fell to approximately 45%. Animals pelletted after 10 weeks of age seldom developed mammary carcinoma.[26]

Table 1

INCIDENCE OF THREE TYPES OF TUMORS IN ESTROGEN TREATED AND
NORMAL, FEMALE AND MALE RATS, FROM 1964 TO 1979 IN 3 AGE
GROUPS

Sex	Treatment	Total Number Rats	Tumors %	6 Months Age		6-12 Months Age		12-18 Months Age	
				Rats (number)	Tumors %	Rats (number)	Tumors %	Rats (number)	Tumors %
				Carcinoma of Adrenal Cortex					
F	EP	10,066	0.56	7,798	0.03	1,875	1.60	393	6.11
F	N	7,343	0.11	4,539	0.02	2,077	0	727	0.96
M	EP	8,389	0.19	6,642	0.02	1,443	0.35	304	3.29
M	N	10,279	0.01	7,371	0	2,015	0.05	843	0
			Breast Fibroadenomas (same groups of rats)						
F	EP		0.78		0.09		2.77		5.09
F	N		1.16		0.22		3.23		9.35
M	EP		0.41		0.05		1.66		2.30
M	N		0.02		0		0		0.20
			Breast Carcinomas (Same groups of rats)						
F	EP		1.40		0.12		3.84		15.27
F	N		0.34		0.02		0.72		1.24
M	EP		0.42		0.06		1.32		3.95
M	N		0.03		0		0.05		0.22

Note: F = Female; M = Male. EP = 90% Estrone Pellet; Age in EP Groups = Months following EP,
(actual age = + 6-8 weeks)

The long time interval which elapsed between the start of treatment and when tumor growth was observed indicates that the initiating change in the cell was a long one, or alternatively, a sudden change in the cell after a prolonged period of treatment affecting the host. The latter alternative seems unlikely. The first transplants of primary hormone-dependent tumors into estrogenized hosts always commence growth very slowly. Successive transplant generations gradually increase their rate of growth.[27] From such figures it is possible to project roughly the time of onset of carcinogenesis in the cells of the primary growth. In the case of most hormone-dependent tumors in Nb rats it is obvious that the carcinogenic process must start at a relatively young age - before maturity. If this is also true for the human, changes initiating hormone dependent growths should be considered as starting in early adolescence.

D. EP Inhibited Tumors

The growth of transplants of a number of pituitary adenoma have been inhibited by estrogen. In two cases growth would not occur in EP rats or in females. Treatment with an EP of males with growing tumors caused prompt and complete regression. Treatment with TPP reduced tumor growth but did not cause regression, although transplants to TPP treated rats did not grow. This type of tumor represents one with a specific inhibited growth response to estrogen which has been retained for many years of transplantation. Tumors may gradually exhibit progression, with a loss of the inhibitory effectiveness of estrogen. Eventually, they become autonomous and are not affected by estrogen.[27]

E. TPP

Androgens, in contrast to estrogens, have rarely been reported to produce cancer or influence the growth of transplants. Kirkman and Algard[28] in extensive research with Syrian hamsters, noted malignant lesions in the ductus deferens and flank organs which followed prolonged testosterone treatment. In Nb rats spontaneous skin carcinoma was more common in males but transplants were not affected by hormones. Recently it has been shown that prolonged treatment with repeated implants of TPP may cause cancer of the prostate in Nb rats. The incidence of carcinoma of the dorsal prostate was 20% compared with less than 1% of rats with the spontaneous disease. The tumors transplanted readily but were not affected by hormones, with a single exception.[29]

F. EP + TPP

Treatment of Nb rats concurrently or sequentially with 2 antagonistic hormones such as androgen and estrogen has resulted in some unusual types of tumors. A hemorrhagic, papillary type of breast carcinoma is of frequent occurrence and develops in animals in which treatment may be started after 2 months of age (60% were noted in males or females after 10 months treatment). Serial transplantation using hormone conditioned hosts has allowed the selection of cells entirely dependent on androgen. Some tumors will not grow in males unless they are also treated with exogenous androgen.[30] Carcinoma of the prostate appears at an earlier age in rats treated with androgen + estrogen than with the former alone, and androgen stimulated sublines of prostate carcinoma have been developed.[31] Transplants of the various tumors tend to "drift" towards estrogen dependency, the female sex hormone apparently having a predominant action. Transplants dependent on androgen may reflect a random selection and concentration of cells by transplantation. Marked stimulation of the bladder epithelium may also occur after androgen in female rats, but malignant transformation has rarely been seen.[32]

IV. TYPES OF TUMORS IN THE NB RAT RESPONSIVE TO HORMONES

A. Spontaneous Tumors

The occurrence of spontaneous tumors in normal female animals may be related to the presence of ovarian hormones or be independent of hormonal influence. Breast fibroadenomas (with varying amounts of stroma) are the most common tumors. Other than the recording of the incidence of fibroadenomas as previously noted in Table 1, the tumors in Nb rats have not been studied further, since extensive observations were made some years ago on fibroadenomas found in Wistar rats.[33] Spontaneous mammary carcinoma on the other hand is unusual in Nb rats, although the incidence may reach 1.24% in females over 12 months of age. One tumor, which grew during successive pregnancies (pregnancy dependent) when transplanted, proved to be a typical estrogen-dependent adenocarcinoma. In females over 1 year of age spontaneous ovarian thecomas were not uncommon, 0.37%. Lymphoma-leukemias and uterine tumors were found in 0.21 and 0.24% of animals of the same age, whereas skin tumors were in 0.10% of animals. Spontaneous tumors of other organs have been noted in female rats but only in one or two instances. Some of these have been transplanted and will be included in subsequent descriptions of the more frequently occurring tumors. In male rats, the spontaneous incidence of all tumors has proved to be low, even in the older age groups. Cancer of the skin or underlying glands and lymphoma-leukemias were the commonest tumors in male rats over 1 year of age - 0.27% in 2908 rats. Cancer of the dorsal prostate has been noted in 4 of 2727 rats killed at an average age of 14 months (12 to 17 months). The maximum incidence therefore was 0.14% of males at the risk age.[34] Interstitial cell tumors of the testes occurred in 4 of 708 animals from 19 to 22 months of age, an incidence of 0.51%.[35] Tumors which have occurred equally in both sexes have not been found to be influenced by hormones, as in the case of 10 nephroblastomas (incidence of 0.04% in 25,000 rats).[36]

B. Primary Tumors
1. Induction Related to Hormone Influence
Adenomas or Hyperplasia — Most normal endocrine tissues are characterized by their limited growth even in the presence of an intense continuing hormone stimulus. Negative feedback mechanisms may allow hypertrophy or an increased growth to occur but not continuing growth or tumor formation. In Nb rats the anterior pituitary, dorsal prostate, and bladder mucosa are exceptional in that continuous steroidal stimulation may cause continuing hyperplasia, but without progression to a transplantable form of malignancy.

Anterior Pituitary — The response of the anterior pituitary gland to continuing estrogen stimulation is unusual. The gland of the normal female rat gradually increases in size in relation to body weight throughout life, in contrast to that of the male which does not change. As found by many workers, the pituitary of estrogen-treated animals of either sex shows a continuous increase in weight until hemorrhagic chromaphobe tumors, up to 250 mg in weight, usually cause the animal's death after a year or more of treatment. Ectopically transplanted pituitaries also grow in the presence of an EP, but not in an untreated rat. Animals with pituitary adenomas do not show any gross biological effects of hormone secretion, although their body weights become plateaued at approximately 160-180 g.[24] Assays of such tumors in hypophysectomized rats similarly did not detect any of the normal hormones (prolactin would not have shown in such tests).[37] In contrast, a single spontaneous pituitary carcinoma was found in an Nb male rat. The animal showed gross stimulation of the mammary and adrenal glands, and subsequent transplants of the tumor continued to be associated with Prolactin, ACTH, and Growth Hormone secretion. The first transplants of pituitary adenomas produced by estrogen grow as carcinomas and are frequently estrogen dependent. Unlike the primary tumor, the transplants immediately commence to produce hormones. This unusual effect associated with transplantation has also been noted by others.[38] It is unlikely that this secretory change is related to a loss of direct connection to the hypothalamus since it was also observed in rats bearing transplants of ectopically situated pituitary tissue.

Bladder Mucosa — A continuous gross hyperplasia of the urogenital epithelium, with or without associated calculi, follows treatment with androgen of female Nb rats. A combined estrogen/androgen stimulus may be important. Despite active proliferative lesions only one transplantable carcinoma of the bladder has been found. Transplants of the hyperplastic mucosa remain viable to form pseudobladders, but progression of transplants to malignancy has not been observed.[32]

Testis — An unusual estrogen-dependent carcinoma of the interstitial cells of the testis was noted in a Nb rat. Animals receiving transplants of this slowly growing testicular tumor initially showed evidence of estrogenization for 4-6 months. As the Leydig cell tumor started to grow, however, it apparently secreted a highly active unknown androgen which eventually overcame the estrogen effects so that the animal becomes strongly androgenized. The prostate was found to be markedly enlarged at postmortem and hyperplasia of the dorsal prostate was severe enough to cause urinary retention. The lesions resembled benign prostatic hyperplasia, and transplants of the tissue, although surviving, never showed evidence of growth in normal or in rats conditioned by various hormones.[34] In contrast, carcinoma of the rat prostate grew readily when transplanted.

Adenocarcinoma of the Pancreas — Tumors of the pancreas have very rarely been reported as occurring spontaneously in rats. Only 4, all in males, were noted out of 1026 males at risk age in Chester Beatty rats.[39] Since first reporting this tumor in Nb rats[24] the numbers have increased to 6 in EP females, 2 in females, an incidence of 2.6% and 0.69% in at risk animals over 1 year old respectively - also 2 tumors occurred in EP male rats. Four of the female animals also had associated primary tumors of the ovary. This unusual incidence suggests that estrogens are implicated in the etiology of carcinoma of the pancreas in Nb rats. Transplants of these tumors, although occasionally slightly influenced by estrogens, have not shown estrogen dependency.

2. Hormone Responsiveness

Transplants of various tumors in Nb rats in many cases have shown some slight response to hormones. These, however, will only be discussed briefly, since estrogen-dependent tumors are more suitable for the demonstration of progression which is emphasized in this paper. Transplants of tumors most frequently observed to be affected by hormones have been thecomas of the ovary, sarcoma of the vagina, leiomyomas or sarcomas of the uterus, lymphomas, and carcinoma of the pancreas.[24] It is likely that in some cases the primary tumors have originally been estrogen dependent, but by the time of transplantation had progressed to a stage where growth occurred slowly without estrogen, but more rapidly in treated animals. Transplants of adenocarcinoma of the prostate which were stimulated by androgen were developed from a transplant of an estrogen-dependent adenocarcinoma of the dorsal prostate.[40,41] The tumor was not androgen dependent, since it grew slowly in castrate male rats. The transplants and metastases have been used extensively by Drago and associates in testing chemotherapeutic drugs which may be of possible value for the treatment of prostatic disease in man.[42,43]

C. Hormone-Dependent Tumors

1. Tumors of Estrogen Target Organs

In contrast to spontaneous tumors, those arising in hormone-treated animals were more frequent, occurred in males and females and showed a markedly increased incidence in older animals. In the case of females hormone treatment appeared to simply exaggerate the incidence of primary tumors of the same type which occurred spontaneously. Transplants of primary tumors usually showed dependence on the same hormone which was used to produce them. Cancer was not confined to target organs of the hormone - (normal tissues which showed trophic or secretory effects of the hormone). Estrogen-dependent tumors of the following tissues have been available for study - adrenal cortex, breast (2 types of carcinoma), anterior pituitary, orbital gland (adenoma), ovary (thecoma), fallopian tube, uterus (carcinoma and leiomyoma), cervix, Leydig cell, and prostate; androgen-dependent tumor - breast carcinoma.

Steroid hormones have been considered in this paper to act directly on the tumor cells. As will be shown, in the case of lymphomas an apparent dependency on estrogen was actually related to the secretion of prolactin produced secondarily to treatment with the steroid. Although no evidence of a similar effect has been shown on other types of tumors tested (salivary gland, pancreas, adrenal, breast, pituitary, testes) the findings are not yet complete.

2. Tumors of Nontarget Organs

Transplants of a number of unusual estrogen dependent tumors which arose in nontarget organs of estrogen-treated animals grew only in estrogenized hosts. Transplanted lines have remained hormone dependent for many years. The tumors include carcinomas of the salivary gland and thymus, a liposarcoma originating in the thymus, liver carcinoma, lymphosarcoma, and reticulum cell lymphomas (T-cell).

3. Cultured Lymphoma Cells

Reticulum cell lymphomas arose in the thymus and involved regional and distant lymph nodes in two estrogenized rats, a female and a male.[24] Transplants of both tumors remained estrogen dependent for some five to ten generations when they became estrogen stimulated, growing approximately twice as rapidly in the estrogenized host. Rats bearing these tumors were used in early studies by Dr. C. T. Beer and associates on the metabolism of the vinca alkaloids - the tumors showing extreme sensitivity to the drug.[44] To extend this work to include cultured lymphoma cells Gout and Beer[45] eventually found a method of readily preparing suspension cultures of these T-cell type lymphomas. The transplanted tumors in rats were noted to grow slowly in males, twice as rapidly in EP rats but most rapidly if the hosts carried transplanted pituitary tumors. As the cells in suspension cultures could conveniently be used to assay hormones which stimulated their growth, it was soon proven that they responded to pituitary prolactin but not to estrogen, the apparent estrogen stimulation in the rat being due to the release of pituitary prolactin.[46] As well as the spontaneous developing lymphomas, 12 other lymphomas have developed at the transplant site of other tumors, replacing them by their more rapid growth. Such lymphomas could also be transplanted successfully and cultured like their spontaneous counterparts.[47] (Normal thymus or lymph node cells did not grow under the same culture conditions).

The cultured rat lymphoma cells have offered a new specific biological assay of pituitary prolactin and placental lactogens. In humans, however, pituitary growth hormone has also been shown to stimulate the cultures. By the use of the respective antisera, prolactin and growth hormone in human blood serum may be assayed separately.[48,49] Cultured lymphoma cells are of particular interest for testing the activity of molecular fragments of pituitary hormones,[50] monoclonal antibodies[51,52] prolactin receptors[53] and in a search for similar but unknown mitogenic substances.[54,55,56]

V. PROGRESSION IN TRANSPLANTS OF HORMONE-DEPENDENT TUMORS

A. Estrogen Dependent

Transplants of all types of estrogen–dependent tumors, irrespective of whether they arose in target organs or elsewhere, behaved in essentially the same manner although the time when growth commenced and the rate of tumor growth showed wide variations in tumors of different organs, but were relatively constant in transplants of the same tumor. The growth of the transplant was directly related to the level of the hormone stimulus. In the presence of a 90% estrone pellet the hormone attains an artificially high level in the body which is above the normal endogenous level. A 20% EP in the male produced few endocrine changes and the animals remain fertile, but a 30% EP interfered with normal testicular function. Estrogen-dependent tumors, therefore, may be subdivided for descriptive purposes as those requiring exogenous levels of the hormone for growth. The use of exogenous high levels of a hormone creates an "artificial" situation since tumors would not normally be encountered under such conditions (i.e., tumor growth would not occur in normal rats). However, it allows a study of growing cells exposed to two levels of the hormone, and exaggerates the length of the stages or progression. Furthermore, it permits the more rapid development of primary tumors and the rate of growth of their transplants. As far as can be determined tumors which progress from an exogenous to an endogenous demand for hormone behave the same as spontaneous tumors which develop from endogenous hormone. Tumor models could represent the clinical situation where a cell becomes abnormally sensitive to the hormone or if a hormone secreting gland became hyperactive. As mentioned previously, the start and rate of growth becomes progressively shorter with successive generations. This also continues as the tumor progresses from hormone dependency towards autonomy. Although the rate of growth in some cases is an indication of the stage of progression it is not an indication of the rate of progression. As will be pointed out, progression proceeds most rapidly in slowly growing cells, and the reverse in rapidly growing cells under EP stimulation. A spontaneous progression of tumor cells to autonomy during growth in one generation is unusual but has been observed in transplants of breast carcinoma maintained by successive transplants in EP rats. Tests for estrogen dependency have been made at intervals to determine if growth would also occur in normal males, indicating a rapid change to autonomy. By 1975 the records of 14 estrogen-dependent breast tumors and numerous sublines indicated that they had experienced 220 transplant generations extending over a summated total of 59 years. During this period transplants had included 430 male rats. Transplants of four different tumors had progressed on one occasion only to autonomous growth during a single transplant generation (0.93%), although this did not take place in other sublines of the same tumors. The four tumors in which the change was noted had been transplanted an average of 22 times over 45 months and had been tested on 160 male rats. Tumor cells which are dependent on an exogenous source of estrogen will not grow in normal females (or males) but remain dormant. In most cases progression will gradually proceed so that growth eventually occurs slowly in females with normal levels of endogenous estrogens. Subsequent transplants then grow more rapidly in normal females. Transplants at this stage maintained in EP rats, even for many generations, do not lose their ability to grow in normal females. It has not been possible, therefore, to reverse progression to the original level in which the tumor would be expected to grow only in the presence of exogenous estrogen. Estrogen dependent tumors such as ovarian thecomas and pituitary carcinomas usually show more rapid progression - within three to ten transplant generations. On the other hand, some estrogen dependent tumors have shown extremely slow progression over many years of successive transplants. For example, a mammary carcinoma and a Leydig cell carcinoma, after 11 years will not grow in normal females but only if they are estrogenized. A carcinoma of the salivary gland maintained for 10 years now grows slowly in unconditioned females, but not in males. Tests at this time have shown that tumor regression still occurs after hormone removal and that subsequent spontaneous regrowth takes place which has progressed to autonomy. Cells also may remain dormant and not die in unconditioned hosts. The responses of the tumors, therefore, are unchanged after some 10 years of transplantation. Immunological drift of tumor cells has been minimal since the above responses in the Nb rat have been identical to those shown by transplants to F1-Nb/Long Evans and in F1-Nb/Furth Wistar, hybrids. Most tumors on the other hand progress more rapidly to the stage requiring only endogenous hormones (similar to spontaneously arising tumors) and continue to show progression, usually at a more rapid rate than that shown in the exogenous hormone stage. Initially they grow in normal females, but do not grow in males or ovariectomized females, but as progression proceeds from hormone dependency to the hormone stimulated type of autonomous tumor growth occurs slowly in untreated males but more rapidly in the estrogenized animal.

Hormone secretion by tumors — Many tumors of endocrine organs secrete steroid or protein hormones or other biologically active substances. Their detection and measurement serve not only as a clinically diagnostic tool but also as an index of the success of treatment. Most secreting tumors, however, show autonomous growth. The secretion of hormones especially by pituitary tumors in different stages of progression has been studied in detail by Furth and collaborators.[57] Although changing patterns of hormone secretion were noted these were variable and not closely related to tumor progression. To preserve the hormone secretory capacity of tumors Furth introduced the extensive use of frozen tumor banks, particularly for prolactin secreting tumors and a unique model (MTW9-MtT) which was specifically permissive for the growth of a transplantable mammary carcinoma (MTW9). Our experience with steroid or protein hormone secretion by tumors has been similar to that of Furth. From general observations it was noted that most tumors after successive transplants tended to lose the ability to secrete active hormones. Conversely, a tumor did not acquire the ability to produce hormones as it progressed. The type of hormone produced by the same pituitary tumor however might change. There seemed to be no consistent relationship to changes in hormone dependency of the tumor and the hormone secreted. An unusual model of a Leydig cell carcinoma was dependent on estrogen for growth and initially for the secretion of androgen. The androgen was readily detected as it caused prostatic enlargement, prevented testicular atrophy due to estrogen and was responsible for the development of large scrotal or femoral hernias.[26] As gradual progression of the tumor took place in serial transplants, it continued to require estrogen for growth but androgen secretion diminished. Ultimately, the Leydig cell tumor grew in the absence of estrogen and did not produce any grossly detectable effects of hormone secretion.

B. Estrogen Inhibited Tumors

As previously noted in Table 1, breast fibroadenomas show the highest incidence in normal females. These unwieldy transplantable tumors showed a remarkably complete range of tumor inhibition by estrogen. In the male, however, estrogen was permissive for the development of fibroadenomas. The elderly normal virgin female developed the highest incidence of tumors, and greater than elderly breeding females.[58] Increased estrogen, as noted, reduced the incidence further in all age groups. Growing fibroadenomas treated with estrogen showed regression (and inhibited tumors progressed to become fibrosarcoma). This was reported many years ago with the note that "continuing tumor growth appeared to ensure benignancy".[59] A novel type of estrogen inhibited tumors has been demonstrated in transplants of a few primary adenomas arising in the pituitary gland after EP treatment. Transplants of two tumors of the pituitary did not grow in estrogenized, but only in normal male rats. This effect was apparent in the first generation, even though the primary tumor was produced by prolonged estrogen stimulation. This type of tumor has been classed as estrogen inhibited, and reflects the mirror image of the estrogen dependent counterpart.[27] Its growth is stopped by estrogen and complete regression follows. Spontaneous tumor regrowth which occurred after long periods of regression was found to be autonomous. Tumor cells transplanted to estrogenized hosts did not grow but remained as dormant viable estrogen - inhibited cells. Removal of the EP even after many months allowed growth to recommence. Estrogen-inhibited cells may initially require dose levels of exogenous hormone to be effective. As progression continues endogenous estrogen may prevent growth, but eventually cells show slow growth in the presence of estrogen. They grow much more rapidly in its absence, a stage referred to as estrogen retarded. Eventually, autonomous growth occurred and treatment had no effect on the growth rate. In this case, therefore, progression was reflected by the tumor cells growing progressively faster with successively lower doses of the hormone, which at first inhibited growth. In the case of dependent tumors, cells also grew progressively faster with successively lower doses of the hormone but in this case the hormone at first had stimulated growth.

C. Androgen-Dependent Tumors

In striking contrast to the number of experimental tumors which have been found to show estrogen dependency is the paucity of reports on androgen-dependent tumors. For unknown reasons the high incidence of androgen-sensitive carcinomas of the dorsal prostate found in man has not been reflected in tumors or the ease of producing similar forms of the disease in experimental animals.[34] A spontaneously arising transplantable mouse mammary Shionogi carcinoma has proven in the past to be the most useful androgen-dependent tumor model available.[60] In Nb rats, as previously noted, an unusual papillary type of breast adenocarcinoma has been found to follow combined treatment with estrogen and androgen. It has been possible, however, to obtain sublines of two different tumors which are dependent on exogenous androgen growth not taking place in untreated males or females. With progression the tumors remain androgen dependent, growing in males but not in castrates or females. (The estrogen-inhibited type of tumor is not androgen dependent since it grows in castrates). The numerous carcinomas of the prostate produced by testosterone treatment have proven to be autonomous. One tumor, however, was shown to be estrogen dependent and led to the production of an androgen-dependent malignancy. It was produced by treating a rat bearing a regressed estrogen-dependent carcinoma of the prostate with TPP implants. Eventually tumor regrowth took place which on transplant grew more rapidly in androgenized Nb males than in females. The tumor was not androgen dependent since slow growth occurred in castrates. It is probably that preferential selection of androgen sensitive cells took place in successive transplants.[41] Drago and associates[61] in collaboration with Gershwin have shown that the various prostate carcinomas showed the same responses to hormones in athymic nude mice as seen in Nb rats.

D. Dormant Cells

Cells from hormone dependent tumors remain viable but do not grow if transplanted into an unconditioned host (see Hadfield,[62] Alsabati,[63] Wheelock et al.,[64]). They may remain dormant throughout the life of the animal even if transplanted into the newborn. Similarly a tumor dependent on exogenous estrogen will not grow if transplanted to a rat with a lower level of the endogenous hormone. The viability of the cells may be shown at any time, even after 15 months, by their growth in response to treatment of the host with estrogen. Progression under such circumstances occurs slowly in the relatively few cells which survive from the transplanted material. In a very few animals - approximately 6% of cases - cells triggered by estrogen to grow after 10 or more months of dormancy were found to have progressed to an autonomous state, growing slowly in unconditioned animals. Apparently they had not progressed to the fully autonomous stage where growth would occur spontaneously. It has been noted repeatedly that it has required a larger dose of hormone to activate the growth of dormant cells than is required to maintain the growth of an estrogen-dependent tumor (demonstrated by the removal of the 90% EP and the substitution of an EP of reduced estrogen content). All types of tumors tested which grow in the presence of a 90% estrone pellet will also grow, although somewhat slower, if a 30% estrone pellet is used. Breast carcinomas required the highest level of estrogen for growth, and the highest level of hormone to activate dormant cells. Some breast tumors will regress in the presence of a 20% estrone pellet. The growth of other carcinomas such as that of the adrenal cortex, Leydig cell salivary gland, and cervix, was not interrupted at a 20% estrone level and in many cases with even a 10% EP. In the case of HD tumors, therefore, the growth rate is related to the level of hormone and changes which may occur with time in any tumor reflect a progression from hormone dependency. Transplanted dormant cells resemble metastases which may circulate from a primary tumor and lodge in the tissues. Hormone-dependent cells would remain dormant until the estrogen level of the host increased, and then grow as hormone-dependent deposits of cells. Those which showed some progression would exhibit slow spontaneous autonomous growth. If the cells were totally autonomous, then growth of spontaneous metastases would occur irrespective of the hormone level. It is possible therefore to have a variation in different stages of progression of cells in the same tumor. This would explain the clinical finding of metastases in a patient which would respond in different ways to hormone treatment. Rats with hormone-dependent tumors may show local or distant metastases. They are found most frequently after transplants of adrenal carcinomas in the liver, lungs, and kidneys, and often target back to the adrenal cortex and corpora lutea of the ovary. Other types of tumors metastasize less frequently and usually to the liver or lungs. Lymphomas spread to adjacent and regional lymph nodes throughout the body and infiltrate the liver. The spleen was seldom found to be enlarged except in leukemias. As far as could be determined, metastases of hormone-dependent tumors have remained dependent, whereas metastases of autonomous tumors have always remained autonomous. The intravenous injection of hormone-dependent cells into unconditioned hosts offered an opportunity to determine experimentally how such dormant cells would be handled by the host. Dr. Heather Watson[65] some years ago injected intravenously cells of estrogen-dependent adrenal carcinomas into male animals. In the absence of estrogen treatment of the host they remained dormant. When EP treatment was commenced from 1 to 5 weeks after injection of the cells, metastatic deposits occurred in lungs, liver, kidney and adrenals in a similar distribution pattern as that noted with spontaneous metastases. After 5 weeks of dormancy the unexpected finding was noted that metastases were not found to develop in the lungs in response to estrogen, although present in other sites. Cells in the lungs had presumably died or been shifted to other areas, but this required a time interval of 5 weeks.

E. Hormone-Stimulated or Retarded Tumors

When a tumor progresses from hormone dependency it will then grow in the absence of the hormone. Its autonomous growth rate in the initial stages of progression may be extremely slow but it remains affected by hormones. As the growth rate increases in successive transplants, the response to hormones diminishes until full autonomy is reached and growth is unaffected by hormones. To assess the growth potential of such a tumor, therefore, requires separate transplantation to both estrogenized and normal hosts so that its growth rate may be compared in both situations. For descriptive purposes this has led to the term for the initial autonomous stage as hormone stimulated. Such a tumor therefore grows slowly in the absence of the hormone but rapidly in its presence. Transplants made from tumors growing in estrogenized hosts progressed slowly but transplants from the unconditioned animal to the normal animal progressed rapidly, usually becoming fully autonomous after 2-3 generations. As previously noted, a hormone-inhibited tumor shows a corresponding but opposite type of autonomous progression to a stage when growth is retarded in the presence of the hormone but is still more rapid in the normal rat. Reference to Figure 1 in the schematic plan of progression shown in section IX will explain the behavior of the different transplants from estrogenized and normal rats. In experimental models it is possible to define autonomy as the final stage of hormonal progression when tumor growth rates are the same irrespective of treatment. Clinically, however, a tumor has to be considered to be autonomous if it shows even minimal growth in the absence of hormones.

F. Progression in Cultured Lymphoma Cells

The finding that cultured rat lymphoma cells were dependent on rat prolactin for mitogenesis presented a unique system for a study of progression in cultured hormone-dependent tumor cells.[8] Furthermore, at any time the cells could be transplanted into hormone conditioned Nb rats and the resulting tumor then be put back into culture, allowing independent and interrelated study of progression of tumor cells, both in vitro and in vivo. This dual model may be envisioned as a double-barrelled shotgun with prolactin the single trigger. Cultured cells fired from the left choke-barrel allow a long range approach to a restricted target, whereas the right barrel offers a wider coverage of the same target in the animal. Cultured cells have shown progression from growing in a medium initially requiring a high prolactin supplement to one with no hormone, so that in both cases mitogenesis eventually took place at the same maximum rate. Progression was produced by passages in successive culture media containing gradually decreasing amounts of prolactin. Conversely, cells showed a stable pattern with little or no progression if maintained in a medium with a high hormone content. This effect was demonstrated in cells derived from two different lymphomas; 2-Node and 4-Node, even though the more dependent 4-Node cells initially required 100 times the dose of the hormone for maximal mitogenesis. Prolactin-dependent cultures do not survive in a medium deprived of the hormone, whereas the autonomous counterparts, in the absence of the hormone survive and grow rapidly. Progression shown by cultured cells was more complete and each step more clear-cut than that shown by tumors maintained in Nb rats with different serum levels of prolactin. Progression was not as readily controlled in vivo as it was in vitro, so that the preservations of stable lines of hormone-dependent cells was more successful in culture. Cultures assayed in media with three levels of prolactin were transplanted to rats with three blood levels of prolactin (exemplified by the normal male, estrogenized male, and pituitary tumor-bearing male). Cultured cells from high prolactin media, when transplanted to the three groups of rats noted above commenced growth in 45, 25, and 10 days respectively. Progression occurred in all three groups but most rapidly in slowly growing tumors in untreated males. It was not possible to prevent progression in vivo or to stabilize it with the same success as with in vitro culture. The growth pattern of cultured tumor cells in different stages of progression, however, closely paralleled their growth in conditioned rats. It has not been possible to reverse progression in cultured cells or those growing in the rat.[8]

VI. PROGRESSION - ITS MODIFICATION OR CONTROL

A. Rapid Progression from Hormone Withdrawal

The initial description in 1941 of the regression of primary mammary carcinomas which followed EP removal in hooded rats included a tumor in which spontaneous regrowth occurred after some weeks of regression. At that time tumors could not be successfully transplanted in random bred rats to establish that the growth was autonomous.[66] It was noted in other experiments, however, that if the growth of transplanted breast fibroadenomas was checked by large doses of estrogen that malignant transformation to fibrosarcoma was frequent and that continuing tumor growth appeared to ensure benignancy.[59] Observations in mice by Andervont, Shimkin, and Canter[67] in 1957 also noted that tumor regression led to autonomous change and led Foulds to conclude that "therapy by suppressing or retarding growth may favor progression from the responsive to the unresponsive, independent state." A matter he noted that was closely relevant to the management of patients on endocrine therapy or chemotherapy.[1] It had previously been noted that estrogen-dependent tumors of the adrenal cortex, salivary gland, prostate, and other organs, showed partial or total regression if the EP was removed. When tumor regrowth occurred it was usually autonomous. The large number of estrogen-dependent mammary carcinomas available in Nb rats suggested that a more complete study of the earlier observations be undertaken. Transplants of 20 different estrogen-dependent mammary tumors growing in 85 male rats were allowed to reach a tumor size varying from 5 to 25 g. The EP was then removed and was followed by partial or complete regression in every case. Cells from the regressed tumors remained viable but dormant for varying periods of time, but regrowth eventually took place. The final tumors were then transplanted and had in all cases become autonomous, growing equally well in normal or estrogenized males. The experiment was then repeated using tumors transplanted to 69 estrogenized female rats. These showed essentially the same growth patterns as noted in males, but only 70% of the final tumor had progressed to autonomy. It seemed likely therefore that the difference in the incidence of autonomous change between the sexes might be explained by the secretion of estrogen by the ovaries in the female.[3]

B. Hormone Replacement vs. Total Withdrawal

It has been noted that if the 90% EP was removed and replaced by a pellet containing less estrogen in a rat with a growing hormone-dependent tumor that regression could be prevented or modified. Whereas tumors of most organs such as the adrenal cortex, salivary gland, cervix, would continue growth in the presence of a 10% EP, breast tumors would continue to regress. Mammary carcinoma required the highest level of estrogen for growth. In most cases regression would continue if a 20% EP was substituted for a 90% EP. In ten male rats transplanted with four different hormone-dependent breast carcinomas complete, regression took place when the 90% EP was replaced with a 10% EP. Tumor regrowth which took place 17-44 weeks later was found in all cases to be autonomous. The substitution of 20-25% EP in ten rats bearing six different tumors was also followed by complete regression but only 40% became autonomous. When only partial regression was produced, however, in 14 animals the tumor regrowth was autonomous in only 14% of animals. In four animals it was possible to maintain a stationary tumor-growth level of the tumors and none became autonomous.[3,68] It was difficult technically to achieve a stationary level of tumor growth as it was frequently necessary to interchange pellets which varied only slightly in estrogen content.

C. Antihormones

In unpublished experiments it was noted that the antiestrogen Tamoxifen, when injected subcutaneously at a dose level of 5 mg weekly effectively blocked the estrogen effects of a 90% EP. The drug was effective with all types of growing estrogen dependent tumors so that regression took place even though the EP was not removed. In contrast, autonomous tumors were unaffected. In some cases tumors responded to a lower dose of 1 mg weekly. In view of the difficulty experienced when using pellets in attempting to reduce the dose of estrogen, similar experiments were conducted but Tamoxifen was used to partially block the action of estrogen. Prolonged regression in male rats during Tamoxifen treatment was followed by a slow regrowth of the tumor. Transplants of such tumors, however, remained estrogen dependent and had not progressed to autonomy. It is possible that Tamoxifen does not completely block all estrogen action so that treated animals resemble those treated with low doses of estrogen. Both the methods described effectively reduced the effect of estrogen, allowing submaximal tumor growth of estrogen-dependent tumors to take place. Under such circumstances progression was prevented or delayed and the tumor remained responsive to hormones. In contrast, ablative procedures to remove all estrogen, although also causing regression, were associated with more rapid progression of residual cells to autonomous uncontrolled growth. The most rational form of treatment for inoperable hormone-dependent tumors therefore would appear to be directed at the control of tumor cell progression rather than at producing total cell death. Once a tumor had already progressed to a semiautonomous state it would grow more rapidly in the presence of the hormone but would respond to estrogen removal in a similar fashion. Regression, however, would be less complete and of brief duration. The stage of progression of breast cancer arising in women after the menopause has alway been an enigma. It seems well-established that the growth of some tumors may be checked by treatment with androgen, estrogen, or antiestrogens such as Tamoxifen. Postmenopausal breast carcinoma, however, resembles in some ways the hormone inhibited tumors described in the Nb rat. Whereas estrogen may inhibit this type of tumor growth, and androgens reduce its growth rate, it has not been found to respond to Tamoxifen (unpublished). Progression occurs in inhbited tumors so that the effect of estrogen is eventually lost.

D. Nonhormonal Drugs

Drago[69-71] has made studies on the comparative effectiveness of a number of chemotherapeutic drugs on autonomous and androgen-stimulated carcinoma of the prostate in Nb rats. Preliminary results suggest that the response of the different tumors varies with the type of chemotherapeutic agent. Lymphomas which arise in Nb rats were shown in our original studies to be extremely sensitive to the Vinca alkaloids.[44] Tumors growing in estrogenized animals were more resistant to treatment. However, this was believed to be a chemical blocking of the action of the drug, since it has been shown that the estrogenized rat is more resistant than the normal to the toxic lethal action of vinblastine.[72] It is now possible to prepare hormone-dependent lymphoma cell lines or those which are autonomous in culture, as previously described. Both types of cells grow in the normal male rat but at different rates. Rats having tumors of the two cell lines were treated with vinblastine (0.4 mg/kg intraperitoneally on 2 successive days). All tumors showed complete regression. The stage of progression of the tumors in this instance did not affect the response to treatment. Characteristically, tumor growth may become resistant to the drug.

E. Monoclonal Antibodies

Cultured rat lymphoma cells have offered a unique model for use in the preparation of monoclonal antibodies. Human growth hormone and prolactin in highly purified form, or as components of normal blood serum, are mitogenic for lymphoma cells. Growth hormone of nonprimates, however, is without action.[49] As more is known about the chemistry of pituitary polypeptides it is increasingly apparent that the specific activity may be confined to one or more specific short polypeptide links in the longer chain.[50] The action of specific monoclonal antibodies to the hormone moieties should prove to be of great interest experimentally, and possibly for eventual therapy of overactivity of the hormones.[51,52] A possible etiological relationship may exist between the functions of prolactin and growth hormone and tumors of the breast and lymphoid tissue, but conclusive findings are not yet available. It is of interest, however, that by using the lymphoma cell assay a "mitogenic factor" for lymphoma cells which does not assay by the routine RIA test for either prolactin or growth hormone has been found in the sera of some patients with breast cancer[73] and in children.[74] Although the significance is at present uncertain, it may be noted that cultured lymphoma cells remain stationary in horse serum and do not grow, but do so in bovine serum. It is curious that spontaneous lymphomatosis in horses is virtually unknown, but not unusual in cattle.

VII. PROGRESSION IN METASTASES

An understanding of the response of metastases to forms of treatment which may be beneficial for primary tumors is essential for a practical form of therapy. Metastases are much more frequent in tumors in man than in animals where they have received less study. Few, if any studies have been possible on metastases of spontaneous hormone-dependent tumors, although the intravenous injection of tumor cells may mimic spontaneous metastatic blood born cells. As noted previously, intravenously injected estrogen-dependent tumor cells did not commence growth in an unconditioned host until it received estrogen treatment. Metastases of primary or transplanted estrogen dependent carcinoma of the adrenal cortex in Nb rats were found in 30-50% of host animals. The occurence was often occasional but most frequent if tumors were allowed to reach a large size. A number of tumors, however, (approximately 10%) individually metastasized in 30-50% of rats bearing the tumor. Since these adrenal tumors exhibited all stages of progression they served as a useful model, although the possible secretion of corticoids might modify the formation and distribution of metastases. Metastases have been most commonly found in the liver and lungs - growth of the former may be roughly estimated by the expanding girth of the abdomen due to a three to fivefold increase in size of the liver. In more than ten cases it was noted that following EP removal the transplanted tumor in the neck stopped growing and slowly regressed. In all cases, however, the liver (abdomen) started or continued to increase in size. Estrogen removal, therefore, did not prevent the growth of liver metastases even though they were from an estrogen-dependent tumor. The impression was formed that EP removal actually enhanced the spread of metastases. Since estrogens are inactivated in the liver the growth of metastases in this organ was assumed to be because they had become autonomous and capable of growth in the absence of the hormone. At autopsy the liver was riddled with metastatic deposits of all sizes. These were transplanted but the unexpected finding showed that in all cases tumors had remained estrogen dependent. (Liver metastases from an autonomous adrenal carcinoma remained autonomous). The observations raise the problem of how can estrogen-dependent tumors grow in the normal liver where estrogens are reputedly inactivated? Why did the liver metastases continue to grow and remain hormone dependent despite EP removal and regression of the primary transplant? Would an antiestrogen such as Tamoxifen cause regression of the metastases in the liver? Could an estrogen metabolite in the liver be responsible for growth? Is there a liver mitogenic factor which could substitute for estrogen? Would the same factors affect hormone-dependent tumors of other organs in the same way? The answers are unknown. It seems unfortunate that these questions could not have been studied in greater detail, since an answer seems vital before methods of treating the metastases of a primary hormone-dependent tumor can be developed. A number of models of carcinoma of the prostate in Nb rats are now available in which metastases are frequently encountered. Tumors growing more rapidly following androgen treatment may also metastasize and are under study by Drago and associates.[43]

VIII. CHEMOTHERAPY OF TUMORS IN DIFFERENT STAGES OF PROGRESSION

A. Sensitivity of Growing and Regressing Tumors

Few studies have been made on the effects of drugs at different stages of progression of tumor cells. It should theoretically be possible in hormone-dependent tumors to produce synchronized cell growth and division. Therapy might be directed at different stages of the cell cycle. Usually, cells in rapid division are more vulnerable to many forms of drug and physical methods of treatment. The response of cells in a regressing tumor to chemotherapy have not been reported, although Manni et al.[71] have attempted to treat human breast cancer in different stages of hormone dependency. A recent report on the DMBA-induced rat breast cancer showed that aniline mustard was twice as effective in causing tumor regression if combined with ovariectomy than was ovariectomy or the drug alone.[75] Tumors in this animal model, however, have been shown by Huggins et al. to be extinguished and cured by hormone manipulation. Drago[43] has tested chemotherapeutic drugs in androgen-stimulated and autonomous prostate cancer in Nb rats, but with little difference in effect. The finding that human pituitary prolactin and growth hormone are strongly mitogenic for malignant cultured lymphoma cells raised the question of a possible relationship in the etiology of the disease. If such was demonstrable, then drugs such as ergot derivatives or monoclonal antibodies might be of value in suppressing pituitary hormone activity. The role of the pituitary, hypothalamus, or higher centers in lymphomatosis is an enigma, since one would have expected some evidence of a physiological action on normal T-cell type lymphocytes or on immunity. Preliminary evidence that the rat lymphomas were of T-cell origin was published.[46] Dr. W. R. McMaster of the Department of Biochemistry, University of British Columbia, has confirmed this finding employing a more sophisticated analysis using monoclonal antibodies and a fluorescence activated cell system.[76]

B. The Dormant Cell and Chemotherapy

The search for drugs or compounds which may destroy cancer cells and prove useful for chemotherapy has been of an immense magnitude over many years. A major problem has been to select tumor models in animals which might be expected to respond in a manner comparable to man. In many cases tests have been conducted on the most rapidly growing tumor systems available. In such cases the effectiveness of drugs was assessed against rapidly growing tumor cells in contrast to cells which remained dormant. One may ask - should a new screening program be considered for testing drugs specifically tailored to affect dormant cells in experimental in vivo or in vitro models? A drug to destroy dormant cells would have to act on processes not necessarily associated with mitogenesis but possibly associated with progression. (Would a preliminary stimulation of the dormant cell to cause growth result in a more effective treatment with contemporary drugs?) The primary objective in hormone sensitive tumors would be not only to kill as many rapidly dividing cells as possible but at the same time make dormant cells responsive to therapy. The assessment of treatment would then emphasize not so much the magnitude of the initial response but rather the duration of regression.

IX. A SCHEMATIC SUMMARY OF PROGRESSION WITH COMMENTS ON CLINICAL IMPLICATIONS

Identifiable stages of continual tumor progression, as outlined in this chapter, are pictured diagrammatically in Figure 1.

The schematic chart is self-explanatory but to be more understandable the concept of progression from a normal to an unresponsive cancer cell may be described. It should be understood initially that the chart shows progression in transplanted tumors as being completed in five generations. In reality, most tumors remain estrogen dependent for many generations over many years and growth may initially be so slow as to require transplantation only after 4-10 months. Once a tumor passes from generation 2 to 3 into the autonomous state progression is much more rapid and tumors require transplanting every 2-3 months. Similarly, progression for generation 3 to 5 may occur within 2 transplant generations. Cells may vary in their rate of progression so that a tumor in any of the stages represented in Figure 1 may consist of cells of greater or lesser levels of progression. The changes shown to occur over 5 generations in the rat, however, may take place in a primary tumor during the life of the animal, and be comparable to those taking place gradually in a human estrogen responsive tumor. The normal cell shown at the bottom of the chart responds to endogenous estrogens, and to exogenous estrogens (an EP), but in the latter case growth becomes plateaued and not continuous irrespective of the dose of the continuous hormonal stimulus. The limitation of response has been thought to be related to the action of

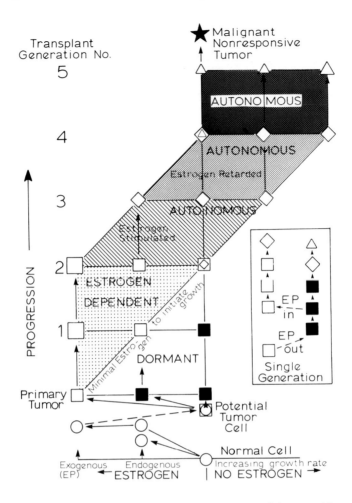

FIGURE 1.   The above drawing attempts to portray the sequence of demonstrable stages of progression of a tumor as it continuously progresses from estrogen dependency, at the bottom of the chart, upwards towards autonomy. Although shown as occurring in 5 transplant generations, the gradual process may extend over many generations. Once tumor growth takes place in the absence of the hormone, as indicated on the right half of the chart, progression is usually rapid. Initially, however, it is still affected by the hormone, growing more rapidly in its presence. Growth of an estrogen dependent cell takes place only in the presence of the hormone, shown on the left half of the chart, but cells have individual threshold levels of the hormone before growth takes place. In the absence of adequate hormone the cell remains dormant and does not grow, although progression towards autonomy may also continue in this state. Cell growth may take place at any stage of progression, indicated by the shaded areas of the chart. As cells grow they shift continuously to the right half of the chart, towards greater autonomy. The rate of cell growth is not indicated, but that of dependent tumors is directly related to the level of the hormone. Once autonomy is reached the growth rate becomes increasingly rapid as progression continues and hormone influence is lost.

negative feedback mechanisms. It is tempting to hypothesize that carcinogenesis may be explained simply as a reflection in a normal cell of changes which are demonstrable in tumor progression.[3] If cancer is a "disease of progression", it would commence in a slowly growing cell and not as an extension of a process involving rapid growth and cell mutation. Cells have an optimal physiological cyclical level of hormone(s) for normal growth and function. If a cell for various reasons does not grow normally but is retarded, an undisciplined maverick, it may become a potential cancer cell. As indicated in Figure 1 repeated fluctuations in the hormone level appears to hasten the process. The evidence suggests that the potential cancer cell exists over a long period of time so that the change may start in adolescence, even during the hormone surges at puberty. Excessive stimulation of a normal cell results in a large mass of cells but allows only a minimal degree of progression towards malignancy. In such hyperplastic areas, however, foci of cells with retarded growth are more prevalent and potential sites for the onset of malignant change. The high incidence of tumors associated with hormone stimulation is therefore fortuitous and not an extension of hyperplasia per se. The potential cancer cell progresses slowly to become a hormone-dependent tumor cell, one which participates beyond its line of physiological duty. Its growth continues indefinitely, provided the critical level of the hormonal stimulus is maintained - the evolution of the primary hormone-dependent tumor. Such a cell cannot be distinguished from a normal one except by its growth response to a continuous high level of hormone. A hormone-dependent tumor cell with minimal progression, however, may remain dormant despite endogenous hormone levels until it progresses to a point where the hormone level is sufficient to initiate hormone-dependent tumor growth. Conversely, at this stage a drop in the level of hormone will return the cell to dormancy. In some cases, if the hormone level is insufficient for growth, progression in a dormant tumor cell may continue through the dependent stage until it eventually emerges as an autonomous estrogen-stimulated tumor (shown at generation 2 level in the chart). As progression continues the estrogen-dependent cell requires diminishing amounts of estrogen to initiate growth until it may grow slowly in its absence, and enter the autonomous stage. As seen in generation 2 to 3, however, it grows more rapidly in the presence of estrogen. As it progresses, it now grows without hormone but more slowly in its presence (generation 3 to 4). To demonstrate this requires the separate transplantation of tumors from estrogenized and normal hosts to both estrogenized and normal rats. Autonomous growth in the absence of hormone occurs after generation 4. It is shown as responsive to progression, however, since successive transplant generations show an increasing rapidity of growth in the normal animal. Finally, (after 5 generations) tumor growth remains autonomous at a relatively constant rate irrespective of hormone treatment.

Progression in rat tumors appears to mimic the behavior of hormone-responsive tumors in humans. To demonstrate the gradual changes of the former, however, requires a panorama seen over many generations of transplants. In man the same changes occur in a primary tumor or its metastases, but are condensed into the lifespan of the individual. The different stages of progression cannot be isolated but have to be visualized from their counterparts, as shown in experimental animals. As noted, potential cancer cells may develop at an early age and progress slowly to the dormant state. Cells may remain dormant and never become tumors in the individual's lifetime, or conversely, they may continue to progress in the absence of adequate hormone levels and emerge as autonomous tumors, omitting the hormone-dependent stage. Such behavior would answer the perennial clinical question of whether autonomous tumors when first diagnosed have passed through a hormone-responsive stage. Dormant tumor cells have individual thresholds of estrogen necessary to initiate and maintain growth as a hormone dependent tumor (the amount of hormone to initiate growth is always the greater). Cells therefore may remain dormant throughout the individual's lifespan and never develop into tumors unless (1) the endogenous hormone level of the host becomes raised to a level which initiates growth (2) exogenous hormone was present in sufficient amounts to increase the endogenous hormone level (3) progression of the dormant cell continued until it reached a point where the existing hormone level initiated growth as a hormone-dependent tumor, or if this did not occur it would eventually emerge as an autonomous growth. It is possible that fluctuations in body estrogen levels may be associated with alternate periods of growth and dormancy in hormone-dependent tumor cells. In rats it has been shown that repeated fluctuations in hormone levels or sequential treatment with antagonistic hormones appeared to hasten tumor progression.[77] Different areas of the same tumor may progress at different rates. If metastases occurred from both areas it would be expected that they would not respond to the same treatment by hormone manipulation - a not uncommon clinical observation.

Hormone-dependent tumors during growth may be subjected to a sudden drop in the hormone level of the host if the surgeon does endocrine organ ablative procedures or if the physician administers antihormone drugs, or if the experimentalist removes the hormone (as indicated in the box in Figure 1). In such a case the tumor may regress completely but residual cells survive and remain dormant. The rate, extent, and duration of regression upon hormone removal is probably related to the degree of hormone dependency of the tumor. The rate of progression in the regressed tumor cells is apparently stimulated by hormone removal so that when spontaneous regrowth takes place it is autonomous, as shown in the chart. Such a finding emphasizes the apprehension emphasized by Foulds that clinical treatment by attempting to remove all tumor stimulating hormones may not be in the best interest of the patient. On the other hand, although the period of regression of a tumor which in the rat may continue for over a year, treatment with an EP starts a rapid regrowth of the tumor. Under such circumstances the tumor cells remain estrogen dependent, as indicated. Its regrowth, however, is always more rapid than the growth of the original transplant, indicating some progression has taken place. On a few occasions, after prolonged regression, treatment of the rat with an EP has resulted in an autonomous growth, apparently cells had progressed to autonomy but did not commence growth until they were stimulated by estrogen. As described in rats, a reduction of the amount of hormone to a point submaximal for tumor growth reduced the rate of progression and lowered the prospect of early autonomous growth. Tamoxifen, an antiestrogen, was equally effective. A similar type of response might be expected in the human, but only if the tumor was estrogen dependent. In premenopausal cases of breast cancer, however, an age when tumor growth would be expected to be hormone dependent, Tamoxifen, with few exceptions, has not been considered to be an effective drug.[78] Such treatment might be expected to prolong the duration of hormone-controlled tumor growth. Unfortunately, the stage of hormone dependency in humans cannot be accurately determined, but only assessed by hormone receptor assays to determine the degree of hormone responsiveness. Most tumors are envisioned to be hormone dependent initially. When first seen, however, many will have progressed to partial autonomy but still may be stimulated by hormones. Since the tumors respond to estrogen, they would also respond to hormone removal, the duration of benefit, however, would be brief as the tumor can grow slowly in the absence of hormone. As progression continues, cells respond to diminishing levels of the hormone until it does not affect the rate of growth.

The growth of hormone-inhibited tumors is not included in Figure 1 as it is not yet certain if they represent an offshoot of some stage of progression from estrogen dependency or a tumor with a different basic response to the hormone. Cells of such tumors do not grow but remain dormant in the presence of the hormone. Removal of the hormone activates dormant cells to grow so that tumor development follows hormone ablation. Similarly, treatment of growing tumors with the hormone causes regression, but progression inevitably follows, so that an escape from estrogen inhibition occurs. It may be noted in Figure 1 that between transplant generations 3 to 4 tumors in estrogenized hosts grow more slowly than in the absence of the hormone. Exogenous estrogen treatment, however, has not been noted to cause regression, so that estrogen inhibited tumors do not seem to be related to this stage of progression. The response of hormone inhibited tumors resembles in some ways that of postmenopausal breast cancer to estrogens - an initial regression of the tumor followed by an escape from the effects of treatment. An understanding of the process by which a cell changes from being stimulated to being inhibited by the same hormone, if such a change does occur, might prove to be of value for treatment.

X. EPILOGUE: PROGRESSION, ESTROGENS, EVOLUTION, TRANSPOSITION, AND NEOPLASIA

Malignant cellular progression and biological evolution have some curiously related characteristics which may catch one's eye and even a bit of one's whims and fancy. Both processes produce a permanent genetic change which usually involves growth or survival. Progression, however, is a gradual local change in phenotypical cells restricted to the lifespan of the host. Evolution is also a slow continuing change, but over many centuries. Both are genetically selfreplicating. Progression of malignancy has deleterious effects on the host in contrast to those of evolution, which are beneficial. One may ask if progression at the cellular level, leading from hormone dependent to autonomous neoplasia is a mirrored reflection of a small fragment of changes which also occur with evolution? Could neoplasia represent a selflimiting type of genetic mistake in the evolutionary scramble for immortality? Cells which are hyperstimulated by a hormone are the foci for increased progression, but this seems related to the stimulation being intermittent. In evolution a superabundance may be followed by a scarcity or restriction which threatens survival. Does this trigger an increased surge in genetic changes towards an altered cell type more adapted to survival? Survival of the fittest but via the unfit.* Progression is not a single event occurring at random, but follows the same consistent pathway in many different types of tumor cells. It is an orderly change and one which may occur in many or all cells. If the same fundamental stimuli have influenced evolution the latter would also have been expected to proceed in many individuals in many identical situations, more or less simultaneously.

Estrogens in mammals produce diverse types of growth stimulation which in some cases are related to the development of malignancy. In rats malignant changes produced by large doses of estrogen may regress initially but then progress more rapidly if the hormonal stimuli is removed. Diethylstilbestrol, a synthetic unnatural estrogen, if given orally may also produce similar cancerous changes in rats.[80] Could the oral intake or absorption of related types of exogenous estrogens have played a part in evolution akin to their role in cellular progression? Estrogenic compounds are widely distributed in nature, being concentrated in such unexpected sources as Dead Sea mud, pussy willows, and subterranean clover. Synthetic estrogens, like many closely related carcinogens, theoretically are synthesizable from carbon, hydrogen, and oxygen under conditions of great pressure and heat. They both may be biologically active orally or through local absorption, and might readily have been formed under earliest prehistoric conditions. Once replicating forms had originated, progression may not have been far behind. Both estrogens and carcinogens cause irreparable changes through progression or mutations. Could evolution have proceeded from the muddy hydrocarbonated ooze which surrounded the primitive earliest unicellular organism to reptiles foraging in the swamps on great quantities of estrogenic plants, but to be weaned to placentate

---

* Many years ago as a fledgling student of J. Arthur Thomson, Regius Professor of Zoology at the University of Aberdeen, I had underlined parts of a paragraph in his Home University Library text book, *Evolution*, published in 1912. We know of some simple units that do their best to get beyond the unicellular state by forming loose colonies. It was probable that body making began in simple organisms unable fully to complete that division into two or more separate units which normally occurs at the limit of growth. "It was perhaps through some weakness that the daughter-units formed by division of a mother-cell remained associated, instead of drifting apart in individual completeness. But out of this weakness - if weakness - strength arose, the strength of animals with a body."

mammals and antediluvian man with endogenous hormones controlling progression? Is it possible that estrogens and carcinogenic hydrocarbons played an essential part in evolution, or is it too steep a step from hydrocarbonated ooze to carbonated booze?

Cairns, in a recent review on the origin of human cancers,[81] concluded that the limited evidence available suggests that most human cancers are not caused by conventional mutagens but are more likely to be the result of genetic transpositions. In a summary of mutagenesis and cancer it was stated that although the arguments are indirect "they do suggest rather strongly that local changes in DNA sequence, produced by conventional mutagens, are probably making only a minor contribution to our national death rates". It has not been possible to attempt to correlate changes in chromosomes in tumor cells in Nb rats related to progression, although the rapidly growing suspension cultures of lymphoma cells in all stages of prolactin dependency would seem to be an ideal model.[8] The remarkably large number of unexpected tumors which developed spontaneously or under hormone influence in many organs of elderly rats suggested that it was not necessary to search for 'outside' etiological factors (see review by Petricciani[82]). Many of the findings relating to genetic transposition would suggest that similar observations might be expected in tumor cells in different stages of progression. Progression of malignancy may be synonomous with cumulative changes in transposition. Transposition is considered a very special form of genetic regulation since it can be programed to occur at any predetermined rate, can be concerned with any desired number of alternative states and can be made virtually irreversible.[81] As previously mentioned, rapidly multiplying bacteria showed only minor mutations from transpositions, whereas a major source of forward mutations was due to transposition in stationary cultures. Many of these features of transposition closely resemble changes associated with tumor progression in Nb rats. It is possible that changes relating to transposition occurs in cells in the earliest stages of progression. More obvious alterations in chromosomes would be expected later in cells as progression continued from hormone dependency to autonomy, and from the diploid to the aneuploid state.

It has been suggested that progression similar to that found in cancer cells may be a continuous gradual process occurring in all normal cells.[3] If this is so, it is an interesting hypothesis that a speeding up of the continuous progression in a normal cell may be a "natural" form of carcinogenesis. Initially, this would lead to a cell which may remain dormant during a normal lifespan or continue progression to one in which growth is activated by and dependent on normal hormone levels of the host. Future research should shed more light on the understanding of progression, the will-o'-the-wisp that flickers in the narrow twilight zone which separates the shadows of hormone-dependent malignancy from the glow of normal cell benignancy and possible cancer prophylaxis.

ACKNOWLEDGMENTS

The research in the Cancer Research Center was supported until 1975 by the National Cancer Institute of Canada. Subsequent grants from the Vancouver Foundation and the B.C. Health Foundation have made possible the maintenance of the animal colony in the Animal Care Centre of the University of British Columbia. Permission to publish quotation from Reference 81 from Nature Macmillan Journals Ltd. is acknowledged.

REFERENCES

1. Foulds, L., *Neoplastic Development*, Vol. 1, Academic Press, New York, 1969, 1.
2. Foulds, L., Tumour progression: a review, *Cancer Res.*, 14, 327, 1954.
3. Noble, R. L., Hormonal control of growth and progression in tumours of Nb rats and a theory of action, *Cancer Res.*, 37, 82, 1977.
4. Wilson, A. C., Bush, G. L., Case, S. M., and King, M. C., Social structuring of mammalian population and rate of chromosomal evolution, *Proc. Natl. Acad. Sci. USA*, 72, 5061, 1975.
5. Bush, G. L., Case, S. M., Wilson, A. C., and Patton, J. L., Rapid speciation and chromosomal solution in Mammals, *Proc. Natl. Acad, Sci. USA*, 74, 3942, 1977.
6. Calos, M. P., Johnsrud, L., and Miller, J. H., DNA sequence at the integration sites of the insertion element ISI, *Cell*, 13, 411, 1978.
7. Arber, W., Iida, S., Jutte, H., Caspers, P., Meyer, J., and Hanni, C., Rearrangement of genetic material in *Escherichi coli* as observed on the bacteriophage PI plasmid, *Cold Spring Harbor Symp. Quant. Biol.*, 43, 1197, 1978.
8. Noble, R. L., Gout, P. W., and Beer, C. T., Progression *in vivo* and *in vitro* of Nb rat lymphoma cells dependent on prolactin for growth, *Proc. Endocrind. Soc.*, 64th meeting, 296, 1982.
9. Beatson, G. T., On the treatment of inoperable cases of carcinoma of the mamma: Suggestions for a new method of treatment with illustrative cases, *Lancet*, 2, 104, 1896.
10. Lett, H., An analysis of 99 cases of inoperable carcinoma of the breast treated by oophorectomy, *Lancet*, 1, 227, 1905.
11. Noble, R. L., Prostate carcinoma of the Nb rat in relation to hormones, *Int. Rev. Exp. Pathol.*, 23, 113, 1981.
12. Noble, R. L., Some aspects of Cancer hormone relationships, *Can. Med. Assoc. J.*, 73, 654, 1955.
13. Foulds, L., Mammary tumors in hybrid mice: growth and progression of spontaneous tumors, *Br. J. Cancer*, 3, 345, 1949.
14. Foulds, L., *Neoplastic Development*, Vol. 2, Academic Press, New York, 1975, 1.
15. Gullino, P. M., Pettigrew, H. M., and Grantham, F. H., N-nitroso-methylurea as a mammary gland carcinogen in rats, *J. Nat. Cancer Inst.*, 54, 401, 1975.
16. Huggins, C. B., *Experimental Leukemia and Mammary Cancer: Induction, Prevention, Cure*, University Chicago Press, Chicago, 1979, 1.
17. Anonymous
18. Furth, J., Pituitary cybernetics and neoplasia, *Harvey Lecture*, 63, 47, 1969.
19. Huggins, C. and Hodges, C. V., Studies on prostatic cancer, *Cancer Res.*, 1, 293, 1941.
20. Dodds, E. C., Golberg, L., Lawson, W., and Robinson, R., Synthetic oestrogenic compounds related to stilbene and diphenylethane, *Proc. R. Soc. London Ser, B.*, 127, 140, 1939.
21. Jensen, E. V., Numato, P. I., Brecher, P., and De Sombre, E. R., Hormone-receptor interaction as a guide to biochemical mechanism, in *The Biochemistry of Steroid Hormone Action*, Smellie, R. M. S., Ed., Academic Press, London, 1971.
22. Noble, R. L., Hormonal regulation of tumor growth, *Pharmacol. Review*, 9, 367, 1957.
23. Noble, R. L., *Tumors and Hormones in The Hormones*, Vol. 5, Academic Press, Pincus, G., Ed., New York, 1964, 1.
24. Noble, R. L., Hochachka, B. C., and King, D., Spontaneous and estrogen produced tumors in Nb rats and their behavior after transplantation, *Cancer Res.*, 35, 766, 1975.
25. Noble, R. L., Pellets of estrogen were 1000 times more effective than daily doses in activating growth of prolactin-stimulated lymphoma cells in Nb rats, *Proc. Am. Ass. Cancer Res.*, 21, 123, 1980.
26. Noble, R. L., A new approach to the hormonal cause and control of experimental carcinomas, including those of the breast, *Ann. R. Coll. Phys. Surg. Can.*, 9, 169, 1976.
27. Noble, R. L. and Hoover, L., A classification of transplantable tumors in Nb rats controlled by estrogen from dormancy to autonomy, *Cancer Res.*, 35, 2935, 1975.
28. Kirkman, H. and Algard, F. T., Autonomous variants of an androgen/estrogen-induced and dependent ductus deferens leiomyosarcoma of the Syrian hamster, *Cancer Res.*, 30, 35, 1970.
29. Noble, R. L., The development of prostatic adenocarcinoma in Nb rats following prolonged sex hormone administration, *Cancer Res.*, 37, 1929, 1977.
30. Noble, R. L., A new characteristic transplantable type of breast cancer in Nb rats following combined estrogen-androgen treatment, *Proc. Am. Assoc. Cancer Res.*, 17, 221, 1976.
31. Noble, R. L., Sex steroids as a cause of adenocarcinoma of the dorsal prostate in Nb rats and their influence on the growth of transplants, *Oncology*, 34, 138, 1977.
32. Noble, R. L., Progressive hyperplastic lesions of the bladder, uroepithelium after hormone stimulation in Nb rats, *Invest. Urol.*, 18, 387, 1981.
33. Millar, M. J. and Noble, R. L., Effects of exogenous hormones on growth characteristics and morphology of transplanted mammary fibroadenoma of the rat, *Br. J. Cancer*, 8, 495, 1954.

34. Noble, R. L., Carcinoma of the rat prostate in relation to hormones, *Int. Rev. Exp. Pathol.*, 23, 113, 1981.

35. Noble, R. L., An estrogen-dependent testicular carcinoma of the rat causing unusual androgen activity, *Proc. Am. Assoc. Cancer Res.*, 13, 121, 1972.

36. Hard, G. C. and Noble, R. L., Occurrence, transplantation, and histologic characteristics of nephroblastoma in the Nb hooded rat, *Invest. Urol.*, 18, 371, 1981.

37. Noble, R. L. and Collip, J. B., Effects of estrogens on the hormone content of the rat pituitary, *Can. Med. Ass. J.*, 44, 82, 1941.

38. Welsch, C. W., Jenkins, T., Amenomori, Y., and Meites, J., Tumorous development of *in situ* and grafted anterior pituitaries in female rats treated with Diethylstilbestrol, *Experientia*, 27, 1350, 1971.

39. Rowlatt, V., Spontaneous epithelial tumors of the pancreas of mammals, *Br. J. Cancer*, 21, 82, 1967.

40. Noble, R. L., The production of Nb rat carcinoma of the dorsal prostate and response of estrogen dependent transplants to sex hormones and Tamoxifen, *Cancer Res.*, 40, 3547, 1980.

41. Noble, R. L., The Development of androgen-stimulated transplants of Nb rat carcinoma of the dorsal prostate and their response to sex hormones and Tamoxifen, *Cancer Res.*, 40, 3551, 1980.

42. Drago, J. R., Goldman, L. B., and Maurer, R. E., The Nb rat prostatic adenocarcinoma model system, in *Models for Prostate Cancer*, Alan R. Liss, Inc., New York, 265, 1980.

43. Drago, J. R., Goldman, L. B., and Gershwin, M. E., Chemotherapeutic and Hormonal considerations of the Nb rat prostatic carcinoma model in *Models for Prostate Cancer*, Alan R. Liss, Inc., New York, 1980.

44. Noble, R. L., Gout, P. W., Wijcik, L. L., Hebden, H. F., and Beer, C. T., The distribution of (3H) Vinblastine in tumor and host tissues of Nb rats bearing a transplantable lymphoma which is highly sensitive to the alkaloid, *Cancer Res.*, 37, 1455, 1977.

45. Gout, P. W., Beer, C. T., and Noble, R. L., Specific culture requirements, including prolactin (PRL) for a number of Nb rat lymphomas, *Proc. Am. Assoc. Cancer Res.*, 21, 67, 1980.

46. Gout, P. W., Beer, C. T., and Noble, R. L., Prolactin-stimulated growth of cell cultures established from malignant Nb rat lymphomas, *Cancer Res.*, 40, 2433, 1980.

47. Gout, P. W., Beer, C. T., and Noble, R. L., Pituitary secretion stimulates growth of malignant lymphomas on Nb rats. Evidence *in vivo* and *in vitro*, *Proc. Am. Assoc. Cancer Res.*, 20, 37, 1979.

48. Tanaka, T., Shiu, R. P. C., Gout, P. W., Beer, C. T., Noble, R. L., and Friesen, H. G., Rapid, sensitive and specific bioassay for lactogenic hormones using a lymphoma cell line, *Proc. Endocrinol. Soc.*, *62nd Meeting*, 267, 1980.

49. Tanaka, T., Shiu, R. P. C., Gout, P. W., Beer, C. T., Noble, R. L., and Friesen, H. G., A new sensitive and specific bioassay for lactogenic hormones: Measurement of Prolactin and growth hormone in human serum, *J. Clin. Endocrinol. Metab.*, 51, 1058, 1980.

50. Mittra, I., A novel "cleaved prolactin" in the rat pituitary, Part I, Biosynthesis, characterization and regulatory control, *Biochem. Biophys. Res. Commun.*, 95, 1750, 1980.

51. Bundesen, P. G., Drake, R. G., Kelly, K., Worsley, I. G., Friesen, H. G., and Sehon, A. H., Radioimmunoassay for human growth hormone using Monoclonal antibodies, *J. Clin. Endocrinol. Metab.*, 51, 1472, 1980.

52. Ivanyi, J. and Davies, P., Monoclonal antibodies against human growth hormones, *Mol. Immunol.*, 17, 287, 1980.

53. Elsholtz, H. and Shiu, R., Biosynthesis of prolactin receptors: Demonstration by density labelling techniques, *Proc. Endocrinol. Soc.*, 63rd Meeting, Bethesda, Md., 221, 1981.

54. Robertson, M. C., Klindt, J., and Friesen, H. G., Ovariectomy leads to major increase in rat placental lactogen (rPL) secretion, *Proc. Endocrinol. Soc.*, *63rd Meeting*, Bethesda, Md., 117, 1981.

55. Kato, N., Differences between Bioassay (BA) and Radioimmunoassay (RIA) values of rPRL secreted in primary pituitary cell cultures, *Proc. Endocrinol. Soc., 63rd Meeting, Bethesda, Md.*, 215, 1981.

56. Klindt, J. and Robertson, M. C., Secretory patterns of rat prolactin (rPRL) as measured by radioimmunoassay (RIA) and bioassay (BA), *Proc. Endocrinol. Soc., 63rd Meeting, Bethesda, Md.*, 217, 1981.

57. Furth, J., Clifton, K. H., Gadsden, E. L., and Buffett, R. F., Dependent and autonomous mammotrophic pituitary tumors in rats: Their somatotropic features, *Cancer Res.*, 16, 608, 1956.

58. Howell, J. S. and Mandl, A. M., The mammary glands of senile Nulliparous and Multiparous rats, *J. Endocrinol.*, 22, 241, 1961.

59. Millar, M. J. and Noble, R. L., The growth characteristics and response to hormones of transplanted fibrosarcoma arising from mammary fibroadenoma in the rat, *Br. J. Cancer*, 8, 508, 1978.

60. Bruchovsky, N. and Rennie, P. S., Classification of dependent and autonomous variants of Shionogi mammary carcinoma based on heterogenous patterns of androgen binding, *Cell*, 13, 273, 1978.

61. Drago, J. R., Gershwin, M. E., Maurer, R. E., Ikeda, R. M., and Eckels, D. D., Immunobiology and therapeutic manipulation of heterotransplanted Nb rat prostate adenocarcinomas into congenitally athymic (nude) mice. I. Hormone dependency and histopathology, *J. Natl. Cancer Inst.*, 62, 1057, 1979.

62. Hadfield, G., The dormant cancer cell, *Br. Med. J.*, 2, 607, 1954.
63. Alsabti, E. A. K., Tumor dormancy (a review), *Neoplasma*, 26, 351, 1979.
64. Wheelock, E. F., Weinhold, K. J. and Levich, J., The tumor dormant state, in *Advances in Cancer Research*, Klein, G. and Weinhouse, S., Eds., Academic Press, New York, 1981, 34.
65. Watson, H. W., unpublished data, 1974.
66. Noble, R. L. and Collip, J. B., Regression of oestrogen induced mammary tumors in female rats following removal of the stimulus, *Can. Med. Assoc. J.*, 44, 1, 1941.
67. Andervont, H. B., Shimkin, M. D., and Canter, H. Y., Effect of discontinued estrogenic stimulation upon the development and growth of testicular tissues in mice, *J. Natl. Cancer Inst.*, 18, 1, 1957.
68. Bruchovsky, N., Rennie, P. S., Van Doorn, E., and Noble, R. L., Pathological growth of androgen-sensitive tissues resulting from latent actions of steroid hormones, *J. Toxicol. Environ. Health*, 4, 391, 1978.
69. Drago, J. R., Maurer, R. E., Gershwin, M. E., Eckels, D. D., and Goldman, L. B., Chemotherapy of the Nb rat adenocarcinoma of the prostate heterotransplanted into congenitally athymic (nude) mice: report of 5-Fluorouracil and Cyclophosphamide, *J. Surg. Res.*, 26, 400, 1979.
70. Drago, J. R., Goldman, L. B., Maurer, R. E., Gershwin, M. E., and Eckels, D. D., Therapeutic manipulation of Nb rat prostate adenocarcinomas. Chemotherapeutic evaluation of autonomous tumors, *Invest. Urol.*, 17, 203, 1979.
71. Manni, A., Trujillo, J. E., and Pearson, O. H., Sequential use of endocrine therapy and chemotherapy for metastatic breast cancer: effect on survival, *Cancer Treat. Rep.*, 64, 111, 1980.
72. Cutts, J. H., Protective action of Diethylstilbestrol on the toxicity of Vinblastine in rats, *J. Natl. Cancer Inst.*, 41, 919, 1968.
73. Emerman, J. T., Leahy, M., Gout, P. W., and Bruchovsky, N., A possible role for growth hormone in human breast cancer, *Clin. Invest. Med.*, 4, 24B, 1981.
74. Leahy, M., Emerman, J. T., Bruchovsky, N., Tze, W. J., Noble, R. L., Beer, C. T., and Gout, P. W., Mitogenic activity of lactogenic hormones in sera from adults and children, *Clin. Invest. Med.*, 4, 15B, 1981.
75. Benckhuysen, C., Hennie, G., Terhart, J., and Van Dijk, P. J., Enhanced cytostatic effectiveness of Analine mustard against 7, 12 Dimethylbenz (a) anthracene-induced rat mammary tumors during regression in response to ovariectomy, *Cancer Treat. Rep.*, 65, 567, 1981.
76. McMaster, R., personal communication.
77. Noble, R. L., Cancer caused by the sequential action of antagonistic sex hormones - as exemplified by the prostate, breast and bladder in Nb rats, *Proc. Can. Fed. Biol. Soc.*, 22, 58, 1979.
78. Wada, T., Koyama, H., and Terasawa, T., Effect of tamoxifen in premenopausal Japanese women with advanced breast cancer, *Cancer Treat. Rep.*, 65, 1981.
79. Fisher, B. & 22 NSABP Investigators, Treatment of primary breast cancer with chemotherapy and Tamoxifen, *New Engl. J. Med.*, 305, 1, 1981.
80. Noble, R. L. and Collip, J. B. The production of mammary tumors in the rat following the oral administration of Diethylstilbestrol over prolonged periods, *Proc. Can. Physiol. Soc.*, October, 1941.
81. Cairns, J., The origin of human cancers, *Nature (London)*, 289, 353, 1981.
82. Petricciani, J. C., On the origin of human tumors, *In Vitro*, 16, 361, 1980.

INDEX

A

Aberrations of chromosomes, 15
Ablation therapy, 145—147, 150
Acceptor sites, 128
    androgen, 110—112, 115
Acentric chromosomal fragments, 7
Acivicin, 29
Actinomycin D, 11
Activation of receptors, 89, 130—131
Adaptive tumor changes, 98
Adenocarcinoma of pancreas, 165
Adenomas, 164
Adjuvant chemotherapy, 37
Adrenal cortex tumor incidence, 161
Adriamycin, 11, 27
Age and estrone pellet, 161—162
Alkaloids, 28
Alkylating agents, 42
Alterations in metabolism, 29—31
Altered androgen acceptor sites, 110—111
Altered drug transport mechanisms, 27—29
Alternation, 73
    protocol, 75
    sequential, 69
    therapy, 66
Amino acids, 143
9-Aminoacridine, 83
Amplification of genes, 8, 11, 15
Androgen, 163
    resistance of, 95—121
    sensitivity of, 100
    transport of, 102—103
Androgen ablation therapy, 145—147, 150
Androgen acceptor sites, 111—112, 115
    altered, 110—111
Androgen-dependent cells, 148
Androgen-dependent tumors, 168—169
Androgen receptors, 101, 105—108, 114, 115
    dysfunctional, 108
    nuclear uptake of, 108—109
Androgen-resistant cells, 101
Androgen-sensitive tumors, 150
Aneuploid tumors, 5
Anterior pituitary tumor, 164
Antibiotics, see also specific antibiotics
    antitumor, 42
Antibodies, 173
Antiestrogens, 130
    pharmacology and, 132—134
Antigenicity of tumor cells, 34—35
Antihormones, 172—173
Antitumor antibiotics, 42
Antitumor drug kinetic classification, 38
Ara-C, 76
L-Asparaginase resistance, 13
Asparagine synthetase, 13
Asparagyl-tRNA synthetase, 13
β-Aspartylhydroxamate, 13

Assays, see also specific assays; Tests
    Courtenay, 41
    Hamburger and Salmon, 41
AT tumors, 152
Autologous bone marrow rescue, 25
Autonomous growth, 170, 177
Autophagia, 98
Autophagic mechanism, 99, 100, 101, 114

B

BCNU, 26
Benign prostatic hyperplasia (BPH), 103, 108,
    112, 113
Binding sites of 17β-estradiol, 131
Biochemical action of estrogen, 125—127
Biological evolution, 179
Bladder mucosa tumor, 164
Bleomycin, 85, 86, 88, 89
Blood-brain barrier, 35
Bone marrow, 33
    autologous rescue of, 25
    toxicity of, 38
BPH, see Benign prostatic hyperplasia
Breakage of chromosomes, 143
Breast tumor, see Mammary tumor

C

Carcinoma
    Leydig cell, 168
    ovarian, 43
    prostate, 96, 106, 140
    Shionogi, 106, 109
Castration, 99, 148, 150
Cell cycle, 56
    drug cytotoxicities dependent on, 40
    kinetic insensitivity in, 31—33
    progression delay in, 31
Cell membrane permeability, 132
Cells
    androgen-dependent, 148
    androgen-resistant, 101
    CEM-C7, 89
    CHO, 5, 8, 9, 13, 28, 85
    differentiation of, 127
    dormant, see Dormant cells
    doubly resistant, 66
    drug-resistance of nucleus of, 12
    drug-resistant, 3
    hemizygous, 6
    homogeneously androgen-dependent, 148
    hormone-dependent, 144
    hormone-independent, 141
    hybrids of, 81, 90—92
    hypoxic, 32
    killing of, see Cytoxicity